Mental Health Service Provision for a Multi-cultural Society

Edited by

Kamaldeep Bhui MSc, MRCPsych
Wellcome Training Fellow
Institute of Psychiatry
and Honorary Senior Registrar
The Maudsley Hospital
London

and

Dele Olajide PhD, FRCPsych
Consultant Psychiatrist
Invicta Community Care NHS Trust
Maidstone
and Clinical Senior Lecturer
Department of Psychological Medicine
Institute of Psychiatry
London

 W.B. SAUNDERS COMPANY LTD
London Edinburgh New York Philadelphia Sydney Toronto

W.B. Saunders
An imprint of Harcourt Brace and Company Ltd

A catalogue record for this book is available from the British Library

ISBN 0–7020–2386–8

Typeset by J&L Composition Ltd, Filey, North Yorkshire
Printed in China
EPC/01

Contents

Contributors

Karla Boyce-Awai RMN
Guy's Hospital, London.

Hindpal Singh Bhui BA, MSc, MA, DipSW
Probation Officer, Inner London Probation Service, London.

Kamaldeep Bhui MSc, MRCPsych
Wellcome Training Fellow, Institute of Psychiatry, and Honorary Senior Registrar, The Maudsley Hospital, London.

Jeff Chandra BSc, MBA, MIMgt, MHSM, DipHSM
Chief Executive, Josam Associates, Slimbridge, Gloucestershire.

Simon Dein
Senior Lecturer, Department of Psychiatry, Middlesex University, London.

Sarah Huline-Dickens BSc, MB BCh, MRCPsych
Specialist Registrar in Child and Adolescent Psychiatry, Douglas House, Cambridge.

Georgina Foulds Dip COT
Day Services Co-ordinator, Hounslow and Spelthorne Community Mental Health NHS Trust, Ashford Hospital, Middlsex.

Joy Francis BA, Cert PEJ
Visiting Lecturer, London College of Printing and Media, and Policy Advisor, Sia – The National Development Agency for the Black Voluntary Sector, London.

Bill (K.W.M.) Fulford DPhil, FRCPsych
Professor of Philosophy and Mental Health, University of Warwick, and Honorary Consultant Psychiatrist, University of Oxford.

Peter Gluckman
Director of Strategic Planning and Consumer Affairs, Lambeth, Southwark and Lewisham Health Authority, London.

Charles Husband
Professor of Social Analysis and Associate Head, Research Unit in Ethnicity and Social Policy, University of Bradford.

Dora Jonathan MSc (Psychol), DipHSM
Director, Jonathan Associates, MHRT.

Satvinder Juss
Harkness Fellow, US Department of Health and Human Services, Washington, DC and Barrister at Law, London.

Frank Ledwith MA, PhD, BA
University College of St Martin, Lancaster.

Kate Loewenthal BSc, PhD, CPsychol, AFBPsS
Reader in Psychology, Royal Holloway College, University of London.

Zenobia Nadirshaw
Lead Clinician and Consultant Clinical Psychologist, Riverside Mental Health Trust, London.

Dele Olajide PhD, FRCPsych
Consultant Psychiatrist, Invicta Community Care NHS Trust, Maidstone, and Clinical Senior Lecturer, Department of Psychological Medicine, Institute of Psychiatry, London.

Sangeeta Patel MB BS, MRCGP, MA (Med Anth)
GP Principal, Balham, and Clinical Lecturer, Division of General Practice and Primary Care, St George's Hospital Medical School, London.

Sonia Preddie RMN
The Maudsley Hospital, London.

Shulamit Ramon BA, MA, PhD
Professor of Interprofessional Health and Social Studies, Anglia Polytechnic University, Cambridge.

Foreword

In 1978 I was asked by World Health Organisation to go to Burma and set up an MSc Course in psychiatry at Rangoon University. The excitement that I had felt on receiving the invitation turned to panic on the day before I left, as I contemplated how little I knew of Burmese culture and symptom experience. One of the patients I saw on my last afternoon in Manchester was a young man who complained that the sparrows at the side of the road were repeating his thoughts. As it happened, the first patient that I saw in Burma complained that the weaver birds in the palm trees were repeating his thoughts. I had come a long way, but some schizophrenic phenomena were invariant, with only trivial modification by the local culture. Subsequent patients had symptoms that were not so easy to interpret, and I often needed to rely on Burmese colleagues to understand the meaning of a symptom.

Since that time, the WHO's international studies of both schizophrenia and depression have demostrated that while both disorders are world wide in their distribution, that both vary in their main manifestations from one culture to another. Since a symptom that is common in one culture may be rare in another, international diagnostic systems (like the 10th revision of the International Classification of Diseases) specify that a person must manifest more than a critical number of phenomena before an abnormal state is diagnosed. Even within a single culture, it may be necessary to do this to take account of the diversity of experiences of distress; but between cultures the need is paramount.

Aubrey Lewis, my teacher and most distinguished predecessor, used to insist that before a phenomenon is regarded as abnormal, one should take account both of the statistical infrequency of the experience and the way in which the symptom was acquired: "if a man expresses an irrational belief – for example that he has been bewitched – we do not call it a delusion . . . unless we are satisfied that the manner in which it was acquired was morbid. This would not be the case if he had been brought up by people who believed in witchcraft . . . but if he is an ordinary 20th century Londoner who has arrived at such a conviction through highly devious, suspicion-laden mental processes, we call the belief abnormal, and the man who holds it unhealthy" (Lewis 1953).

Such niceties are often lost when today's young psychiatrists refer to their diagnostic criteria, and merely make a count of the abnormal phenomena present without making allowance for the way in which they were aquired. This mindless application of lists I have found to be just as common in India and Pakistan as it is in England, so that the process of trying to understand the nature of the patients experience becomes lost in the hurry of declaring that the patient "has" diagnosis A, perhaps even "co-morbid" with diagnosis B!

In Chapter 8 of this volume, Satvinder Juss argues that "the definition of mental health for ethnic minorities may be broader because of the impact of discrimination, poor housing, poor education, poverty, lack of employment, and social isolation leading to increased psychological and emotional difficulties". Would it apply to a young Irishman brought up in London, who had experienced all these disadvantages? Would it not be better to say that all these factors make the development of a mental disorder more likely, and that they are especially true among ethnic minorities? It is certainly the case that all these features (except discrimination) are also very common among young white patients with schizophrenia, and this should make use more aware of the social factors that may make the manifestation of schizophrenic forms of experience more likely – in whites as well as blacks.

It is not helpful to make a simplistic equation between these kinds of social disadvantage and racism: we must remember that Asians have been indiscriminately subjected to violence, and earlier Jews were also severly discriminated against, but neither of these groups developed higher rates of schizophrenia. It is of course true that the disadvantages experienced by black minorities can often be traced to racism in the majority population – but it is the disadvantages to which this leads which are harmful, rather than the racism itself – repugnant as this always is.

The chapters that follow nonetheless make uncomfortable reading for members of the ethnic majority, most of whom are aware that the services that they offer to minorities are often viewed as oppressive and are resented. It is essential that services in areas containing ethnic minorities become "culturally compliant", and it is unhelpful to describe the hiring of staff from ethnic minorities as "tokenism". In a multicultural society, mental health services should make every effort to see that the ethnic mix of staff they employ roughly corresponds to the population that they serve. This is not tokenism, it is good practice.

As a society we are now spending somewhat more than we used to of our GDP on health, but there has not so far been a corresponding increase in our spend on mental health. All of us who work in the mental health services have to endure an under-resourced service, in which innovation is much more difficult than it should be. The services for ethnic minorities described in Chapter 9 sound exciting – but for the foreseeable future black patients will still need to be admitted to hospitals, and it is important to ensure that the sevices they receive are as good as they can possibly be, within the restraints that are imposed upon us.

At a time when the rest of medicine is being urged to become "evidence-based", it is important that the efficacy of non-medical treatments that may be introduced are subject to the same scrutiny as medical treatments, if they are to be purchased with public money.

Finally, should we be studying schizophrenia among our black patients? In Chapter 1, the authors have their doubts, but in my view it would be reckless to abandon this line of research, which seems very likely to advance our understanding about the forms of social disadvantage that make psychotic illnesses likely to arise. Now that we know that the prevalence of schizophrenia is no higher in Jamaica than it is among whites in England, and remembering that cannabis is freely available in Jamaica – we have to go beyond either genes or cannabis in finding an explanation for the increased rates. It is my hope that reserach in the next few years will throw important light on the nature of these environmental factors. When this has occurred, the new knowledge will be just as important for disadvantaged whites as it will be for disadvantaged blacks.

David Goldberg
Institute of Psychiatry
King's College, London

Reference

Lewis, A. (1953) Health as a social concept. *British Journal of Sociology* **4**: 109–124.

Preface

The Oxford English Dictionary defines **society** as "the social mode of life, the customs and the organization of an ordered community; participation in hospitality, companionship and the association of persons united by a common aim or interest in people." What characterizes care in our society? How do people of diverse languages, customs and folklore modify our notions of society? There are few occasions when common aims and hopes have led to action in the provision of mental health services suited to all ethnic, cultural and linguistic groups. Society ought to have a view that recruits commonsense notions of justice and care. Health care should emerge from the aspirations and expectations of "society" as much as by political imperatives and economics.

Britain is a multi-cultural society. Diversity of culture, ethnicity, race, language, skin colour, preferred dress and diet, leisure, play and prayer reflect an enriched society. It is only recently, however, that the larger society has respectfully acknowledged that difference may exist and that this is not accompanied by threat. Those who are culturally different are indeed just as significant in their contribution to our society as those who show less divergence from the stereotypical British person. This requires a re-evaluation of what constitutes **British identity** for society and its various agents. Only then will public services truly serve a multi-cultural and multi-ethnic society.

The mentally ill have always been the focus of suspicion and fear in societies; add to this their unusual behaviours which deviate from societal norms and we obtain a potent brew of distrusts (mistrusts) across the mental health divide. Community care as a policy has been implemented incrementally since the 1960s. In the public arena, it has become conspicuous only in the context of headline incidents which have reinforced the fears and prejudices of the public. The politics of race, class and culture further constitute a treble jeopardy which black and ethnic minority mentally ill patients have to overcome in order to obtain professional assistance. They have done so in order to survive a system of mental health care which they perceive as largely unattractive, inflexible and unresponsive to their needs. They have done so with little support or encouragement from service providers, policy-makers and in a climate of increasing hostility from the general public. This is no longer a viable position for society to adopt.

This scenario inspired the writing of this book. It is written by people with special experience of humanity, suffering and its alleviation in the broadest context. We have deliberately encouraged a multi-professional re-conceptualization of the central issues that are relevant to the provision of mental health care for a multi-cultural society. The contributors have performed this task by bringing new insights from quite different historical, theoretical, research and experientially informed strategies for the management of suffering in both its narrow and wider sense. We aim to contribute to, and further stimulate, critical debate in this area of mental health care. The book can serve as a resource as well as a manual; we hope it ultimately equips all members of society to do their best for the mental health needs of not only their friends, family and colleagues but also people with whom they do not share cultures, religions, health beliefs, world views, skin colour, languages, sense of self-identity and group belonging.

KB and DO

Part I
Introduction

1

Context and Consensus

Kam Bhui and Dele Olajide

Ethnic minorities represent 6.2 per cent (Peach, 1996) of the UK population; in some regions they make up 40–50 per cent of local populations. If current demographic trends persist, black and ethnic minority people will comprise a greater proportion of the British population in the next century. Those of mixed race and ethnicity are under-represented in demographic data and in public health surveys, which makes meaningful evaluation of their health care needs rather difficult. New groups arriving in this country are often not recognised as citizens requiring a service, despite their economic contribution (McKee, 1997). New ethnicities and cultural identities are emerging without due attention to the dynamic nature of their health care needs. The evidence points out ethnic differences in the epidemiology and management of coronary heart disease, stroke, breast cancer, lung cancer, suicides, and undetermined deaths and accidents (Balarajan, 1995) as well as mental ill-health (Bhui, 1997). There is a great deal of literature about black and other ethnic minority groups' unsatisfactory experience of mental health services (Wilson, 1993; NHS Executive, 1994). Research evidence also consistently demonstrates differences in their treatments and pathways into mental health services (Lloyd and Moodley, 1992; Cole *et al.*, 1995). These data strongly suggest inequitable, oppressive, or poor management of mental ill-health amongst black and ethnic minority people. Yet, there has been no systematic implementation of pragmatic changes in the delivery of care or in the training of the professionals charged with providing care to these populations.

A great deal of hospital-based research has focused on the incidence and prevalence of mental illness, especially schizophrenia, amongst African and Caribbean peoples (Wessely, 1991; Glover *et al.*, 1994; Bhugra *et al.*, 1997). Research has focused on the empirical examination of putative aetiological factors which may be significant in the high prevalence of schizophrenia in this population (Glover *et al.*, 1994), without any serious attempt to understand better the pathogenesis of schizophrenia in general or to mobilise services to treat the high-risk populations. In some instances, investigators appeared to be preoccupied with exploring hypotheses that are specific to black and ethnic minority populations to the exclusion of other groups with a similarly higher prevalence of psychosis – such as the Irish (Bracken *et al.*, 1998). This mode of inquiry (which is mainly biological in orientation) inadvertently supports the perception that the causes of mental ill-health among black and ethnic minorities differ in totality from those that occur in the "white" populations. It pathologises and exoticises black people's beliefs, behaviour and life-style, such that a separatist solution is envisaged to be necessary to handle the unfamiliar. Consequently, mainstream mental health services do not accommodate the needs of all British citizens; separate services for black and ethnic minority groups emerged to deal with the crisis noticed by culturally diverse populations themselves. Black and ethnic minority workers are actively engaged in a political solution as well as a pragmatic approach to develop an alternative style of service that incorporates a biopsychosocial understanding of mental ill-health and effective interventions. Statutory sector professionals seem reluctant to effect the drastic changes required to provide a service that users and their carers perceive as relevant to their needs.

The challenge is to examine and evaluate interventions which range from specific clinical treatments to service configurations and policy. The findings of a higher incidence of psychosis amongst ethnic minorities has not motivated any greater attention to the management of these populations. Those at high risk of developing a specific illness should be the subject of targeted and preventive policies. This has not happened. There is a political and social imperative to scrutinise and correct injustice where this compounds social oppression of ethnic minorities in Britain. There is now a convergence of attention from all the major mental health charities, the King's Fund Institute, the Department of Health and the Royal Colleges. All are in pursuit of pragmatic solutions but there is a paralysis of any corrective intentions because of conflicting definitions of mental ill-health, and competing views about the contribution of racism. Teasing out the responsibilities of each professional body, as well as the charities, is essential to ensure co-ordinated change. Hence the General Medical Council, the Royal Colleges of Psychiatry, Nursing and Occupational Therapy, the British Psychological Society, the Association of University Teachers, the Confederation of Health Authorities and Trusts, Purchasers and Providers, to name but a few, all seem to be struggling in their response to the unequivocal data.

The purpose of this book is to examine critically the contributions of professionals involved in the care of mentally ill people from black and ethnic minority groups. All contributors have a special perspective on mental ill-health and its alleviation. Although the volume is intended to be a pragmatic guide to service development, other crucial theoretical issues of medical ethics, philosophy, political and economic dilemmas are also scrutinised. Moffic and Kinzie (1996) present a critique of the historical development of cross-cultural services (Table 1.1). We strongly recommend Phase 5 of Moffic's model as the focus for service planners and providers in Britain:

> These seek innovation in service structures and styles of care delivery such that the service optimally manages distress in the targeted cultural groups.

It is possible that these five stages can co-exist interchangeably depending on the most recent political and economic stance taken at local and national level in the UK. Nonetheless, the theoretical and practical issues examined

Table 1.1 Cross-cultural mental health services: historical developments.

Phase 1: Recognition of difference	An awareness that minority ethnic populations have different health care needs.
Phase 2: Treatment variations	That desired treatments vary across racial and ethnic groups and that there is a differential use of services.
Phase 3: Treatment changes	Altering staff and service characteristics. Using bilingual staff and non-Western modes of healing.
Phase 4: Cultural biology	Demonstrated that not only are some groups psychologically and culturally different but they have unique race and culture based responses to interventions. This can be understood not only from a biomedical model (different rates of metabolism of drugs) but also from a socio-cultural response (different expectations and degrees of adherence to interventions).
Phase 5: Newer directions	These seek innovation in service structures and styles of care delivery such that the service optimally manages distress in the targeted cultural groups. Thus the involvement of family, offering physical investigations and assessments, services suited to specific refugee groups which are still integral to generic service. Essentially broadening the remit to achieve more effective outcomes.

Source: Moffic and Kinzie (1996).

are relevant for service development initiatives globally. Debates of theory, policy and practice rarely accommodate the unique perceptions of the individual who suffers with emotional distress, that is the service user. Service planners and providers rarely acknowledge the expertise and insights that patients (and their carers) possess with respect to their mental ill-health. All mental health service policy must attend to this omission (Chapter 2). Professionals are unaware that their training does not capture the totality of the sufferer's experience. Resource rationing and evidence-based medicine do not accommodate lay value systems of society at large. Professional ethics and value systems are closed and self-supporting, encouraging great resistance to alterations of practice, let alone a change in empirical attitudes about the competent and comprehensive provision of health care (Chapter 3). All organisations harbour contradictory institutio-nalised procedures and policies that are detrimental to the very people the organisations intend to serve (Chapter 16). The voluntary sector emerged in response to statutory sector inertia and addresses the needs of black and ethnic minorities, but it has never been properly supported (Chapter 5). Community care developments have appeared without due consideration of their impact on ethnic minorities; any future policy initiatives must understand the historical and cultural context of people from ethnic minorities in order to appreciate fully this perpetuation of indifference (Chapter 15).

Data clearly illustrate ethnic variations in the use of psychotropic drugs and application of mental health legislation (Takei *et al.*, 1998); yet again this appears not to have mobilised concerns. The consultant psychiatrist's role of leading the community mental health team is a crucial point of influence for better services (Chapter 6). The need for psychotherapy services by ethnic minorities is not matched by their level of use of such services; indeed even where ethnic minorities do utilise psychotherapy services there are special issues to do with training and models of healing that seem to be obfuscated. The professions of nursing (Chapter 11), occupational therapy (Chapter 10), psychology (Chapter 12) and social work (Chapter 14) are essential to the effective and comprehensive provision of mental health care; the cross-cultural limitations of accepted practice and organisational priority within each of these professions are being addressed assertively.

Psychiatric practice has received serious and critical attention as its diagnostic and treatment procedures are clearly ethnocentric (Chapter 4); anthropology as a discipline critically questions the psychiatric profession's limited appreciation of more global approaches to healing and dealing with emotional distress. For example, service provision for distinct religious groups raises some specific diagnostic and spiritual concerns for providers (Chapter 5). Psychiatric and legal organisations ensure that mentally disordered offender patients from black and ethnic minorities continue to receive treatment and detention without an analysis of the contribution of culture and race to notions of criminality and forensic service provision (Chapters 7 and 8; Bhui *et al.*, 1998).

Government policy has restructured the relationship between GPs, patients and specialists but the opportunity to include primary care interventions specific to the mental ill-health of black and ethnic minorities has been missed (Chapter 13). GPs, purchasers and the public seek better management of health services to improve the quality, effectiveness and quantity of service provision for a multi-cultural and multi-ethnic Britain. Few providers know how to respond to, or even take the trouble to face, the challenge of honouring their commitments to all citizens (Chapter 17). The purchaser (or commissioner)/provider split offers a unique opportunity to revitalise service development initiatives and then to ensure the quality of service provision (Chapter 18). The machinery for pursuing progress by influencing purchasers and commissioners is complex, but it does ensure that central funding is tapped rather than specialist, limited or marginalised, and hence vulnerable, source of funding.

There remains a diversity of ideologies and policies which are differentially emphasised by distinct professions. In the final chapter (Chapter 19) we integrate the experiences of all contributors in order to outline essential service strategies. Each requires careful exploration and adaptation to suit local population profiles, distinct service specialities and specific professional and legislative imperatives.

References

Balarajan, R. (1995) Ethnicity and variations in the nation's health. *Health Trends* **27**(4): 114–119.

Bhugra, D. Leff, J., Mallet, R. *et al.* (1997) Incidence of schizophrenia in Afrio-Caribbeans and Asians in London. *Psychological Medicine* **27(4)**: 791–8.

Bhui, K. (1997) London's ethnic minorities and the provision of mental health services. In: Johnson *et al.* (ed.) *London's Mental Health*. London: King's Fund Institute.

Bhui, K., Brown, P., Hardie, T. *et al.* (1998) African Caribbean men remanded to Brixton Prison. Socio-demographic and forensic characteristics and outcome of final court appearance. *British Journal of Psychiatry* **172**: 337–344.

Bracken, P.J., Greenslade, L. *et al.* (1998) Mental health and ethnicity: an Irish dimension. *British Journal of Psychiatry* **172**: 103–105.

Cole, E., Leavey, G., King, M. *et al.* (1995) Pathways to care for patients with a first episode of psychosis. A comparison of ethnic groups. *British Journal of Psychiatry* **167**: 770–776.

Glover, G., Flannigan, C., Feeney, S. *et al.* (1994) Admission of British Caribbeans to mental hospitals: is it a cohort effect? *Social Psychiatry and Psychiatric Epidemiology* **29**: 282–284.

Lloyd, K. and Moodley, P. (1992) Psychotropic medication and ethnicity: an inpatient study. *Social Psychiatry and Psychiatric Epidemiology* **27**: 95–101.

McKee, M. (1997) The health of gypsies. Lack of understanding exemplifies wider disregard of the health of ethnic minorities. *British Medical Journal* **315**: 1172–1173.

Moffic, H.S. and Kinzie, J.D. (1996) The history and future of cross-cultural psychiatric services. *Community Mental Health Journal* **32**(6): 581–592.

NHS Executive (1994) *Black Mental Health: a dialogue for change.* London: NHS Executive.

Peach, C. (1996) The ethnic minority populations of Great Britain. In: Peach, C. (ed.) *Ethnicity in the 1991 Census.* Vol II. London: Office for National Statistics, HMSO.

Takei N., Persaud, R. *et al.* (1998) First episodes of psychosis in Afro-Caribbean and white people. An 18-year follow-up population based study. *British Journal of Psychiatry* **172**: 147–153.

Wessely, S. (1991) Schizophrenia and Afrio-Caribbeans: a case control study. *British Journal of Psychiatry* **159**: 795–801.

Wilson, M. (1993) *Britain's Black Communities.* London: NHS Management Executive, Mental Health Task Force and King's Fund Centre.

Part II
Beliefs and Values

2

Unanswered Questions: a User's Perspective

Anonymous Mental Health Service User

Sleepless nights, enveloping despair – guilt
Guilt at being me – black, female, poor,
Part of a large family –
Part of an even larger society
Resounding with racism and rejection.

Valium, psychiatrists, falling more into the abyss
Of white man's medicine.
Hospital, enforced activity, constant cajoling
To fit their categorisation of me,
All the time denying me my pain, my hurt, my confusion.
Reinforcing my "badness" at feeling these things.
Isolating me – alone – with my problems,

Unexpressed anger, increasing guilt,
The silence growing louder.
Largactil, locked doors, ECT, eventually stillness.
Sinking deeper and deeper into the sanctuary of insanity:
Beautiful – silent – still – feelingless – internal death;
Pushing back the screaming agony
Before I infect them with my poison –
The poison of my blackness, my culture, my very being;
All wrong, all contradicting the norms of their society,
All disrupting their ordered world.

And in the end I saw it their way, the guilt was *mine.*
So I tried – and battled – and pulled my self out of it –
And buried myself deeper, keeping me inside,
Smiling nicely, acting right, colluding with them,
Ensuring their equilibrium was maintained,
So I have the privilege of existing in their world –
Of experiencing their values, their beliefs,
Their prejudice, their power.
What does it matter that I died in the process?

What does it matter? One more black, crazy female,
One more drain on society, what does it matter?
To them nothing –
And ultimately to me it must mean nothing too,
Otherwise even existence becomes impossible
And internal death can only be mirrored in external reality.

(Survivors' Poetry, 1992)

At the present time, many different terms are used by people to describe themselves in relation to the mental health services, e.g. patient, user, client, consumer, survivor, the one/ones selected for use usually being those that feel comfortable or correct. For many of us, the various terms may each represent a particular political perspective, and we may use different terms in different contexts. The use of one term (in this chapter "user") does not exclude the validity of any other.

Introduction

Much has been written in the last decade about mental health, race and culture. Issues have been hotly debated in the pages of learned journals and at academic conferences and in planning meetings by a myriad of professionals, but relatively few black users of mental health services have ever been actively involved in discussions about black mental health. Partly this is because many black users, given the punitive and degrading treatment they have received at the hands of the statutory mental health services, do not wish to participate in any way with proponents of the "system". For those who do, the ways in are frequently blocked by high-minded officials or judgmental and patronising attitudes which keep users firmly in the position of "passive psychiatric patient" rather than as human beings with useful and relevant powers of evaluative thought and creativity. Yet unless black users can find some way of opening up communication and pass on their knowledge and experience to establish more appropriate and acceptable mental health services for their communities, we will continue to be the losers. The problems will continue to be seen as ours and all occurrences of mental and emotional distress will continue to be treated through diagnosis, incarceration and medication, irrespective of their origin or their wider social and political contexts (Fernando, 1995). But each black user has to determine their own position and assess how comfortable they would feel working with the (predominantly white) statutory institutions and services. Meaningful partnerships depend on attitudes and practices. It is not yet clear, however, whether individuals and institutions involved in mental health are prepared to change their current attitudes and practices, or whether society as a whole will ever accept responsibility for mental well-being, rather than dumping it at the door of psychiatry.

In writing this chapter, I do not claim to represent anyone other than myself. Obviously there are issues which others recognise and which can unite us in supportive and political action but each of us has our own unique story. Reclaiming our voice to tell that story (often after many years of damaging treatment) and owning it are still some of the hardest challenges we face. Here, I have decided to use the poem printed above to illustrate my own personal experiences of the mental health system over 20 years. I certainly do not deny that mental illness exists as a real phenomenon, but I do question very strongly how it is defined, and how it (correctly or incorrectly diagnosed) is treated and perpetuated in isolation from its cultural, social and political contexts. Whether such questions will ever be addressed remains to be seen.

Why Does Psychiatry Continue to Lock Us into Diagnosed Mental Distress?

The poem quoted at the start of this chapter was not, as might appear, written in a moment of despair and despondency, but rather at a time of startling realisation. A realisation that the system that I truly believed had helped and sustained me in times of utter madness and distress was actually, with each hospital admission, locking me more and more firmly into my mental illness. Maybe the psychiatric system, not understanding the distress that I as a black person brought to it, could work only by transforming it into a more familiar medicalised form – translating it into neat text-book diagnoses and subjecting it to relatively straightforward physical treatments. While I do acknowledge that this approach did often provide me with some instant "knockout relief" at the time, in the long term each hospital admission only compounded my original distress, denying its emotional, spiritual and social contexts, adding even more layers to my already blurred sense of self (*"isolating me, alone with my problems"*).

   Although enlightening, such cognisance about a system that I had truly believed had helped and sustained me in times of utter madness and despair was terrifying. I knew there were times when, all too desperately, I needed help, support and asylum (in the best sense of the word) and since the system was, in my experience, all there was at such times, what would happen if I began to doubt it? Who would be there to hold me (for better or worse) the next time, and the next, and the next. But perhaps that was the very point – somehow psychiatry, by not addressing the true issues, always ensures there *will* be a next time. On deeper reflection, I began to see how this could be interpreted, not in terms of care, but, sinisterly, in terms of social control. So society seems to have invested the essentially biological discipline of psychiatry with moral and legislative powers which enable it effectively to remove those emotionally and mentally distressed people who it sees as having no useful role in society. But how can psychiatry alone be responsible for such decisions? Other institutions are likely to have equally (or more) important contributions to make, e.g. education, housing, social welfare, employment, but for whatever reason society has chosen to involve only psychiatry to act as society's alienists.

Why Does Psychiatry Invalidate Our Collective and Individual Identity?

Identity is defined in *The Oxford English Dictionary* as "the condition of being a specific person" and a clear and positive sense of identity is essential for mental well-being. For many from minority ethnic communities, identity may be even more important, with a strong cultural identity being the lynch-pin which facilitates meaningful survival in an often hostile and racist environment. However, developing such an identity is not easy. Cross (1978) and Jackson and Hardiman (1983) have both suggested models of black identity development, each involving several dynamic but inter-related stages (Table 2.1). For those of us who have a fragile sense of self, negotiating these stages and the various reactions they might provoke in the majority community can bring about emotional and mental crises. It is often these that bring us (voluntarily or involuntarily) to the attention of the mental health system.

However, ethnicity and culture (while being central) are not the only determinants of our identity. Other factors such as gender, class, sexuality, religion, political convictions or occupation also play a role in shaping who we are. For those of us who encounter the psychiatric system, this rich, multi-faceted complex is, however, often denied as we are treated either in a culture-blind way or stereotyped according to our ethnicity. Both may be equally damaging.

Culture-blindness

In the culture-blind approach to psychiatry, it is usually proudly pro-nounced that all users are treated in the same way, i.e. assessed, diagnosed and treated in terms of Western culturally determined and historically based norms. Such a patronising and judgmental approach discounts that people from different cultures may have very different (but equally legit-imate) value systems, social structures and religious beliefs. All of these influence their expressions of distress and their perception of what would help them. In addition, the culture-blind approach completely negates the damaging experiences many from ethnic minority communities face in an essentially hostile society and the devastating effects that they can have on our psyche. For me, a lot of the symptoms of my distress were related to such experiences but the pressure to deny them and conform to Western

Table 2.1 Jackson's model of black identity development theory. (Jackson and Hardiman, 1983)

Stage 1	**Naivety** in which the individual has no awareness of themselves as a black person.
Stage 2	**Acceptance** in which the individual thinks of themselves as non-white but defines his identity in relation to the other so that white is construed as the correct way of being and individual may therefore be highly subservient and co-operative (Uncle Tom).
Stage 3	**Resistance and naming** in which the individual recognises that being black is an identity in itself and encounters blackness and its full meaning in an often racist society.
Stage 4	**Redefinition and reflection** in which the individual continues to develop a firm black identity in its own right.
Stage 5	**Multiperspective internalisation** in which the individual becomes a black person with pride in himself and an awareness of others, recognising the worthwhile dimensions of the dominant culture and fighting those aspects which represent racism and oppression, viewing the world through multiple frames of reference.

norms was enormous (*"all the time denying me my pain, my hurt, my confusion; reinforcing my badness at feeling these things"*).

And in the end, because I was desperate for help, I colluded with them (*"smiling nicely, acting right, colluding with them, ensuring their equilibrium was maintained"*) even though it meant losing the little that was there of my own sense of self. Thomas (1995) discusses a similar concept in psycho-therapeutic relationships, in which clients/users seek to protect themselves from rejection by projecting a proxy self which is usable by anyone but is actually devoid of any real meaning. While this can partly be seen as a protective device for the individual user, it provides false solutions and inevitably causes even further disintegration to their sense of self as negative self-images become perpetuated (*"before I infect them with my poison, the poison of my blackness, my culture, my very being"*).

Ethnic Stereotyping

Equally as damaging is ethnic stereotyping in psychiatry, since it assumes every member of a particular ethnic or cultural group has exactly the same identity. But this is not so. While a person's cultural group may say something about the mental health needs of the majority of people seen as belonging to that group (in the same way as a residential address may do so in terms of housing, deprivation, etc.), it can say no more. Each individual's identity will vary according to their personal interpretation of their cultural traditions and beliefs, their degree of assimilation to Western values and their membership of other groups in society. Discounting these variations inevitably leads to pigeon-holing users into purely ethnic categories and, for those of us who already have difficulties with establishing our true identity, this can be extremely damaging (*"one more black, crazy female, one more drain on society"*).

While undoubtedly important on an individual level, adherence to either a culture-blind or stereotyped approach in psychiatry may be even more important on a societal level, because society has endowed psychiatry with legislative powers to determine what is and what is not acceptable in society. But rather than taking the opportunity to draw attention to the inequality and injustice in society and develop constructive ways of dealing with it, psychiatry all too often confirms and reinforces many of society's racist ideas. It constructs a perceived reality in which Western is normal and anything else abnormal (*"my very being, all wrong, all contradicting the norms of their society"*) and effectively removes many potentially useful people from mainstream society for ever (*"and buried myself deeper, keeping me inside"*).

Why Do Biological Perspectives Monopolise Emotional Distress in Black People?

While it is popularly accepted that physico-biological factors are an important primary cause of mental illness, very extensive research has so far failed to identify any definitive links between biological constructs and the mental, emotional and spiritual components of the human psyche. This does not, however, seem to stop a mainly biological approach being taken in psychiatry, based on a purely Western medical model of diagnosis and treatment, with only cursory regard to social factors and usually no regard to cultural or spiritual ones. With sectioning and forced medication always in the picture and power very firmly in the hands of the professional, the user is essentially forced into complying with this physico-biological approach, whatever their perception of their own distress. As time goes on the user either becomes more resistant and bitter about the treatment they are receiving or just agrees with what they are told in order to avoid continual damaging confrontations about diagnosis and any accompanying treatment.

Thereafter, absolutely any further distress in the user's life can be conveniently attributed to their diagnosed mental illness, regardless of its origin, with for example anger and aggression at racist practices or to losing personal liberty being seen as purely pathological signs of illness rather than a normal and healthy response to injustice. At the same time as all emotional and psychological features are attributed to physico-biological causes, it is interesting that real physico-biologically based phenomena (e.g. side-effects of drugs or electro-convulsive therapy, ECT) which users have to endure are too often dismissed as insignificant or even assigned to psychological causes!

For me, medicalisation resulted in me abandoning my own truth and taking on completely the label of chronic psychiatric patient, with all its sequelae (*"hospital, constant cajoling to fit their categorisation of me . . . and in the end I saw it their way"*). After a few hospital admissions it became easier and I fell easily into the pattern of blocking everything out with medication or ECT and became increasingly dependent on the psychiatric system (*"sinking deeper and deeper into the sanctuary of insanity – beautiful, silent, still, internal death"*). Assigning my symptoms to a biological cause also led me to think of myself as a helpless victim who had little control over their own life and certainly carried no responsibility for its course. Repeated and long hospital admissions inevitably followed, each serving gradually to wipe out my past links with society and severing all hope of my ever having any useful future within it (*"one more black crazy female, one more drain on society"*).

That is not to say, however, that these admissions did not at the time provide some relief from severely disabling distress, but rather that nothing followed (*"so I battled and pulled myself out of it and buried myself deeper, keeping me inside"*). The original distress was never explored and any personal resources I had were not used to help me address my own crises (*"what does it matter that I died in the process"*). Maybe in that respect medicine, with its emphasis on biological treatments, showed me that, while it may have a place, it is not necessarily the only or best medium to help people manage or understand their own madness and pain. In other cultures mental distress is addressed in ways that do not involve biological medicine, e.g. through shamans[1] and obeah[2] (see Chapter 12). While

---

[1] A form of traditional healer.
[2] Magic and witchcraft.

these may not be wholly appropriate in this society, they do suggest that links between mental distress and other aspects of self may well warrant further investigation. Perhaps, then, rather than focusing on the development of newer and "more effective" biological treatments, we should be looking at mental distress in a wider context and perhaps re-examine how medicine came to take on responsibility for control of the psyche in the first place.

Why is Psychiatry Solely Responsible for Emotional and Mental Well-being?

Medical concepts of madness grew about 300 years ago when a need to control people who (for whatever reason) were disturbing social order through "lunatic behaviour" was linked to an increasing interest in Europe about biological concepts of the mind. For black people, such linking was particularly important since it evolved at a time when powerful myths of racism, slavery and colonialism were being integrated into imperialist European cultures. This meant that, even though there were relatively few black people in Europe at the time, racism became central to the development of psychiatry, with the minds and life-styles of people from other cultures being used to illustrate the superiority of the European races.

And, although not so blatant, racism remains firmly embedded within psychiatry; with its firm adherence to Eurocentric norms, its invalidation of the positive ideologies about life and its problems that come from black world views and the too frequent pathologisation of black expression of emotion, psychiatry continues to perpetuate the myth of the superior Western mind. And now, at the end of the 20th century, the psychiatrist and their team still play the role of society's custodian and alienist, fulfilling an uncaring society's requirements through enforced hospitalisation, compulsory medication and supervision registers.

The "Caring" Profession of Psychiatry Terrifies the Black Community: Why?

When considering the way Western psychiatry treats black users, it is also necessary to consider the impact that it has on black communities. It is perhaps particularly ironic that black people, who in the 1950s were invited half way across the world to work in an under-staffed British health service and worked long and hard to build up that service, now fear certain aspects of it (Prins *et al.*, 1993). Many who once extolled the virtues of the British health system are literally terrified of their families having any contact with psychiatric services, since they have experienced or heard about the punitive and degrading ways in which black people are so often treated. Because of such fears, black people are voting with their feet and essentially giving up their statutory rights to (what they consider to be inappropriate) mental health care, struggling against all odds to contain distressed individuals within the family or community, with no external help. If the crisis cannot be contained or deepens, outside agencies (e.g. neighbours, the police) may, however, call on the statutory services who confirm the family's fears by sectioning, hospitalising and medicating the individual. The often high-handed and punitive way in which this is done evokes many diverse feelings; for the individual concerned feelings of betrayal, rejection and anger, and for the family feelings of failure and guilt. So a vicious cycle is set up in which black people fear the power of white services and yet are often forced into them. This inevitably breeds more distrust and fear, and impacts on black–white relationships in other areas of society.

Why Are Useful Partnerships Between Psychiatry and Black Users So Often Impossible?

User involvement in health service development is now enshrined in law, with The Community Care Act 1990 stating that users' needs should be at the centre of service planning and the NHS Executive's Patient Partnership Strategy calling for active user participation in both individual patient care and overall service development. To some extent this is beginning to happen in some Trusts with national and/or local user organisations becoming more actively involved in shaping mental health service delivery. But these liaisons tend to be predominantly white, with little participation from black users.

Certainly this is not because the statutory services and the (predominantly white) user organisations, with their ideology of equal opportunities, do not wish to be seen to be involving them. The black user is frequently seen as a valuable commodity and actively nurtured and encouraged to express their views on issues of common concern to both black and white users. This may, however, be more difficult when black users articulate differences between the white and black user experience, both within and outside the mental health system. Sassoon and Lindlow (1995) have described how issues of the inequality of power in society and its consequences, racism and internalised oppression may all make it easier for black users to work with other black users rather than in a mixed group. In addition, although black and white users both strive for empowerment (gaining control over one's life), the basis for this may differ markedly according to cultural differences, i.e. black users may seek control in harmony and in consideration of the family and community while white users may be more inclined to seek control from a more individual, autonomous stance. If mixed user organisations and partnership institutions cannot accommodate such differences, black users may be silenced and their experiences invalidated. Alternatively, there may be patronising sympathy and a plea for the black user to educate the organisation or institution about black culture and values, again effectively silencing them with regard to what they actually want to say.

Transformations

Both scenarios describe the black user withdrawing, often with bitter self-recriminations that they have allowed themselves to be drawn once more into a situation where their true voice could not be heard. In many cases the organisation or institution may proclaim it has tried its best for the black user and lay the blame for any problems firmly with them, continue to claim its commitment to equal opportunities and then essentially carry on as before without any useful change. My own plight might have been similar if it were not for four specific factors. First, meeting other users with similar and dissimilar experiences of dissatisfaction were vital validating experiences. I was not alone and my grievances were not part of a "dysfunction" or "illness". Second, mental health conferences which demonstrated genuine support for the user's voice were a source of hope, inspiration and constructive anger. The professionals at these conferences who clearly had the user in mind were social workers and voluntary sector staff. Rarely did psychiatrists have a sensitive receptivity to users' dissatisfaction. It is therefore paradoxical that the third critical experience was meeting a psychiatrist. He saw me as a person and treated me with the dignity and respect due to any human being. He helped me see that my personhood, sense of self and humanity were not superseded by illness. The continuing existence of other aspects of my personality were recognised by him when I no longer knew of them. I had stopped valuing the healthy and illness-unrelated aspects of me. The final instrumental experience was a writing course for women. This encouraged, shaped and understood emotional expression to any level of intensity without drawing immediately on the language of psychiatry or the classifications of illness. All of these events took place within a two-year period and freed me to think and be a person with an illness rather than an illness bereft of human existence.

Conclusions

The solution to all these questions challenges the authors in this volume. We seek collectively to examine the philosophical, political, managerial, theoretical, inter-personal and spiritual dimensions of mental health care. Individual professions are limited in their scope of influence; the society-based approach to mental health care taken in this volume is sadly rarely replicated in the majority of services. The problems are complex and require more than a rhetorical commitment to anti-oppressive/anti-racist practice, which is all too often directed at white audiences rather than at black users in need of more effective services. What we want are services that respond positively to our own needs, recognise our strengths as well as our distress and take far more serious account of our varied spiritual, cultural and social traditions (see Webb-Johnson, 1991). The institution of psychiatry needs to examine its agenda honestly and assess whether it is concerned with care or control and, if the former, whether it is prepared to give up some of its power in order to provide better care. If it does this, then society as a whole must start taking responsibility for the rising numbers of black people entering the mental health services, with a strong political commitment to involving other institutions in preventing and dealing with the causes and consequences of mental distress. Whether we ever have a society that truly cares about the mental well-being of **all** of its communities, deals with mental distress in appropriate, acceptable and accountable ways, and accommodates all the rich complex of identities equally, remains to be seen.

References

Cross, W.E. (1978) The Thomas and Cross models of psychological nigrescence: a review. *Journal of Black Psychology* **5**(1): 13–31.

Fernando, S. (1995) *Mental Health in a Multi-ethnic Society.* London: Routledge.

Jackson, B. and Hardiman, R. (1983) Racial identity development: implications for managing the multicultural workforce. In: Vitivo, R. and Sargent, A. (eds) *The NTL Managers' Hand Book*, pp. 107–119. Arlingon, Virginia: NTL Institute.

Prins, H., Blacker-Holst, T., Francis, E. and Keitch, I. (1993) *Big, Black and Dangerous.* Report of Committee of Enquiry into the death in Broadmoor Hospital of Orville Blackwood and a review of the deaths of two other Afro-Caribbean patients. London: Special Hospital Services Authority.

Sassoon, M. and Lindlow, V. (1995) Consulting and empowering black mental health system users. In: Fernando, S. (ed.) *Mental Health in a Multi-ethnic Society*, pp. 89–106. London: Routledge.

Survivors' Poetry (1992) In: Bangay, S. Bidder, J. and Porter, H. (eds) *From Dark to Light*. London: Survivors Press.

Thomas, L. (1995) Psychotherapy in the context of race and culture. An intercultural therapeutic approach. In: Fernando, S. (ed.) *Mental Health in a Multi-ethnic Society*, pp. 172–190. London: Routledge.

Webb-Johnson, A. (1991) *A cry for change. An Asian perspective in developing quality mental health care.* Confederation of Indian Organisations, UK.

3

From Culturally Sensitive to Culturally Competent

K.W.M. Fulford

In cross-cultural aspects of their work, psychiatrists find themselves caught between a rock and a hard place. Here, above all, it is important to engage directly with real people, with the values and beliefs of unique individuals located in particular social and cultural contexts. Yet the very authority of psychiatry as a scientific medical discipline seems to require an impersonal stance, an approach that is objective and decontextualised.

The tension between subjectivity and objectivity, although surfacing at different times in different guises, is not new to psychiatry. Karl Jaspers, one of the founding fathers of descriptive psychopathology, repeatedly emphasised the need for empathic understanding as well as for scientific explanations in psychiatry (Jaspers, 1913a); and recent developments in AI (Artificial Intelligence) and neuroscience have prompted some ingenious attempts to reconcile meanings and causes by way of modern representational theories of mind (Bolton and Hill, 1996). In this chapter, however, we will be concerned with this tension primarily as a *practical* problem. We will explore the skills, philosophical as well as practical, required to navigate successfully between the rock of subjective values and the hard place of objective facts. These skills, as we will see, are required not only for cross-cultural psychiatry but for psychiatry generally. Hence the take-home message of the chapter will be that a psychiatry which is not merely culturally *sensitive* but culturally *competent* is a competent psychiatry.

The Structure of the Chapter

Because this chapter is concerned with philosophy and practice, it is presented in the form of a seminar. It can be read as an ordinary chapter. But the best way to read it is in the spirit of taking part in the seminar, thinking about the points raised for yourself, and in particular trying out the "Questions for the Reader" as you go along.

The seminar is divided into three parts, each of approximately half an hour. Part I covers a case history (the case of Simon) and a diagnosis. Part II introduces some ideas from philosophy, specifically from linguistic analysis and value theory. These offer a set of "thinking skills" for understanding some of the difficulties thrown up by the diagnosis in Simon's case in Part I. Part III then looks at the practical consequences of the new understanding of Simon's case given to us by the philosophy introduced in Part II. These consequences, although drawn initially in respect of psychiatric diagnosis, are important also for a wide range of other issues, not only in cross-cultural psychiatry but in psychiatry generally.

PART I: CASE HISTORY AND DIAGNOSIS

Questions for the reader: *Read through the following case history with two questions in mind: 1. what is the diagnosis; 2. what steps did you go through to reach your diagnosis?*

A key contribution of philosophy to good practice in mental health is to help us develop new "thinking skills". Hence it is important to think about and to answer these questions **for yourself** *– whether as a doctor or a user, a nurse, a social worker, a manager, or whatever –* **before** *reading on. We learn new skills by trying them out actively for ourselves and getting feedback, not by sitting back and passively watching others! So, write down a few words about, 1. the diagnostic possibilities* **you** *would consider, and 2. your reasoning, i.e. how* **you** *would come to a diagnosis.*

The Case of Simon

Simon, aged 40, was a senior, black American professional, from a middle-class, Baptist family. Before the onset of his symptoms, he reported sporadic, relatively unremarkable, psychic experiences. These had led him to seek the guidance of a professional "seer", with whom he occasionally consulted on major life events and decisions.

Presenting history

Recently, his hitherto successful career had been threatened by legal action from a group of colleagues. Although he claimed to be innocent, mounting a defence would be expensive and hazardous. He responded to this crisis by praying at a small altar which he set up in his front room. After an emotional evening's "outpouring", he discovered that the candle wax had left a "seal" (or "sun") on several consecutive pages of his bible, covering certain letters and words. He described his experiences thus. "I got up and I saw the seal that was on my father's bible and I called x and I said, you know 'something remarkable is going on over here.' I think the beauty of it was the specificity by which the sun burned through. It was . . . in my mind, a clever play on words." Although the marked words and letters had no explicit meaning, Simon interpreted this event as a direct communication from God, which signified that he had a special purpose or mission. From this time on, over a period of some months, Simon received a complex series of "revelations" largely conveyed through the images left in melted candle wax. He carried photos of these, which left most observers unimpressed, but were, for him, clearly representations of biblical symbols, particularly from the book of Revelations (the bull, the 24 elders, the arc of the covenant, etc.). They signified that "I am the living son of David . . . and I'm also a relative of Ishmael, and . . . of Joseph". He was also the "captain of the guard of Israel". He found this role carried awesome responsibilities: "Sometimes I'm saying – O my God, why did you choose me, and there's no answer to that". His special status had the effect of "increasing my own inward sense, wisdom, understanding, and endurance" which would "allow me to do whatever is required in terms of bringing whatever message it is that God wants me to bring".

He expressed these beliefs with full conviction. "The truths that are up in that room are the truths that have been spoken of for 4000 years". When confronted with scepticism, he commented: "I don't get upset, because I know within myself what I know."

He also described experiences of thoughts coming into his head: "If you're sitting and watching television, and then somebody turns on the vacuum cleaner, and the TV goes on the fritz, it's like that . . . the things that come are not the things I have been thinking about . . . they kind of short circuit the brain, and bring their message."

Simon's Case – How do your Conclusions Compare with those of other Seminar Groups?

I have tried out Simon's case history, exactly as described above, with several groups of trainees in different parts of the United Kingdom. Working in pairs, I ask them to write down answers to the above two questions and we then "compare notes". You may have come up with different answers, but most groups come up with something along the following lines:

Question 1: *What is the diagnosis?* A typical list of diagnostic possibilities is "schizophrenia, schizoaffective disorder, hypomania, organic disorder (?drug-induced), hysteria". Most groups decide on schizophrenia, or possibly schizoaffective disorder, as the diagnosis.

Question 2: *What is the diagnosis based on?* Following the conventional two-step (medical) diagnostic process, we first identify Simon's symptoms and then fit them to a diagnostic category. Thus, most trainees quickly pick out a clear first-rank symptom of schizophrenia, i.e. a delusional perception (in Simon's reading of meanings into the wax seals). They also identify possible thought insertion (in Simon's mind "going on the fritz" – both symptoms are described further below).

As to a diagnostic category, the strongly positive affective colouring to Simon's experiences, and his somewhat "grandiose" thinking, suggest hypomania; but the first-rank symptoms make schizophrenia, or perhaps schizoaffective disorder, a more appropriate category. First-rank symptoms may also occur in organic disorders (such as dementia) but Simon shows, apparently, no "clouding of consciousness" (i.e. reduction in the level of consciousness), though drug-induced psychoses may occur in clear consciousness. Organic disorder would thus have to be borne in mind, but is unlikely, particularly given the extended duration of Simon's history without intellectual decline. Similarly for hysteria: it can be very difficult to distinguish hysteria from genuine psychosis, but the symptoms are so specific as to make this unlikely. The better trainees, however, note that careful monitoring of Simon's mental state and physical condition over an extended period will be important in this respect, since even genuine hysterical symptoms may turn out to be only the first warning of more serious underlying disorder, organic or functional. All in all, though, on the story as presented, schizophrenia and schizoaffective disorder are the most likely diagnoses.

At this point in the seminar, we go back to Simon's case history to look at the outcome of his history.

Simon's case – outcome

Simon's experiences gave him the strength to take on and win the lawsuit that was being mounted against him. A lawyer himself, this restored his self-confidence as a high-achieving black person working in an area where racism was still rampant. His career flourished and he used some of the large amount of money he made to set up a new charitable foundation. Through all this, his revelations had continued, and he now saw his purpose in life to bring about a reconciliation of Christianity and Islam.

Simons' Case – Back to the Differential Diagnosis

Questions for the reader: Does this outcome change your view about Simon's diagnosis? Can we still make a diagnosis of schizophrenia? Can we say that he is ill at all? Again, think about these questions for yourself before reading on.

The outcome of Simon's story generally provokes a lively debate. One reaction, perhaps the most common, is to say that he had a "benign form" of schizophrenia. The counter to this is that he was not ill at all, but, despite appearances, was undergoing a religious experience. Either way, the surprisingly positive outcome of his story is a shock to the psychiatric diagnostic system. Indeed, in the context of a training seminar, Simon's story might seem unduly subversive. After all, it would be grist to the mill of the anti-psychiatrists, those who argue that there is no such thing as mental illness. Thomas Szasz, now an Emeritus Professor of Psychiatry at Upstate University, New York, remains the exemplar of the view that mental illness is a myth, and Simon's story might seem to offer support for his claim that mental disorders are, really, moral problems ("problems of living", as he called them; Szasz, 1960, 1987) rather than medical problems. Psychiatrists of a more conventional persuasion, on the other hand, have reacted strongly to such views. Asserting the reality of mental illness (Roth and Kroll, 1986), they have argued that mental illness is, really, no different from physical illness (Kendell, 1975). Specifically in the case of religious experience, this has led some to subsume it *en bloc* to psychopathology (Group for the Advancement of Psychiatry, 1976).

Leaving aside these extremes, however, Simon's case – presenting with apparently clear-cut symptoms of severe mental illness, yet issuing in a highly adaptive rather than pathological outcome – prompts us to look more carefully at the diagnosis, and in particular at how we differentiate between spiritual experience and psychosis. The sometimes close similarities between religious or spiritual experience and severe psychiatric illness have been well recognised for many years. William James, a philosopher–psychologist and one of the founding fathers of cultural anthropology, described "delusional insanity" as "religious mysticism turned upside down" (James, 1902). That there should be close links between spiritual experience and psychopathology is not in itself surprising. *All* symptoms, after all, physical as well as mental, merge with experiences and/or behaviour that are normal or indeed highly adaptive – pain, nausea, rumination, conviction, to take four very different examples, are all in some contexts normal and adaptive.

Just how pathology should be characterised, however, has generated a voluminous literature, from anthropologists (e.g. Littlewood and Lipsedge, 1989) and sociologists (e.g. Fitzpatrick *et al.*, 1984), psychiatrists (e.g. Fulford, 1989) and indeed philosophers (e.g. Flew, 1973). The possible criteria for identifying the genuinely pathological suggested in this literature are both general and specific. As to general criteria, pathology is said to have a certain intensity and duration – for instance, a very mild and brief pain is unlikely to be experienced as a symptom of illness. In the case of ruminative and other obsessional phenomena, to take another example, these very general characteristics of pathology are diagnostically central (minor obsessional phenomena, like getting a tune "stuck in your head", being normal). Clearly, though, further and more specific criteria are required to distinguish between spiritual experience and psychotic symptoms, since both may, as in Simon's case, be intense and enduring. These more specific criteria, in descriptive psychopathology, define the form and content of particular symptoms. We owe the notions of form and content to the 17th century Prussian philosopher, Immanuel Kant. They have come down to us in psychiatry through the work of Karl Jaspers in his foundational *General Psychopathology* (1913b). It is by form and content, then, that the first-rank symptoms of schizophrenia (including, as in Simon's case, delusional perception and thought insertion) are defined and identified.

So, what has gone wrong in Simon's case? Given the positive outcome of his story, we have had to extend the diagnostic possibilities to include, at worst, a remarkably benign form of schizophrenia, at best, a healthy and adaptive religious experience. Yet neither possibility was suggested originally, i.e. when we had only his presenting story to go on. Has our diagnostic reasoning been defective, then? Have we been careless about the precise form and content of first-rank symptoms, perhaps; or clumsy in applying the diagnostic concepts based on these symptoms?

The need for careful definition both of the symptoms and syndrome of schizophrenia is well recognised. In the International Pilot Study of Schizophrenia (WHO, 1978), for example, loose diagnostic criteria were shown to have led to widely different diagnostic practices in different parts of the world. In some cases, notoriously in the former USSR, this was a factor leading to the abusive misdiagnosis of political dissent as schizophrenia (Bloch and Reddaway, 1977). The development of standardised diagnostic schedules with high degrees of reliability (i.e. of consistency between users) has taken us a long way towards putting psychiatric diagnosis on a firmer scientific footing. The Present State Examination, or PSE, was among the first structured interview schedules aimed at precise definition of symptoms, reflecting best practice in the clinical examination of the mental state (Wing *et al.*, 1974). Similarly, the World Health Organisation's ICD-10 (International Classification of Diseases, Edition 10; WHO, 1992), and the American Psychiatric Association's DSM-IV (the Fourth Edition of their Diagnostic and Statistical Manual; APA, 1994), have given us detailed inclusion and exclusion criteria for all the main categories of psychiatric disorder, including schizophrenia.

So, again, what has gone wrong in Simon's case? Are we heading towards the conclusion that the standard instruments fail to distinguish religious experience from psychopathology, "Simon the Seer", as we could now call him, from "Simon with Schizophrenia"? Given philosophy's reputation for subversive activities, we might expect so. Socrates, who was voted the poisoned chalice by his fellow citizens in 399BC for corrupting the youth, was known as "the gadfly of Athens"! And the standard diagnostic instruments, after all, *have* been accused of being "culturally insensitive". The ICD (although consciously aiming at world-wide acceptability) and the DSM (although expressly addressing cross-cultural issues) have both been accused of reflecting a distinctively white and Western, not to say male, paradigm (Radden, 1994). Modern classifications, it has been said in their defence, do include the so-called "culture-bound" syndromes; but this very term, so the argument goes, implies that there are conditions that are *not* culture bound – it denies the essentially culture-bound nature of psychiatry.

Questions for the reader: *At this point, think about Simon's diagnosis one final time. If you have access to them, look up the criteria for schizophrenia in ICD-10 and DSM-IV. 1. Are they different? 2. Does this make a difference to how we should understand Simon's experiences?*

Surprisingly, perhaps, the seminar is certainly *not* heading towards undermining psychiatric diagnosis. Despite the fact that most seminar groups fail even to think of the possibility of normal religious experience, "Simon the Seer" *can* be distinguished from "Simon with Schizophrenia" using only the criteria in the standard classifications. The distinction can indeed be made quite straightforwardly. Thus, our initial diagnosis was based on the presence of at least one first-rank symptom, persisting for a month or more. In the absence of evidence of organic disorder, this is sufficient according to the ICD-10 criteria (which reflect the traditional diagnostic concept) for a diagnosis of schizophrenia (or of schizoaffective disorder). The problem, though, as we have seen, is that the ICD-10 criteria fail to distinguish schizophrenia from religious experience. The American DSM-IV, however, adds a further criterion (criterion B) which makes the distinction relatively straightforward. In the DSM-IV, in addition to persistent first-rank symptoms, a diagnosis of schizophrenia requires that there be "social/occupational dysfunction," i.e. deterioration in one or more areas "such as work, inter-personal relations or self-care" (American Psychiatry Association, 1994, p. 285). Simon showed no such deterioration. Hence, far from having schizophrenia, even in a benign form, he did not have schizophrenia at all.

We may wish to discuss further just *how* Simon's experiences should be understood. But his own view, that they were revelations from God, a view which many would share, cannot be discounted as merely pathological. God may of course work through pathology, but Simon's beliefs that his experiences were revelations cannot, according at least to the DSM criteria, be simply written off as symptoms of schizophrenia. For according to DSM-IV, whatever he "had", he did not have schizophrenia.

Questions for the reader: *What do you think about criterion B, as above? Does it fit the DSM's self-image as a scientific classification concerned only with objective facts?*

So, is it QED for medical psychiatry? Well, criterion B from DSM-IV certainly does make the distinction between "Simon the Seer" and "Simon with Schizophrenia". But, as you may have spotted, there is a sting in the (philosophical gadfly's) tail! The sting in the tail is that the crucial criterion in the differential diagnosis of schizophrenia is (or depends on) a **value judgement**. According to DSM-IV, for a diagnosis of schizophrenia it is not sufficient to establish the fact that the person concerned has one or more first-rank 'symptoms' (together with other facts about duration, etc.); it is not sufficient even to establish the fact that there has been a change in life functioning; for a diagnosis of schizophrenia, a value judgement has also to be made about the course of the person's life, i.e. about whether or not there is deterioration in life functioning, a change for the worse. This becomes clear if we look carefully at the words actually used: "social/occupational *dys*function"; functioning *"below"* previous levels; *"failure* to achieve" expected levels (all DSM-IV, p. 285, emphases added). From the perspective of a conventional medical–scientific model of psychiatry, then, this value judgement is a potentially lethal sting in the philosophical gadfly's tail. For it seems flatly to contradict the key requirement for a scientific psychiatry, that psychiatric diagnosis should be based on objective facts.

PART II: PHILOSOPHY

In this part of the seminar we are going to take a step back from Simon's case for a few minutes, to consider how philosophy can help us to understand the kind of problem with which he presents. To do this, we need to look first, in a general way, at philosophy itself – at what philosophers do and how they go about doing it. We will find that there are no fewer than four important points of contact between philosophers and mental health practitioners. We will then go on to look at philosophical work specifically on facts and values, and at how this can help us towards a clearer understanding of the meanings of concepts of disorder, such as illness and disease. What we will find is that philosophy gives us what amounts to a set of tools for thinking more clearly about psychiatric diagnosis. In the last part of the seminar, we will come back to Simon's case, and the practical implications of thinking more clearly about psychiatric diagnosis.

What is Philosophy and what do Philosophers do?

Questions for the reader: *Think about these two questions for yourself – just what* **is** *philosophy; and just what* **do** *philosophers do? You may have done some philosophy or you may not. Either way, you will have ideas of your own if you reflect on these questions for a moment or two. So, write down a few brief notes in answer to both questions, again, before reading on.*

To many practitioners, if philosophy means anything it means "playing with words". It is ironic that among psychiatrists this description is often intended pejoratively ("philosophy is *merely* playing with words"). For words are a key tool in psychiatry: as Simon's case illustrates, many of our most acute practical difficulties are difficulties about meanings, about how mental disorder itself should be understood; and unlike more technological areas of medicine, our effectiveness in every aspect of mental health practice depends critically on effective communication. Word use, moreover, is a skill, and, as the format of this seminar emphasises, skills development depends on practice (on play!).

So philosophers and mental health practitioners have an important point of contact in their shared concern with language. Good practice in mental health depends on being sensitive to meaning; and philosophy, correspondingly, as William James put it, is "an unusually stubborn effort to think clearly". This indeed places philosophy at the very coal face of psychiatric practice. There is, moreover, a way of doing philosophy, of pursuing the search for clear meaning, which is highly concordant with the case-based experience of practitioners, in that it starts not from abstract reflection on definitions but with the *actual words we use* in everyday language. This method, employed most explicitly by J.L. Austin, as Professor of Moral Philosophy in Oxford in the period after the Second World War, is called linguistic analysis (Austin, 1956–57). Austin urged philosophers to get out of their libraries and to examine real cases in the real world.

Linguistic analysis, then, with its emphasis on cases, provides a second point of contact between philosophy and psychiatry. The rationale for this method provides yet a third point of contact. Austin, building on the ideas of the Austrian philosopher Ludwig Wittgenstein (who worked mainly in Cambridge), pointed out that we are better at using words than defining them: a favourite philosophical example is "time" – we use the word time all the time, yet we would be completely stumped if asked to define it. And all this, to a psychiatrist, should make excellent sense developmentally; for we learn the meanings of words largely by shared use in a social context rather than by reading dictionaries full of definitions.

The results of philosophical work of this kind, the practical results to which it leads, provide a fourth point of contact with psychiatry. Austin, again building on Wittgenstein, described philosophy (of this linguistic analytical kind) as giving us a more complete picture of the meanings of the concepts with which we are concerned (Austin, 1956–57). The point here is that we are so good at just using words that we have become relatively blind to their full meanings. Explicit definitions, as in dictionaries and textbooks, thus tend to reflect only partial, and often biased, interpretations of meanings. Looking at the way words are actually used, on the other hand, can help us to break through what Austin called the "veil of ease and obviousness" by which their full meanings are often obscured. Linguistic analysis, therefore, is in this respect like psychoanalysis. Both help to make hidden meanings explicit. As the late Sir Denis Hill, then Professor of Psychiatry at the Maudsley Hospital, once put it, both are "consciousness raising exercises" (personal communication). And both kinds of analysis, linguistic and psychoanalytical, having brought hidden meanings into full consciousness, allow us to deal with them more effectively.

In starting this chapter with a case, with the story of Simon, we were true to Austin's philosophical method. The key point, moreover, on which the practical difficulty presented by Simon's differential diagnosis turned, was a philosophical difficulty. It was a difficulty of meaning, of how his experiences of revelation should be interpreted or understood. Our initial list of diagnoses failed to include normal religious experience; and the ICD-10, indeed, consistently with the traditional concept of schizophrenia, failed to allow for this diagnostic possibility. We can now see this failure as reflecting a kind of Austinian "incomplete view". Deeply influenced as we all are by the medical–scientific model of psychiatry, we assumed that religious revelations of this kind, conforming to the standard factual criteria for first-rank symptoms, *had* to be pathological. At first glance, the DSM-IV, as a scientific classification, appeared to provide an escape route for the medical–scientific model. For the DSM-IV included an additional criterion for schizophrenia, criterion B, that as well as first-rank symptoms there should be a deterioration in life functioning. However, when we focused, with a J.L. Austin-sharpened eye, on the words actually used in expressing this criterion, it suddenly became evident that the criterion expressed not a matter of scientific fact, but a value judgement.

So the whole of the first part of this seminar, although presented as an exercise in practical diagnosis, could equally well have been an exercise in linguistic analytical philosophy. We tackled a problem of meaning by starting with an actual case; then, by looking carefully at the words actually used, we broke through Austin's "veil of ease and obviousness", in this case represented by the definitions in (what takes itself to be) a scientific classification (the DSM-IV); and we found that the diagnosis in the original case turned on a value judgement. Consciousness-raising with a vengeance, then; but where do we go from here?

Fact, Value and the Case of Mental Disorder

The discovery of a value judgement at the very heart of the diagnosis of schizophrenia was described at the end of the first part of this seminar as a potentially lethal sting in the philosophical gadfly's tail. The sting was only lethal, however, to a conventional medical–scientific model of psychiatry, one in which it is assumed that our core diagnostic concepts have to be defined in terms of value-free scientific facts. Interestingly, work in the philosophy of science has shown the extent to which much of science itself (even our choice of theories) is driven by values (see, for example, Hesse, 1980, for a balanced treatment of the "theory ladenness" of science). So the conventional medical model may be hitching itself to a false, or at any rate over-simplified, picture of science. All the same, the model has been highly influential, and not least in the long-running "debate about mental illness'.

We touched on this debate in Part I of the seminar. Szasz (1960), we noted then, representing one pole of anti-psychiatry, argued that mental illnesses are, really, moral (or life) problems. The force of Szasz's argument, however, we can now see, arises from a feature of mental illness that is acknowledged equally by pro-psychiatrists, namely that the concept of mental illness is *prima facie* more value-laden than the concept of physical illness. In Part I of the seminar, the pro-psychiatry position was represented by authors such as Kendell (1975). For these authors, too, the "problem" was that mental disorders are closer than physical disorders to moral problems – alcoholism is close to drunkenness, for example, psychopathy to delinquency, and so on. Hence the difference between anti- and pro-psychiatry positions came down to whether or not the value-ladenness of mental disorder, acknowledged by both sides, can be defined away. Szasz argued that it cannot; Kendell, on the other hand, argued that it can. "Mental disorder," he suggested, "is in this respect just like "physical disorder;" it implies the presence of "biological dysfunction"; and this apparently evaluative notion ("biological *dysfunction*"), Kendell concluded, can be redefined in terms of straightforwardly factual criteria such as reduced life and/or reproductive potential.

What has philosophy to offer here? The general philosophical method of linguistic analysis is important. It shows, for example, that even those most committed to a value-free definition of disease continue to use the term with clear evaluative connotations (Fulford, 1989, Chapter 3). In this instance, though, substantive philosophical work on the logical properties of value terms and their relationship to factual terms offers specific insights into the debate about mental illness, insights which, we will see, are directly relevant to our understanding of psychiatric diagnosis. A full discussion of this would take us beyond the scope of this seminar (but see Chapters 2–5 of Fulford, 1989). There is one point, however, that we do need to look at in more detail, namely just *why* mental disorders are more value-laden than their bodily counterparts. Philosophy offers an explanation for this which, although seemingly rather theoretical, is in fact the key to understanding the practical implications of the value judgements implicit in psychiatric diagnosis.

Why Mental Disorder is more Value-laden than Physical Disorder

Questions for the reader: *Why do you think mental disorder is more value-laden than physical disorder? Is it because psychiatry's scientific base is less well developed than the scientific base of physical medicine? Or is there some other reason? Spend some time thinking about this for yourself. We are coming to a key point of understanding. You will grasp the point far more effectively if you have a go at thinking it through for yourself before reading on.*

Most people, certainly most doctors, faced with the more value-laden nature of mental illness, assume that this is a result of psychiatry being based on a primitive or under-developed science. Certain philosophers have thought this too, the American philosopher Christopher Boorse, for example (Boorse, 1975). Other philosophers, though, working in the linguistic analytical tradition on the relationship between facts and values (this branch of philosophy is sometimes called "theoretical ethics"), have come up with a quite different explanation; or rather, they have given us an insight into the logical relationship (the relationship of meaning) between facts and values, which allows us to understand the more value-laden nature of mental illness, and correspondingly the *less* value-laden nature of physical illness, in a quite different way.

The key point can be developed thus: Kendell's redefinition of (the evaluative) "biological dysfunction" in terms of (the facts of) reduced life and/or reproductive expectations can be understood as a form of what in philosophical value theory is called **descriptivism**. Descriptivism has a long and honourable tradition of philosophical work behind it. The Oxford philosopher, Geoffrey Warnock (1971), for instance, argued that in some circumstances evaluative terms (like dysfunction) can indeed be redefined in factual terms (like life/reproductive expectations). Other philosophers, however, have taken the opposing or *non-descriptivist* line, that there is an insuperable gap of meaning between facts and values (or between descriptions and evaluations). Non-descriptivism, in one form or another, also goes back a long way, at least as far as the 18th century Scottish empiricist philosopher, David Hume (McNabb edition, 1962). The essence of Hume's non-descriptivist argument is that to get values out of an expression, you have to put values in ("no ought from an is" is the slogan). Descriptivism, non-descriptivists argue, appears plausible in some cases, but this is only for *psychological*, not logical, reasons. The key point, then, to get to it at last, is this: that values may appear to be redefinable in terms of facts, but *only when the factual criteria for the value judgement in question are widely settled or agreed upon.*

Clear? Not very, as yet. An example which many find helps to make the point clearer was given by another Oxford philosopher, R.M. Hare (e.g. in Hare, 1981). Hare pointed out that an evaluative expression like "good eating apple" appears to be redefinable in terms of facts like "clean-skinned, sweet, etc." But, he continued, does it follow from this that "good eating apple" really means "clean-skinned, sweet, etc. apple"? If it does, then it would be self-contradictory to say of an apple that it is "a *good* eating apple" but *not* "clean-skinned, sweet, etc.". This test, of self-contradiction, is a useful test of meaning. "Bitch", a standard philosophical example, means "female dog"; and in this case it really is self-contradictory to say of an animal that it is a bitch but is *not* a female dog (metaphorical meanings aside). By contrast, though, it is not self-contradictory to say of an apple that it is a *good* eating apple but is *not* clean-skinned and sweet. It would be unusual to say this. Our psychology (the psychology of our taste in eating apples) is such that most people judge clean-skinned, sweet apples to be good eating apples. But it would be psychologically eccentric, not logically self-contradictory, for someone to evaluate apples differently. Hence "good eating apple", although fact-laden rather than value-laden, does not mean "clean-skinned, sweet, etc.". Hence "good eating apple" cannot be redefined solely in terms of these facts.

This somewhat theoretical argument goes to the heart of what is distinctive about psychiatry compared with physical medicine. Descriptivism, the attempt to redefine values in terms of facts, *looks* persuasive where the criteria (the factual, or descriptive, criteria) are widely agreed upon. This is true of "good eating apple", and it is true of Kendell's "biological dysfunction" (most people value longer life and greater fecundity). It is also true of the symptoms typically associated with physical illness – pain, nausea, shortness of breath, etc., if severe and prolonged, are, most people agree, bad. But now, what about psychological medicine? Can the same be said to be true of the symptoms typically associated with mental illness? Surely not. For in psychiatry we are concerned, characteristically, with the "higher" functions, such as desire, belief, wish, volition and appetite. And in respect of these higher functions, far from being widely settled or agreed upon, our values differ widely.

The bottom line, then, is that people's values differ, and differ legitimately, more widely in the areas of human experience and behaviour with which psychiatry is typically concerned (desire, beliefs, etc.) than in the areas with which physical medicine is typically concerned (pain, nausea, etc.). It is individual human variation, then, not an underdeveloped psychiatric science, which is the explanation for mental disorder being more value-laden than physical disorder. And importantly, therefore, the diversity of our values, and hence the importance of values in psychiatry, is not something that will be changed by future scientific advances. Under the influence of the medical–scientific model, it is widely assumed (at least by psychiatrists) that as the scientific base of psychiatry develops, so the importance of values in psychiatric diagnosis will diminish. If, however, the philosophical account of values just given is right, this is something that we must fervently hope future scientific advances will not be *allowed* to change. For the diversity of our values in the areas of human experience and behaviour with which psychiatry is concerned is an important aspect of our very distinctiveness as individual human beings.

PART III: PUTTING THEORY INTO PRACTICE

Questions for the reader: *What are the practical consequences of recognising and facing up to the importance of values in psychiatry? Think about Simon's case here; but think also, more broadly, about classification and diagnosis generally in psychiatry; in particular, 1. Does recognising the importance of values make good science redundant? 2. What is the significance of this for our understanding of the concept of "mental illness", and of its relationship with "physical illness"? 3. If values are important, how should they be handled practically?*

The first and in some ways the most important point to make about recognising the importance of values in psychiatry is that it in no way undermines the importance of good science. This may seem odd; after all, Kendell's attempt to redefine (medical) value judgements in terms of facts, and similar attempts by other authors both in general medicine (e.g. Campbell *et al.*, 1979) and in philosophy (e.g. Boorse, 1975), have all had the aim of placing psychiatric diagnosis on a firm scientific footing. Remember, though, that in non-descriptivist ethical theory, as developed by R.M. Hare, value judgements are actually based on descriptive (or factual) criteria. Hence all the clinical skills required for carefully eliciting and describing the relevant facts about a patient's experience and behaviour (history taking, mental state examination, and so on) are no less important in a non-descriptivist model of diagnosis than in the conventional medical model.

The effect of philosophical theory, therefore, is not to substitute a value-only model for the conventional medical fact-only model. It is rather to require us to work with a model in which fact and value are equally important. This is consistent with the general picture of philosophy developed earlier in the seminar, as giving us a more complete understanding of the meanings of the concepts with which we are concerned. The medical model reflects an incomplete understanding of the medical concepts (disease, illness, etc.), focusing as it does only on the factual element in their meanings; a fact-plus-value model represents a more complete understanding, a more complete picture. This is Figure 3.1.

The addition of values to facts (in a fact-plus-value model) gives us a quite different way of understanding the concept of "mental illness" and its relationship to "physical illness". In the old debate about mental illness, you will recall, both sides, consistently with the medical model, assumed that the concept of "physical illness" is value-free. The anti-psychiatrists, however, like Szasz, took "mental illness" to be essentially value-laden (and hence not a genuine *medical* concept), whereas the pro-psychiatrists, like Kendell, argued that the evaluative element in the meaning of "mental illness" could be redefined in terms of facts (and hence that mental illness *is* a genuine medical concept). A non-descriptivist (fact-plus-value) model suggests, contrary to both sides, that "illness" itself is a value term. Hence the relevant difference between physical illness and mental illness is that the values relevant to physical illness can be ignored (because they are widely agreed upon and hence are not problematic – acute appendicitis and

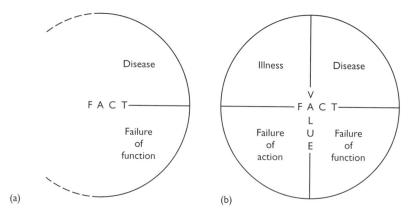

Figure 3.1   From a half-field to a full-field model of medicine. The traditional "medical" model (a) offers a limited (or half-field) view of the conceptual structure of medicine and psychiatry. Linguistic analytical philosophy gives us a more complete (or full-field) view: it adds values to facts, the patient's experience of illness to medical knowledge of disease, and an analysis of the experience of illness in terms of failure of action (or incapacity) to the analysis of disease in terms of failure of function (the value-based model, b). In this chapter we focus on the significance of values for psychiatry. The theoretical basis of this is discussed in Fulford, 1989, Chapters 1–5. For a detailed account of the significance of the patient's experience of illness analysed in terms of failure of action, especially for our understanding of psychopathological symptoms (such as delusion), see Fulford, 1989, Chapters 6–10.

pneumonia are bad conditions for everyone), whereas the values relevant to mental illness *cannot* be ignored (because they are *not* widely agreed upon and hence they *are* problematic). Values, therefore, are important in principle in diagnosis in all areas of medicine, but they are important also in practice in diagnosis in psychiatry.

This is well illustrated by Simon's case. Leave out the values expressed by criterion B in DSM-IV, and we have no way of distinguishing between the (positively evaluated) religious experience and the (negatively evaluated) schizophrenic symptoms. In Simon's case he avoided being "labelled" schizophrenic; he was careful to whom he spoke about his experiences. But recent epidemiological work has shown the extent to which many people feel that their spiritual and religious experiences are misunderstood by psychiatrists (Jackson, 1997). Nor is the importance of values limited to this particular area of differential diagnosis. I have shown elsewhere that if we look carefully, as J.L. Austin recommended, at the actual words used in our standard classifications, values are almost as much in evidence as facts (Fulford, 1994). A failure to recognise this, moreover, is no mere theoretical oversight. It is a failure to recognise what is crucially difficult about psychiatric diagnosis. This failure, as several chapters in this volume show (e.g. Chapter 2), is central to the problems of assessment and diagnosis in cross-cultural psychiatry. It has also been a major contributory factor in the development of grossly abusive practices, such as the misdiagnosis of political dissidence as schizophrenia in the former USSR (Fulford *et al.*, 1993).

Values, then, are a central and inescapable element in the practical problems of psychiatric diagnosis. They are there in principle in all areas of medicine. They are important in practice in psychiatry because of the diversity of human values. Surely, though, someone may now say, if we give up the medical-model ideal of a value-free science of psychiatry, does this not raise the spectre of unfettered relativism, of "anything goes", of ethical (and indeed diagnostic) chaos. Relativism, however, is no more and no less of a spectre here in medicine than in other areas of human activity in which the place of values is more widely recognised, such as the law. Human values, although indeed diverse, are not, after all, chaotic. Neither then is the law; and neither need medicine be.

On the other hand, a clear implication of a fact-plus-value model is that the values of particular people, be they individual or cultural values, must weigh centrally in psychiatric diagnosis. So how are we to handle this practically? The key to this is good communication as a basis for, 1. a more patient-centred approach to diagnosis, and 2. a wider role for the multi-disciplinary team.

The importance of a more patient-centred approach to diagnosis can be appreciated by analogy with the notion of "patient autonomy" as it has come to be understood in traditional medical ethics. In medical ethics it is now widely accepted that patients should be centrally involved in treatment choice. A fact-plus-value model of diagnosis shows that, important as this is, patients' values must also come into how their problem is diagnosed in the first place, i.e. before we even get to treatment. Patients, that is to say, must be involved in deciding not just how they should be treated but how they are *understood* (I owe this clear way of putting the point to Dr V. Y. Allison-Bolger). But understanding depends on communication. Hence one essential for handling the values in psychiatric diagnosis is good communication skills. The importance of good communication in medical ethics is increasingly recognised (Hope *et al.*, 1996). Its importance in different aspects of cross-cultural mental health care is emphasised by several authors in this book (for example, in managing the stress of cross-cultural encounter; see Chapter 16). In diagnosis, the importance of good communication skills has traditionally been thought to be limited to the skills required to elicit the facts of the patient's history and of their mental state. In physical medicine, this may be sufficient, to the extent that the relevant values are shared, and, hence, unproblematic. In psychiatry, though, according to a fact-plus-value model, as well as eliciting the facts, understanding the patient's values is critically important to diagnosis.

Diagnosis, then, in psychiatry, should be in this rather specific sense more "patient centred" (Fulford, 1995). Contrary, though, to a consumer model of patient choice, it does not follow that the patient's values should necessarily trump everyone else's. A fact-plus-value model does not substitute a patient-hegemony for the old medical-hegemony. Of course, if values conflict, if the patient's values conflict with those of others, we have no hard and fast rule, no algorithm, for resolving them. What is important practically in these circumstances, though, is that there should be a *balance* of values. It is this which the multi-disciplinary team can help to provide. In an exclusively scientific model of psychiatric diagnosis, the multi-disciplinary team, representing as it does a range of treatment skills, is important in the management of mental disorders. In a fact-plus-value model, the multi-disciplinary team, representing as it does a range of value perspectives, is important, also, in diagnosis. For it is through this range of value perspectives that the diagnostically crucial balance of values can be achieved.

It is perhaps worth emphasising the extent of the practical importance of this balance. We noted earlier that, in the former Soviet Union, the vulnerability of psychiatry to abuse arose directly from unbalanced political values. An exclusively scientific model of psychiatric diagnosis gave to Soviet values the authority of objective science (Fulford *et al.*, 1993). A similar process has recently been shown to have been important in the abusive uses of psychiatry in Nazi Germany (Herbert, personal communication). These were high-profile cases. But the literature from the user movement in psychiatry (Campbell, 1996), from sociological studies (Rogers *et al.*, 1993), from work on how religious experience is handled by psychiatrists (Jackson, 1997), and perhaps above all in cross-cultural psychiatry (see Chapters 2 and 16), all show the extent to which abusive misdiagnoses are driven by unbalanced values, be they political, ideological or indeed medical. In a fact-plus-value model of psychiatry then, a well-functioning multi-disciplinary team, representing a balance of value perspectives, is essential as much to the initial diagnostic assessment as it is to its more traditional roles of implementing treatment in psychiatry.

Not, it should be added, that recognising the importance of values in psychiatric diagnosis is unimportant to treatment. In all areas of health care we should try to come to a shared understanding of "the problem" as the basis for effective treatment. But this is especially important in psychiatry (cognitive behavioural approaches, for example, actually engage with and start from the values and beliefs of individual patients); and it is especially important above all in cross-cultural aspects of psychiatry. As the author of Chapter 2 so vividly portrays, treatment approaches that, with the best of intentions, are based on the values and beliefs typical of one culture may be highly abusive if transferred to a culture with quite different values and beliefs. The user in Chapter 2, and Simon in the first part of this seminar, both illustrate the importance of values in the management of psychotic disorders; a corresponding point has been made by Bracken *et al.* (1995) in relation to the management of trauma.

Some final questions for the reader: *1. Why do you think we have concentrated in this seminar on diagnosis (and related aspects of treatment)? 2. In what other aspects of psychiatry could values be important? 3. How does cross-cultural psychiatry differ from other areas of psychiatry in respect of the importance of values?*

The importance of values in psychiatry has traditionally been emphasised for treatment (as in medical ethics) and in the diagnosis of overtly value-laden conditions at the margins of medical psychiatry, such as personality disorders and the paraphilias (disorders of sexual object choice). Simon's case, combined with philosophical work on the concept of illness, has shown us that values are important, too, to the diagnosis of conditions (like schizophrenia) at the very heart of medical psychiatry.

If values are important even here, then, at the diagnostic heart of psychiatry, how much more important will they be in other more peripheral areas of the subject. We can see this in a general way, i.e. from the reinforcement the value-dependence of diagnosis gives to the idea that psychiatry, through and through, must engage with people's values as well as with scientific facts. It follows though, also, and more rigorously, from the philosophical insight that the very concept of illness is, essentially, an evaluative concept. According to a fact-plus-value model, diagnosis in general (i.e. not just in psychiatry) involves a negative value judgement (it involves much else besides, of course; see above, pp. 33–36, and Fulford, 1989, Chapters 6–10). The key difference, though, you will recall, between the diagnosis of mental illness and that of physical illness is not that one is value-dependent while the other is value-free, but that the relevant values are more often contentious (and hence problematic) in the case of mental illness. But diagnosis is the gate-keeper to everything else in health care. Hence if the values involved in diagnosis in psychiatry are, in this sense, open and problematic, it is vital that the values of users, individually and collectively, are fully incorporated also into every other aspect of the provision of mental health care.

The importance of values is of course well recognised in other aspects of psychiatry, many of which, as described in this book, are critically important to cross-cultural issues. If treatment choice in general should reflect patients' values, the greater diversity of values in cross-cultural psychiatry means that psychiatrists must be even more alert to the values of patients from cultural groups other than their own (see Chapter 2). Similar considerations apply to such "macro" issues as health service management and resource allocation. There are well recognised difficulties involved in "measuring" patients' needs and values, but, as Ledwith and Husband note (Chapter 16), the importance of involving users increasingly in all aspects of service planning and delivery in mental health is now widely accepted.

More surprisingly, perhaps, besides these practical aspects of psychiatry, recognising the significance of values in psychiatric diagnosis is important also for several areas of research. It is important, for example, for research in descriptive psychopathology. The standard fact-centred medical model, as a framework for descriptive psychopathology, tends to exclude positively evaluated counterparts of negatively evaluated symptoms: the positively evaluated experiences just never come to medical attention. It is important for similar reasons in epidemiological research. Random sampling, fieldwork, and so on, can reduce selection biases, but so long as we fail to recognise the importance of values the very comprehensiveness of good epidemiological research design will result in very different conditions being conflated: a design powerful enough to pick up all "first-rank" experiences will simply roll together spiritual and pathological varieties. This conflation follows through even into the neurosciences. In dynamic brain imaging studies, for example, if two very different kinds of condition (positively and negatively evaluated) are treated as one, the findings, however high powered technically, will be to an extent spurious (Jackson and Fulford, 1997).

This last point also shows that cross-cultural psychiatry, although traditionally associated with the social sciences, could make a crucial contribution in its own right to research in the neurosciences. The very diversity of human experience and behaviour represented by different cultures is, on a fact-plus-value model of psychiatry, a rich resource for research in the neurosciences. Traditional biological psychiatry, operating with an exclusively fact-based model of mental disorder, seeks results which are culture-neutral. But as the survivor in Chapter 2 puts it, this is to be culture-*blind*. The form of this blindness, a fact-plus-value model suggests, is a kind of tunnel vision, an excessively *intra*-cultural perspective. And the cure for this tunnel vision, then, is research in the neurosciences which is not intra-cultural but *inter*-cultural in design.

Conclusions – Learning Points from the Seminar

In this seminar we have been considering the practical importance of values in psychiatric diagnosis. In the first part of the seminar we started with a case, the story of Simon. Simon had first-rank symptoms of schizophrenia but, far from being ill, he was going through an empowering religious experience. The relevant diagnosis (normal religious experience) did not occur to us initially, and it was indeed precluded by the ICD-10 classification. "Simon the Seer" was distinguishable from "Simon with schizophrenia" in the DSM-IV. But this turned out to be only because, contrary to the DSM's claimed scientific status, it included an evaluative criterion (criterion B) in the diagnosis of schizophrenia, namely that the patient had to show a *deterioration* in life functioning.

In Part II of the seminar we looked at how philosophy can help us to understanding Simon's case. The contributions of philosophy were both general and specific. The general contributions of philosophy were four points of contact between philosophy and psychiatric practice: 1. both are concerned with problems of meaning; 2. both focus on real cases; 3. both recognise that meanings are learned primarily through shared use in a social context; and 4. both aim to raise our awareness of meanings as a first step towards handling them more effectively.

The specific contributions of philosophy were through value theory. Attempts to re-define the values inherent in psychiatric (and indeed medical) diagnostic concepts in terms of facts were shown to be a form of descriptivism. Descriptivism relies on shared values. What is distinctive about psychiatry, though, compared with physical medicine, is that it is concerned with areas of human behaviour and experiences in which our values are *not* shared. People differ far more widely over the way they evaluate the higher functions with which psychiatry is concerned (belief, desire, volition, etc.) than over the lower functions with which physical medicine is concerned (pain, in our earlier example, if intense and enduring, being a bad thing for almost everyone). Hence what is needed in psychiatry is a model in which values and facts are on an equal basis, a fact-*plus*-value model to replace the fact-centred biomedical model.

This led, in Part III of the seminar, to a whole series of practical consequences. The essential point was that whereas values can be ignored for practical purposes in diagnosis in physical medicine (because, being widely shared, they are largely unproblematic) they cannot be ignored in diagnosis in psychiatry (because the values themselves, being diverse, are often part of the problem). This, however, 1. did not mean that science was any less important – a fact-plus-value model of diagnosis adds values to facts rather than replacing facts with values. Hence all the standard clinical skills of history taking, mental state examination, and so on, are as important as ever. By the same token, though, 2. values, as well as facts, have to be taken seriously: we had a series of examples of situations in which failures to take values seriously had led to abusive practices (in the USSR, in Nazi Germany, and in everyday psychiatry). Neither side, therefore, in the traditional "debate about mental illness" was completely right; science is important in psychiatry (*contra* Szasz and the anti-psychiatrists), but so also are values (*contra* Kendell and the pro-psychiatrists).

The fear that letting values into diagnosis would lead to "anything goes" was shown to be misplaced. Differences in human values are real but not random. Recognising that differences in values are, nonetheless, real differences led to a number of further practical points; 3. that good communication skills, as well as being important for eliciting symptoms, are essential in coming to a shared understanding of values as the basis for a more patient-centred approach to diagnosis; 4. that in this process the multi-disciplinary team, in offering a balance of evaluative perspectives, has a crucial role to play; 5. that a shared understanding of the problem is crucial to treatment (especially to cognitive-behavioural approaches); and 6. that the diversity of human values is important even in research, notably in descriptive psychopathology, in epidemiology, and in neuroscience.

We began this seminar with a psychiatry caught between the rock of subjective values and the hard place of objective facts. This predicament, we noted, although general to psychiatry, is especially acute in cross-cultural contexts. Yet we have been concerned here with the importance of values (alongside facts) not just in cross-cultural psychiatry but in psychiatry as a whole. This is no coincidence. In a fact-centred biomedical model, an essentially "Western" perspective on mental disorder, hidden behind a mask of scientific objectivity, offers a favoured vantage point. Such a psychiatry aspires to "cultural sensitivity". The psychiatry of a fact-plus-value model, by contrast, while equally scientific in the genuinely scientific aspects of the subject, offers no such favoured vantage point.

Hence a fact-plus-value psychiatry must be competent to express the values of peoples of *all* cultures. Such a psychiatry, therefore, being culturally competent, is indeed, as we anticipated, a genuinely competent psychiatry.

Acknowledgements

The case described in Part I of the seminar was reported by Dr Mike Jackson in a study of religious experience and psychopathology (Jackson, 1997); the implications of these and similar cases for our understanding of psychopathology were explored in Jackson and Fulford (1997). Figure 3.1 appeared in print in Fulford (1991) and Bloch and Chodoff (1991) and I am grateful to them for permission to reproduce it here.

References

American Psychiatric Association (1994) *Diagnostic and Statistical Manual of Mental Disorders*, 4th edn. Washington, DC: American Psychiatric Association.
Austin, J.L. (1956–57). A plea for excuses. *Proceedings of the Aristotelian Society* **57**: 1–30. Reprinted in White, A.R. (ed.) (1968) *The Philosophy of Action*. Oxford: Oxford University Press.
Bloch, S. and Reddaway, P. (1977) *Russia's Political Hospitals: The Abuse of Psychiatry in the Soviet Union*. Southampton: The Camelot Press.
Bolton, D. and Hill, J. (1996) *Mind, Meaning and Mental Disorder: The Nature of Causal Explanation in Psychology and Psychiatry*. Oxford: Oxford University Press.
Boorse, C. (1975) On the distinction between disease and illness. *Philosophy and Public Affairs* **5**: 49–68.
Bracken, P.J., Giller, J.E. and Summerfield, D. (1995) Psychological responses to war and atrocity: the limitations of current concepts. *Social Science and Medicine* **40**: 1073–1082.
Campbell, P. (1996) What we want from mental health services. In: Read, J. and Reynolds, J. (eds) *Speaking Our Minds: An Anthology*, pp. 180–183. London: Macmillan Press.
Campbell, E.J., Scadding, J.G. and Roberts, R.S. (1979) The concept of disease. *British Medical Journal* **2**: 757–762.
Fitzpatrick, R., Hinton, J., Newman, S., Scrambler, G. and Thompson, J. (1984) *The Experience of Illness*. London: Tavistock Publications.
Flew, A. (1973) *Crime or Disease?* New York: Barnes and Noble.
Fulford, K.W.M. (1989) *Moral Theory and Medical Practice*. Cambridge: Cambridge University Press (Reprinted in paperback in 1995).
Fulford, K.W.M. (1991) The concept of disease. In: Bloch, S. and Chodoff, P. (eds) *Psychiatric Ethics*, 2nd edn, Chapter 6. Oxford: Oxford University Press.
Fulford, K.W.M. (1994) Closet logics: hidden conceptual elements in the DSM and ICD classifications of mental disorders. In: Sadler, J.Z., Wiggins, O.P. and Schwartz, M.A. (eds) *Philosophical Perspectives on Psychiatric Diagnostic Classification*. Baltimore: The Johns Hopkins University Press.
Fulford, K.W.M. (1995) Concepts of disease and the meaning of patient-centred care. In: Fulford, K.W.M., Ersser, S. and Hope, T. (eds) *Essential Practice in Patient-Centred Care*, Chapter 1. Oxford: Blackwell Science.
Fulford, K.W.M., Smirnoff, A.Y.U. and Snow, E. (1993) Concepts of disease and the abuse of psychiatry in the USSR. *British Journal of Psychiatry* **162**: 801–810.
Group for the Advancement of Psychiatry (1976) *Mysticism: Spiritual Quest or Psychic Disorder?* New York: GAP Publications.
Hare, R.M. (1981) *Moral Thinking: Its Levels, Method and Point*. Oxford: Clarendon Press.
Hesse, M. (1980) *Revolutions and Reconstructions in the Philosophy of Science*. Brighton, UK: Harvester Press.
Hope, T., Fulford, K.W.M. and Yates, A. (1996) *The Oxford Practice Skills Course: Ethics, Law and Communication in Health Care Education*. Oxford: Oxford University Press.

Hume, D. (1962) *A Treatise of Human Nature.* Edited by D.G.C. Macnabb, Glasgow: Fontana/Collins.

Jackson, M.C. (1997) Benign schizotypy? The case of spiritual experience. In: Claridge, G.S. (ed.) *Schizotypy; Relations to Illness and Health.* Oxford: Oxford University Press.

Jackson, M.C. and Fulford, K.W.M. (1997) Spiritual experience and psychopathology. *Philosophy, Psychiatry and Psychology* 4: 41–66 (Commentaries by Littlewood, R., Lu, F.G. *et al.*; Sims, A; and Storr, A; with response from authors, pp. 67–90).

James, W. (1902) *The Varieties of Religious Experience.* New York: Longmans.

Jaspers, K. (1913a) Causal and meaningful connexions between life history and psychosis. In: Hirsch, S.R. and Shepherd, M. (eds) (1974) *Themes and Variations in European Psychiatry.* Bristol: John Wright and Sons.

Jaspers, K. (1913b) *Allgemeine Psychopathologie.* Berlin: Springer. English edition: Hoenig, J. and Hamilton, M.W. (1963) *General Psychopathology.* Manchester: Manchester University Press.

Kendell, R.E. (1975) The concept of disease and its implications for psychiatry. *British Journal of Psychiatry* 127: 305–315.

Littlewood, R. and Lipsedge, M. (1989) *Aliens and Alienists: Ethnic Minorities and Psychiatry,* 2nd edn. London: Routledge.

Radden, J. (1994) Recent criticisms of psychiatric nosology: a review. *Philosophy, Psychiatry and Psychology* 1: 193–200.

Rogers, A., Pilgrim, D. and Lacey, R. (1993) *Experiencing Psychiatry: Users' Views of Services.* London: Macmillan Press.

Roth, M. and Kroll, J. (1986) *The Reality of Mental Illness.* Cambridge, UK: Cambridge University Press.

Szasz, T.S. (1960) The myth of mental illness. *American Psychologists* 15: 113–118.

Szasz, T.S. (1987) *Insanity: The Idea and its Consequences.* New York: John Wiley.

Warnock, G.J. (1971) *The Object of Morality.* London: Methuen.

Wing, J.K., Cooper, J.E. and Sartorius, N. (1974) *Measurement and Classification of Psychiatric Symptoms.* Cambridge, UK: Cambridge University Press.

WHO (1978) *Report of the International Pilot Study of Schizophrenia, Vol. 1.* Geneva: World Health Organisation.

WHO (1992) *The ICD-10 Classification of Mental and Behavioural Disorders: Clinical Descriptions and Diagnostic Guidelines.* Geneva: World Health Organisation.

Further Reading

A detailed analysis of the concepts of illness and disease, focusing particularly on the way values are important to our diagnostic concepts in psychiatry, is given in Fulford, K.W.M. (1989), reprinted in paperback (1995) *Moral Theory and Medical Practice,* Cambridge University Press.

A useful review of early theories of the meaning of the concept of mental illness is Clare, A. (1979) "The Disease Concept of Psychiatry", in Hill, P., Murray, R. and Thorley, A. (eds) *Essentials of Postgraduate Psychiatry.* New York: Grune and Stratton.

Many of the most important classical papers in the debate about the validity of mental illness are to be found in the edited collection, Caplan, A.L., Englehardt, T. and McCartney, J.J. (eds) (1981) *Concepts of Health and Disease: Interdisciplinary Perspectives.* Reading, MA: Addison-Wesley.

These sources are brought up to date in Fulford, K.W.M. (1998) "Mental Illness: Concept of", in Chadwick, R. (ed.), *Encyclopedia of Applied Ethics.* San Diego: Academic Press.

A number of important articles are to be found in Sadler, J.Z., Wiggins, O.P. and Schwartz, M.A. (1994) *Philosophical Perspectives on Psychiatric Diagnostic Classification.* Baltimore: The Johns Hopkins University Press; and in an issue of *The Journal of Medicine and Philosophy,* edited by

Kopelman, L. (1992), on "Philosophical Issues Concerning Psychiatric Diagnosis" (Vol. **17**, no. 2).

Articles on the importance of values in all areas of psychiatry appear regularly in the international journal, *Philosophy, Psychiatry and Psychology*, edited by Fulford, K.W.M. and Sadler, J.Z. (published by the Johns Hopkins University Press); examples include, Dickenson, D. and Jones, D. (1995) "True Wishes: The Philosophy and Development Psychology of Children's Informed Consent", Vol. **2**, pp. 287–315 (with commentaries by Eekelar, J., McCormick, S., Murray T.H., Parker, M. and Wells, L.A.); Jackson, M. and Fulford, K.W.M. (1997) "Spiritual Experience and Psychopathology", Vol. **4**, pp. 41–66 (commentaries by Littlewood, R., Lu, F.G. *et al.*; Sims, A. and Storr, A., with Response by authors, pp. 67–90); Kopelman, L.M. (1994) "Normal Grief: Good or Bad? Health or Disease?", Vol. **1**, pp. 209–220 (commentaries by Dominian, J. and Wise, T.N., pp. 221–224; response by Kopelman, pp. 226–227); Marshall, M. (1994) "How Should We Measure Need? Concept and Practice in the Development of a Standardised Assessment Schedule", Vol. **1**, pp. 27–36 (commentaries by Crisp, R. and Morgan, J., pp. 37–40); Moore, A., Hope, T. and Fulford, K.W.M. (1994) "Mild Mania and Well-Being", Vol. **1**, pp. 165–192 (commentaries by Nordenfelt, L. and Seedhouse, D.); Sadler, J.Z. (1996) "Epistemic Value Commitments in the Debate over Categorical vs. Dimensional Personality Diagnosis." Vol. **3**, pp. 203–222 (commentaries by Livesley, W.J. and Luntley, M., pp. 223–230); Sadler, J.Z. and Agich, G.J. (1995) "Diseases, Functions, Values, and Psychiatric Classification", Vol. **2**, pp. 219–232; Wakefield, J.C. (1995) "Dysfunction as a Value-Free Concept: a Reply to Sadler and Agich", Vol. **2**, pp. 233–246.

4

Mental Health and the Anthropologist

Sarah Huline-Dickens and Simon Dein

Introduction

Anthropology is an essential discipline for the examination of cross-cultural mental health care. Anthropological research methods have brought into focus the assumptions accepted unquestioningly about mental illness, and have emphasized that socio-cultural factors are of primary importance in the understanding of abnormal mental states. Furthermore, the study of culture now includes description and analysis of Western professions and institutions with a recognition that "culture" is constantly being produced by human action in response to the material conditions of life. Examination of the role of ritual, symbol and systems of value is an important part of studying any culture.

What constitutes "normality" in different cultures clearly varies, and hence what is perceived as mental health or mental illness will vary also. It has often been overlooked that implicit cultural models shape the perception of mental disorder not only among lay populations but among those professionals involved in their care. It is for this reason, and in an attempt to redress the balance of ethnocentrism, that there has been an increasing interest in research into folk beliefs and classifications.

The Western view of "self" as a well-defined and distinct entity reflecting a philosophy that the individual is an autonomous social agent contrasts sharply with that held in some non-Western cultures, such as Asian, African and Pacific cultures, where clear boundaries do not exist between the organic and non-organic, or the physical and mental. Similarly, in the West, emotions are regarded as internal and physiological and are frequently diagnosed and treated as a closed system, whereas in many Asian cultures (e.g. in Samoa) emotions are considered to be more closely integrated with inter-personal relations and somatic processes.

A further important distinction is found when ideas of responsibility and causality are considered, Western explanations tending to locate the cause of mental disorder within the individual psyche, whereas Asian, African and Pacific ideas are more likely to consider that independent somatic processes, supernatural forces or social relations are causative. Clearly, such beliefs have important consequences for the reactions of others to the afflicted (White and Marsella, 1982). A further complexity is introduced into the discussion when it is realized that traditional beliefs are more likely to be held by the older generation, and modified forms by acculturated Africans and Asians.

There has been much interest in "culture-bound syndromes" in the past, a term used to describe those folk illnesses that were thought to be unique to particular cultures or geographical areas, and dozens have been described (see Simons and Hughes, 1985). Littlewood (1990) considers that local patterns of behaviour which failed to correspond to Western psychiatric classifications were often called "culture-bound syndromes", and that many authors have argued the term to be meaningless, as many reactions of distress are to some degree culturally determined. Simons and Hughes have suggested the alternative term **folk diagnostic categories**. Others have proposed that a number of common behaviours can be regarded as Western culture-bound syndromes such as anorexia, obesity, premenstrual syndrome, type-A coronary prone behaviour (Helman, 1994), overdosing with tablets, agoraphobia, exhibitionism and certain kinds of shoplifting (Littlewood and Lipsedge, 1987).

Current studies by psychological anthropologists examine child-rearing practices, the socialisation of emotion, the linguistics of emotion, and violence and sexual abuse (Scheper-Hughes, 1987). Ethnographic studies have attempted to clarify how patients understand psychotropic drugs, how relatives understand schizophrenia, and have investigated traditional or lay healers. They have also been used to study the process of psychotherapy in other cultures. For example, Lock (1982) describes how, in Japanese society, avoidance of verbal analysis of psychological problems, the desire to protect one's inner self from exposure and the popular belief that personality is a fixed structure are traditional values. It is therefore unlikely that psychotherapy as practised in the West would be acceptable. Indigenous Japanese therapies which employ meditation techniques (**Naikan therapy**) and diary keeping (**Morita therapy**) are aimed at achieving adaptation through accommodation rather than resolving internal conflicts. Insight in Naikan therapy is associated with a discovery of relations of responsibility, obligation and dependency, which represent the reality of social life in Japan, and the goal of Naikan is *sunao*, an important value in Japanese culture which implies honesty, humility, docility and simplicity (Murase, 1982).

There has been increasing interest recently in the effectiveness and validity of indigenous healing, and the WHO has recommended that traditional medicine be promoted, developed and integrated where possible with modern scientific approaches (WHO, 1978). Is this interest in traditional healing provoked by a realisation that Western services are failing to provide appropriate care to ethnic minorities who need it?

The extent of use of traditional healers in Britain is not known. Karmi (1995) estimated that at least 35 per cent of a Sikh population in Southall took traditional remedies but Aslam (1979) claimed that so many people consulted traditional healers (*hakims*) that a parallel system of care co-existed alongside the NHS. Commenting that hakims may have a useful role as a kind of medical social worker, Aslam also highlighted several areas of concern, such as their use of toxic substances containing heavy metals, and herbal medicines which were often harmful, and recommended that these practitioners should be properly registered and controlled.

In China and India, where established, parallel systems of health care co-exist, these difficulties have to some extent been overcome. A fundamental principle of Chinese medical practice is the psychological aetiology of disease, but somatisation of physical problems is considered to be characteristic of Chinese patients and studies have shown that "talk therapy" is distrusted (Kleinman and Lin, 1980), whereas treatments with physical ingredients such as herbs or food are welcomed (Lee, 1980). Treatment of both psychological and physical disorders in Chinese medicine has been through use of acupuncture, moxibustion and other measures to restore internal harmony (Crozier, 1968).

The Current State of Service Provision

The process of migration naturally affects mental health significantly. Migration is a stressful event, involving insecurity, isolation, helplessness, language difficulties and hostility from the host population (Littlewood and Lipsedge, 1989). Severance from the culture of origin, a process described as "cultural bereavement", and cultural disorganisation may ensue when a folk community moves to an urban centre. Struggles with immigration laws and the traumas suffered by some refugees clearly exacerbate these difficulties. Studies have shown higher rates of mental illness requiring admission to hospital in migrant populations, specifically first-generation immigrants, and there is some evidence that the rate may be particularly high for women (Carpenter and Brockington, 1980).

Yet there is abundant evidence that minority groups under-utilise mental health services. It has been found, for example, that Asian-Americans, American Indians and people from other minority groups terminate counselling significantly earlier than white Americans (Pedersen, 1982). Cultural and language barriers and class-bound attitudes have been cited as explanations for this phenomenon by some writers, but others have suggested that mental health services are perceived as alien by the minority group and are thus avoided in an effort to maintain personal (cultural) identity (Dinges *et al.*, 1981). Racism may be another important factor (see below).

This under-utilisation of services appears to extend to child and adolescent clinics also. In their study, Hillier *et al.* (1994) found that, of those Bangladeshi parents in East London who did bring their children to the clinic, many complained that they were given no somatic explanations of their child's symptoms nor any medicines, and would have preferred to see Bangladeshi professionals. Hillier and Rahman (1996) suggest that lack of traditional sources of help, fear of possible legal consequences of seeking help and lack of awareness of services, together with parental disempowerment, mean that many children from this ethnic minority will not be receiving the help that they need.

Commander *et al.* (1997a), applying the model of "pathways to care", recently found that, in agreement with a number of other studies in inner city areas with high proportions of people from ethnic minorities, only half of those individuals consulting their GP with psychiatric morbidity had their problems recognised. Yet there were high rates of compulsory detention for black people and the majority of admissions to the Regional Secure Unit were young black men with psychotic disorders. It is clear from this study, and a companion paper (Commander *et al.* 1997b), that people of African-Caribbean descent are over-represented in specialist services, and are more likely to be compulsorily detained, and yet psychiatric morbidity among this group is not being detected and treated at the primary care level. There is also evidence that this population is more likely to be treated with high doses of anti-psychotic drugs (Cole and Pilisuk, 1976). Various explanations have been offered to account for the high rate of compulsory admissions of people of African-Caribbean descent: higher rates of psychotic illnesses, and/or late intervention such that emergency services are involved; stigma such that there might be delays in seeking help; or racial stereotyping so that young African-Caribbean men are perceived as being more threatening (see Littlewood and Lipsedge, 1989).

Whilst it is unclear whether compulsory admission is associated with lack of involvement of a GP, social isolation, misdiagnosis, socio-economic disadvantage, poor housing or unemployment, there is little doubt that social and political considerations are important, for example that African-Caribbean people have been oppressed and marginalised historically, and continue to experience racism. Furthermore, there is evidence that second-generation African-Caribbean children suffer from disproportionately higher rates of psychotic disorders (Goodman and Richards, 1995), a finding that has implications for child and adolescent services.

It is striking that, viewed cross-culturally, distress is far more commonly manifest in *somatic* than *psychological* form (Kleinman, 1986). However, Western professionals continue to consider somatic presentations of distress as somehow deviant, perhaps because such syndromes cannot be easily accommodated in the rather inflexible Western classifications of mental disorder. It is important to bear in mind that the notion of emotional differentiation has been historically highly developed in Western cultures and poorly so in non-Western cultures. Somatisation is a phenomenon influenced not only by cultural categories, but also systems of health care (how much help people can expect to get) and the stigma of mental illness.

Depression is considered to be everywhere more common in women than in men, and in Britain women immigrants from Asia (India, Pakistan and Bangladesh) appear to suffer disproportionately. These groups have been found to experience higher rates of attempted suicide than women in their countries of origin (Burke, 1976) and, as more recently found, higher rates of completed suicide than the general population of women of corresponding ages, and higher rates than for Indian men (Soni Raleigh *et al.*, 1990). Burke considers that the explanation for this may be the language difficulties faced by women, as they are more likely to remain isolated within the home. Soni Raleigh *et al.* (1990) consider that stress, social isolation, inter-generational and marital conflict arising from restricting relationships and pressures to conform are important factors, and that this high rate is an index of large numbers of vulnerable and distressed young people.

Anorexia nervosa has been considered a Western culture-bound syndrome by several writers, and although this point continues to be debated it is becoming clear that rates are increasing in other ethnic groups and in lower socio-economic classes than those originally thought to be at risk. The reports of an increase in anorexia among African-Caribbean adolescents by Pumariega *et al.* (1984), for example, suggest that a greater awareness of the condition, improved case detection and changes in socio-economic and cultural patterns (so that there is a widespread adoption of the Western ideal body shape) may be aetiologically significant. But the research by Lee (1991) conducted among Hong Kong Chinese adolescents of lower socio-economic classes showed that the supposedly characteristic fear of fat and distorted body image were not present, and that there was a cultural stigma against thinness, which was considered to be associated with ill-health and bad luck. These findings have also been demonstrated in India (Khandelwal and Saxena, 1990) and in Nigeria, where there are pre-nuptial rituals of fattening girls among the Calabar people.

Whilst the role of asceticism in the aetiology of anorexia in different cultures is the subject of continuing research, Littlewood (1995), in his examination of the relationship between modernisation and eating disorders in South Asian societies, suggests that through bodily denial women may achieve some degree of self-determination. Self-starvation, in a similar way to spirit possession or dissociative states, can be looked upon as an expression of women's limited personal agency, shaped and legitimised by religious or medical practice. Yet at a recent international conference attended by one of us (SHD), the cross-cultural aspects of eating disorders were not discussed at either a theoretical or clinical level, which is a surprising omission in view of the increasing numbers of sufferers from ethnic minorities.

In order to understand why people from ethnic minorities are failed by existing services, it is crucial to examine their experiences and perceptions of these services. There may be a disbelief in their right to help, feelings of alienation, and suspicion about legal issues and unequal power relationships. There may also be distrust of psychiatric systems which may be associated with the police and other agencies of social control. In some cases a history of colonialism and slavery will influence perceptions, and in others there may be first- or second-hand experience or misunderstanding, lack of facilities in hospital, discrimination or stigma.

How then can services be made more appropriate?

Future Developments

We believe that services must become far more flexible and acceptable to people from ethnic minorities. A new culture of mental health care must be created, led by need and not by the expectation that patients "fit". Measures are needed at every level – from the doctor–patient interaction to models of treatment and service provision – to achieve these goals.

The Doctor–Patient Relationship

The doctor–patient interaction is a well-studied phenomenon in the sociology of medicine, and a crucial process to instigate therapeutic change. In cross-cultural settings, it is important that the determinants of help-seeking are appreciated and languages of distress understood, whether they are verbal or non-verbal, somatic or psychological. There can be no therapeutic success without consensus achieved through understanding, communication and negotiation. A useful paradigm developed in this area is the **explanatory model** of illness (Kleinman, 1980), described by Helman (1994). The explanatory model is used by the patient to explain the current episode of ill-health in his or her terms of aetiology, symptoms, physiological changes, natural history and possible treatments. As such, the model can be viewed as the narrative of the patient's illness, influenced by personality, cultural factors and a number of idiosyncratic meanings. An understanding of a patient's explanatory model is necessary if successful therapy is to occur. The use of culturally fair tests as diagnostic tools is also essential.

In addition to the standard psychiatric history, information should be gathered on the patient's perspective and cultural identity, cultural factors relevant to the illness and social functioning, and cultural factors in the clinician–patient relationship. Information from community workers or others familiar with the culture will be important here.

The assessment may need to be based in a community mental health centre or in the patient's home, wherever the patient feels comfortable, and naturally may involve an interpreter specially trained in mental health. The patient may also want an advocate to be present. The assessment may take longer and has an important function in engaging the patient in the therapeutic process. Regular consultation meetings with community workers who are familiar with the culture could be arranged at the weekly team allocation meeting as a further measure to increase understanding.

There often needs to be involvement of the family. Culture is transmitted trans-generationally, and the family system can protect from or engender mental illness. Families can expect to be the focus of at least some therapeutic intervention. Furthermore the interest in recent years in systems theory has led to novel and flexible ways to approach problems which focus on relationships within the family, or system, rather than on the individual.

Bringing About Change

More training and supervision in medical anthropology may help to enrich clinicians' practice; alternatively, authropologists could be consulted by clinicians. **Advocacy anthropology** is the activity whereby an anthropologist works with community organisations to represent the views or needs of the community, and **cultural brokerage** the process of mediation between two cultures, so that cultural appropriateness of services is increased and the resources of the community enhanced (Van Willigen, 1986, describes how these models have been employed in America). Public policy statements (emphasising the need for professionals to be familiar with their clients' ethnic and cultural background), special funding for research on cross-cultural mental health issues, and accreditation of culturally sensitive training programmes (Pedersen, 1982) are helpful developments.

The providers of mental health services have a role in monitoring, by means of audit, the acceptability of treatment at local day centres and in hospital by both trusts and health authorities. In the community, there needs to be greater emphasis on support by community workers, and specific types of psychotherapies by trained professionals. Attention to culturally appropriate food and facilities on hospital wards and the availability of items for the care of skin and hair, for example, are important features which are often overlooked. Information should be translated into appropriate languages, and special attention should be paid to education about the use of medication and associated adverse effects.

The provision of culturally appropriate psychotherapy is also important. For this to be achieved, different models and a more flexible approach may need to be used so that, for example, a patient can choose a therapy or therapist, and an advocate can be present if so desired. The essential condition of psychotherapy is that the relationship between the therapist and patient is used to help make sense of, and alleviate, the patient's distress; for this relationship to be effective there must be consideration of the culture of the patient. The Nafsiyat Intercultural Therapy Centre in London provides therapy particularly adapted to the cultural context of the client, but elsewhere such provision is rare. Racism also needs to be addressed at an individual and institutional level, as it is possible that black people are not being referred for psychotherapy owing to negative stereotypes. Unless racism is openly discussed in the training of therapists, systems of more equal access to psychotherapy devised, and more therapists from ethnic minorities trained, this situation is unlikely to improve.

Culturally Appropriate Psychotherapy

Culturally appropriate psychotherapy:

- necessarily requires the therapist to understand the system of values, rituals and symbols of the patient's culture;
- involves an awareness of the racial and cultural aspects of mental health problems and of unequal power relationships;
- occurs in a setting which is congenial to the patient, such as a local community centre;

- begins by identifying what the therapist needs to know in order to respect the patient and his or her culture;
- more frequently engages the family and other members of the community and may be based on family and group therapies rather than on individual therapies;
- may be based on techniques other than verbal expression, such as art or drama;
- involves therapeutic goals which may be different for differing cultures and which may not, for example, include enhanced autonomy or individuation.

Although it may be a good strategy to support some kinds of traditional healers, it cannot be assumed that non-Western practices are necessarily beneficial to health, nor that they are always holistic. Some traditional practices may not only be physically injurious, but are unable to accommodate changing views on the patterns of ill-health, and indeed may be supporting a social order that is unhelpful or unjust. Furthermore, traditional healing methods cannot be assumed to be preferred by individuals, as Western systems are often perceived as more prestigious.

Finally, services need to be planned and developed in conjunction with community groups. This has been successfully achieved in the services provided by Leicester Social Services, for example, where community representatives have been recently involved in planning the refurbishment of a residential home for elderly Asian women. Among other initiatives, which have been suggested by the communities themselves, are a user group, the Black Mental Health Shop and a special team for black children. Equality targets, and a policy statement that every citizen of Leicester receives a service based on immediate need, have guided the development of service provision.

Case Study: The Vietnamese Mental Health Project

The Vietnamese Mental Health Project, an initiative established in partnership with community organisations, provides mental health care for a population of Vietnamese refugees in London, many of whom have been traumatised by war. The aims of the project are to increase access to health and social care, provide counselling and information for patients, and training for non-Vietnamese professionals about Vietnamese culture. In addition, a drop-in centre, support for carers, and leaflets in Vietnamese on mental health services are available.

The success of this project would appear to stem from a commitment to acknowledgement and support of Vietnamese cultural beliefs and practices as far as possible. Many of these beliefs, however, are not aligned with Western views. For example, the belief that illness is caused by a loss of balance in the "hot" and "cold" elements suggests the remedy of taking a special food to restore harmony; neuroleptic drugs are considered "hot" for the body and thus are thought to work against nature. Furthermore, it is held that Western medicine, to some extent endowed with magical properties, should be effective in a few days, and there is therefore a natural resistance to the concept of long-term treatment. In a similar way, compliance may be poor with antidepressant treatment, as the delayed onset of action of these drugs means that adverse effects very often appear before clinical improvement.

A belief that supernatural forces cause mental disorder and the stigma of mental illness, which may affect the entire family, leads families to conceal patients at home whilst trying other remedies. Emotions are frequently controlled and complaints are seldom expressed; thus, talking as part of the treatment may seem alien to the patient and his or her family.

The mental health project recognises the need to involve the entire family in the therapy, and that relatives and friends are often the most appropriate people to provide emotional support, without assuming that extended families can be left to look after themselves. The negotiation of change can occur within the context of the support that already exists, and with an understanding of the cultural factors and beliefs that are important for a sense of individual and community identity.

The example of the Vietnamese Mental Health Project illustrates some of the fundamental principles that are necessary to the establishment of an acceptable and flexible service, namely the partnership with community organisations, a willingness to understand cultural beliefs that are not shared by the majority population and constant awareness that services need to be adaptable if they are to be used by those that need them. This example of good practice could be adapted for other ethnic groups.

Conclusion

People from ethnic minorities frequently face multiple stressors, such as language difficulties, loss of status, discrimination, unemployment, poor housing, poverty and social isolation. It is therefore of paramount importance that these factors are not disregarded in examining the relationship between culture and mental health. These factors are likely to exacerbate or prolong the mental health problems of people from ethnic minorities, and evidence has shown that people from ethnic minorities are less likely to receive the care that they require. There is clearly a need to deliver culturally appropriate mental health care, and at the same time to examine why people from ethnic minorities are failing to receive appropriate care.

It is possible that research into the field of traditional healing, the practitioners who use it, how individuals gain access to them and how effective they might be, would give interesting information on patterns of consultation and provide a means of collaboration with general practitioners and psychiatrists. It may also be useful to examine the benefit of joint approaches to care. It should be recognised that all kinds of healing involve powerful symbols and imagery, and that goals of treatment are likely to be different in different cultures.

Greater use of patients' explanatory models could help to improve communication between patients and health care workers, and lead to developments in liaison psychiatry. It is recommended that more consideration be given to different kinds of treatments, preferably using resources and knowledge that communities already possess, which may be more relevant. There needs to be greater availability of culturally appropriate psychotherapy, that is, psychotherapy which is culturally sensitive and considers the historical and political context of the patient.

Providers of services need to consider strategies of prevention as well as delivery of care. There are clearly problems facing mental health services in delivering care to all the ethnic minorities in Britain, but the consequences of failing to meet this challenge are untreated mental health problems. The culture of health care needs to change so that services are perceived as acceptable. Barriers to progress are failing to recognise that existing services are not acceptable for a variety of reasons, a lack of flexibility in approach and a failure to attend to the context of mental distress. Local initiatives such as the Vietnamese Mental Health Project illustrate what it is possible to accomplish when an informed and culturally sensitive approach is adopted in the development of a service that is acceptable, flexible and led by need.

References

Aslam, M. (1979) The practice of Asian medicine in the United Kingdom. Unpublished PhD thesis: University of Nottingham.

Burke, A.W. (1976) Attempted suicide among Asian immigrants in Birmingham. *British Journal of Psychiatry* **128**: 528–533.

Carpenter, L. and Brockington, I.F. (1980) A study of mental illness in Asians, West Indians and Africans living in Manchester. *British Journal of Psychiatry* **137**: 201–205.

Cole, J. and Pilisuk, M. (1976) Differences in the provision of mental health services by race. *American Journal of Psychiatry* **46**: 510–525.

Commander, M.J., Sashi Dharan, S.P., Odell, S.M. and Surtees, P.G. (1997a) Access to mental health care in an inner-city health district. I: Pathways into and within specialist psychiatric services. *British Journal of Psychiatry* **170**: 312–316.

Commander, M.J., Sashi Dharan, S.P., Odell, S.M. and Surtees, P.G. (1997b) Access to mental health care in an inner-city mental health district. II: Association with demographic factors. *British Journal of Psychiatry* **170**: 317–320.

Crozier, R. (1968) *Traditional Medicine in Modern China*. Cambridge, MA: Harvard University Press.

Dinges, N., Trimble, J.E., Manson, S.M. and Pasquale, F.L. (1981) The social ecology of counselling and psychotherapy with American Indians and Alaskan Natives. In: Marsella, A. and Pedersen, P. (eds) *Cross-Cultural Counselling and Psychotherapy*. Elmsford, New York: Pergamon.

Goodman, R. and Richards, H. (1995) Child and adolescent psychiatric presentations of second-generation African-Caribbeans in Britain. *British Journal of Psychiatry* **167**: 362–369.

Helman, C.G. (1994) *Culture, Health and Illness*, 3rd edn. Oxford: Butterworth-Heinemann.

Hillier, S. and Rahman, S. (1996) Childhood development and behavioural and emotional problems as perceived by Bangladeshi parents in East London. In: Kelleher, D. and Hillier, S. (eds) *Researching Cultural Differences in Health*. London: Routledge.

Hillier, S., Loshak, R., Rahman, S. and Marks, F. (1994) An evaluation of child psychiatric services for Bangladeshi parents. *Journal of Mental Health* **3**: 327–337.

Karmi, G. (1995) *Traditional Asian Medicine in Britain: A Survey of Traditional Practices in a West London Community*. Wisbech: MENAS Press.

Khandelwal, S.K. and Saxena, S. (1990) Anorexia nervosa in people of Asian extraction. *British Journal of Psychiatry* **157**: 784.

Kleinman, A. (1980) *Patients and Healers in the Context of Medicine*. Berkeley: University of California Press.

Kleinman, A. (1986) *Social Origins of Distress and Disease: Depression, Neurasthenia and Pain in Modern China*. New Haven: Yale University Press.

Kleinman, A. and Lin, T.Y. (1980) *Normal and Abnormal Behaviour in Chinese Culture*. Dordrecht, Holland: Reidel.

Lee, R.P.L. (1980) Perceptions and uses of Chinese medicine among the Chinese in Hong Kong. *Culture, Medicine and Psychiatry* 4: 345–375.

Lee, S. (1991) Anorexia nervosa in Hong Kong: a Chinese perspective. *Psychological Medicine* **21**: 703–711.

Littlewood, R. (1990) From categories to contexts: a decade of the "new cross-cultural psychiatry". *British Journal of Psychiatry* **156**: 308–327.

Littlewood, R. (1995) Psychopathology and personal agency: modernity, culture change and eating disorders in South Asian societies. *British Journal of Medical Psychology* **68**: 45–63.

Littlewood, R. and Lipsedge, M. (1987) The butterfly and the serpent: culture, psychopathology and biomedicine. *Culture, Medicine and Psychiatry* **11**: 289–335.

Littlewood, R. and Lipsedge, M. (1989) *Aliens and Alienists: Ethnic Minorities and Psychiatry*, 2nd edn. London: Unwin Hyman.

Lock, M. (1982) Popular conceptions of mental health in Japan. In: Marsella, A.J. and White, G.M. (eds) *Cultural Conceptions of Mental Health and Therapy*. Dordrecht, Holland: Reidel.

Murase, T. (1982) Sunao: a central value in Japanese psychotherapy. In: Marsella, A.J. and White, G.M. (eds) *Cultural Conceptions of Mental Health and Therapy*. Dordrecht, Holland: Reidel.

Pedersen, P. (1982) The intercultural context of counselling and therapy. In: Marsella, A.J. and White, G.M. (eds) *Cultural Conceptions of Mental Health and Therapy*. Dordrecht, Holland: Reidel.

Pumariega, A.J., Edwards, P. and Mitchell, C. (1984) Anorexia in black adolescents. *Journal of the American Academy of Child Psychiatry* **23**(1): 111–114.

Scheper-Hughes, N. (1987) *Child Survival: Anthropological Perspectives on the Treatment and Maltreatment of Children*. Dordrecht, Holland: Reidel.

Simons, R.C. and Hughes, C.C. (1985) *The Culture-Bound Syndromes*. Dordrecht, Holland: Reidel.

Soni Raleigh, V., Bulusu, L. and Balarajan, R. (1990) Suicides among immigrants from the Indian Subcontinent. *British Journal of Psychiatry* **156**: 46–50.

Van Willigen, J. (1986) *Applied Anthropology*. South Hadley MA, USA: Bergin and Garvey.

Vietnamese Mental Health Project (1996), *The Vietnamese Perspective in Mental Health*. Booklet available from: 49 Effra Road, Units 21 and 23, Brixton, London SW2 1BZ.

White, G.M. and Marsella, A.J. (1982) Introduction: Cultural conceptions in mental health research and practice. In: Marsella, A.J. and White, G.M. (eds) *Cultural Conceptions of Mental Health and Therapy*. Dordrecht, Holland: Reidel.

WHO (1978) *The promotion and development of traditional medicine*. WHO Tech. Rep. Ser. 622. Geneva: World Health Organisation.

5

Religious Issues and their Psychological Aspects

Kate Miriam Loewenthal

Professional and Historical Perspective

For cultural minority groups in the so-called Western world, religion may be far more salient than it is in the dominant, host culture. Religion is often the most important and heavily invested aspect of identity, and threats to religious beliefs and practices strike to the heart of the individual. This is important because mental health providers may offer such threats, even though they do not usually intend to.

As a psychologist interested in religious issues in mental health, I am struck by the fact that, with mental health in cultural minority groups, the crucial issues are often *religious*. Here are a few examples; all have important implications for uptake of mental health services, and for training and clinical practice.

Religious Behaviour as Psychopathology

To put it bluntly, in the eyes of someone from another social/cultural/religious group religious behaviours and beliefs can seem psychopathological. But to the believer, they are not only sane, but sacred, and they embody all that gives life meaning and purpose. A perennial problem is where to draw the line beyond which psychopathology lies.

For instance Mr X, an orthodox Jew, has been causing his family concern for some time. He has no job and, although not very scholarly, he spends hours immersed in the mikveh (ritual bath) and at prayer, fasts a great deal, and is over-scrupulous about what he eats. He denies being depressed or ill in any way, and says that his behaviour is inspired by hasidic (mystical) teaching; he goes to the doctor with great reluctance, only to please his family (Littlewood and Lipsedge, 1989). Mr Z, another orthodox Jew, has also been causing his family concern. He is overly concerned about mixtures of milk and meat food (prohibited by religious law) and washes his hands up to thirty times a day to avoid the risk of forbidden mixture. Unlike Mr X, he feels that his behaviour and concerns, although along the right religious lines, are excessive (Greenberg, 1987).

The apparent "madness" of religious behaviour was shown clearly in the widely quoted 19th-century case of a cult convert (Schwieso, 1996), who was confined in a private asylum on the grounds that her "religious opinions were irreconcilable with soundness of mind", even though she was "competent, calm and rational". Another case (Evarts, 1914) involved a young African-American woman, confined to a psychiatric hospital with a diagnosis of dementia praecox, apparently solely on the basis of her religious behaviour and beliefs. She prayed and read her bible "all day long", and believed that the institution and its food were unholy.

These cases illustrate two important points: first, that religious beliefs and behaviour can be readily seen as psychopathological, and second, precisely because of their sacred character, these beliefs and behaviours are held to most strongly. Note that a person may be considered mad (by outsiders to the religious group) *on the basis of religious behaviour alone.*

Eileen Barker has recently (1996) stated the alternative case most boldly, implying that *no* religious belief or behaviour need indicate mental illness. She asks: "How . . . could any except the mentally deluded believe that they are going to live for ever? That by chanting some weird mumbo-jumbo we can store spiritual energy from outer space? That a chubby little boy can give us instant enlightenment . . . ?" Barker suggests that " . . . 'strange beliefs' should not be taken by themselves as being an indicator that the person is mentally ill".

Perhaps they should not. They may be erroneous, morally doubtful, and otherwise wrong. But they are often taken as mad, and the culturally alien are particularly frightened that their religious behaviour and beliefs will be misjudged. A white Briton might consult his/her doctor when under stress, and will probably not be too afraid of being judged as psychiatrically disturbed if the doctor becomes aware, for instance, that he/she gets up very early on Sunday morning to attend a ritual in which he/she drinks wine believed to be the blood of the son of God . . . this is normative, acceptable Anglo-Christian behaviour and belief. But Hindu patients who get out of hospital beds to die on the floor, orthodox-Jewish boys who sway back and forth as they pray and study sacred texts, Pentecostalists who speak in tongues – these may all be seen as psychologically disturbed (Loewenthal, 1995). These and other minority groups have a healthy fear of seeking professional help for psychological problems for fear of misjudgment. There may be other religious reasons for avoiding mental health professionals, as we shall see. But so far we have arrived at a contrast, between in-group and out-group views of religious behaviour.

The problem is that sometimes religious behaviour can be a manifestation of psychological disturbance, and professionals need guidelines to enable them to recognise when this might have happened. There are three important needs for training and practice:

1. **Information** about the normative religious practices and beliefs in the client's religious group, and the range of variation;
2. **Contact(s)** within the client's religious group, who are able to evaluate whether a particular piece of "religious" behaviour is seen as disturbed by other members of the group;

3. **Diagnostic criteria**: patients with religious "symptoms" may not have other symptoms of psychopathology. There may be a danger of clinicians losing sight of standard diagnostic criteria, such is the force of the often "bizarre", dramatic manifestations of religion.

Sin, Spirit Possession and Madness

Beliefs about spirit possession illustrate the conflicts between in-group and out-group views. In malign possession, the afflicted person feels distressed, may suffer bodily pains, may undergo dissociative states in which strange things are said in a strange voice, may see horrific visions, and above all believes that they are the victim of a malign spiritual force, sometimes a possessing demon, sometimes the victim of witchcraft or sorcery. Thus Dein (1996) describes a young Nigerian woman with violent abdominal pains which she believed were caused by witchcraft practised by a disappointed admirer. The psychiatrist may see the affliction in terms of inner psychic forces, externalised or projected as persecutory agencies. Benign possession, as in glossolalia (speaking in tongues) may be sought after, but in the first half of this century the standard psychiatric view was that it was a form of mass hysteria or psychosis (Grady and Loewenthal, 1997). Possession is the archetypal case in which traditional-religious and medical-scientific metaphors and models confront each other in apparent conflict, with different treatment implications.

An important variation is the belief that afflictions are caused by personal failings (sin, wrongdoing). Psychologically, the sufferer believes or fears that they themselves are the cause of their afflictions. This has important implications for the kind of help sought. The sufferer may seek to find an atonement or correction for their wrongdoing. Perhaps more commonly, the sufferer may feel some shame: "a truly good Muslim/Christian/Jew should not feel depressed", for example. Illness may be denied (and no treatment will be sought). Or illness may show in a form that does not imply personal failing.

Implications for practice are stated simply:

1. Beliefs about possession or sin should not be dismissed as insubstantial superstitions, or seen as necessary signs of pathology;
2. Many professionals will work in liaison with traditional religious healers, if this is what suits the patient.

Beneficial and Other Effects of Religion

So far I have written as if there were a conflict between traditional-religious and medical-scientific views of mental illnesses. In fact there is much scope for collaboration (Bhugra, 1996; Turbott, 1996).

For example there is much scientific and medical interest in the tendency for high levels of religious activity to be associated with better mental health. Bergin (1983), Levin (1994), Loewenthal (1995) and others summarise some of this material. The association between religion and better mental health appears to hold for some minority groups, although not all minority groups have been examined.

How might these effects come about? There are several possibilities; one is that religious groups provide good social support, which has been shown to have a stress-buffering effect. Additionally there are many cognitive aspects of religion – for instance beliefs about God's care and providence, meditation, contemplation and prayer – which may have stress-buffering effects; these need much further investigation. However, religion may also be used as a justification for abuse (Capps, 1992), but this has received little systematic attention.

The most obvious implication for practice is that religious practices which are reported to be helpful in alleviating distress should not be too readily dismissed. Mental health service providers may wish to consult or refer to sources of relevant help.

With this background we turn to current provision and practice.

Current State of Service Provision

In existing legislation and practice it is hard to discover explicit guidelines about religious issues. The Mental Health Handbook (Drew and King, 1995), a current layperson's guide to resources, does not index religions or religious issues at all. However, a number of mental health helping agencies have a religious impetus, continuing the tradition pioneered by the Quaker, Tuke.

There are many reasons – some of them quite good ones, some less so – for psychiatry's "neglect" of religion (Neeleman and Persaud, 1995; Bhugra, 1996). The French pioneer of humane psychiatric treatment, Pinel, for instance, feared that encouraging religious practices in psychiatric institutions might increase delusions and hallucinations. We do not know whether this might happen, but there is a danger that religion is an issue that could be mishandled by mental health professionals. Religion has often been swept under the carpet, leaving religious issues for pastoral counsellors and the clergy for whom there are few opportunities to liaise with mental health professionals concerning the progress of any given patient. Religious issues are beginning to be attended to in the training of mental health professionals, especially where multicultural issues are salient, and some professionals may cross-refer or cooperate with religious healers or counsellors. In cities with significant ethnic-minority populations, there may be culture-specific help-lines, crisis centres, refuges and other mental health-promoting services with funding from local government; such centres known to this author encourage the use of a range of religious help and self-help methods.

Religious Behaviour as Psychopathology

The historical account of confusion between religious behaviour and psychiatric symptoms is not just of academic interest. Recent experience throws up:

- a Jewish man treated with fluvoxamine because he was troubled by his wish for a religiously forbidden marriage. There were no clinical symptoms of anxiety, depression or (other) psychopathology (Jacobsen, 1995);
- the mother of a child paralysed by meningitis was legally ruled to be paranoid-schizophrenic, and denied access to the child. The sole grounds were apparently that she "fasted, and prayed for his recovery, and attributed the illness to demonic forces" (Redlener and Scott, 1979);
- in two recent cases brought to the author's attention, attempts have been made to deprive divorcees of custody of their children on the grounds of psychiatric testimony that the parent is suffering from "religious fanaticism". No (other) evidence of psychopathology has been brought forward, and the children's wishes in both cases have been to remain in the custody of the "religious-fanatical" parent;
- the leader of a small Trinidadian religous group was found to have "paranoid ideas and delusions", "evidence of psychosis" and "relapsed schizophrenia", although there was "no difficulty in communicating with her" and "her affect was quite appropriate". The only evidence of psychosis was her "untidy dress" and "bizarre ideas", for instance that she is Mother Earth and that the sun is coming closer to the earth and that there would be a fire. Both sets of "symptoms" were derived from her religious beliefs (Littlewood, 1993).

These are all clear examples of confusion between religious behaviour and psychiatric symptoms: psychopathology was inferred *solely on the basis of religious behaviour*. But perhaps the religious behaviour was really in some way disturbed?

Observers of religious behaviour and beliefs have a long-standing tradition of distinguishing between "healthy" and "unhealthy" religiosity (e.g. Allport, 1950; Jung, 1958; Loewenthal, 1995). How to make this distinction continues to be a matter of concern.

In the classic *Aliens and Alienists* (Littlewood and Lipsedge, 1989), most of the cases involve religious issues. For example, Evadne, a West Indian medical orderly and an enthusiastic member of a Pentecostal church, became very agitated while at work, complaining of unfair treatment, and was referred to the psychiatrist. The psychiatrist wondered whether her incoherent babbling, interspersed with enthusiastic hymn-singing and the like, might be glossolalia (speaking in tongues, a rhythmic speech, mainly incoherent, believed to be a gift of the spirit and particularly encouraged in Pentecostal and some charismatic Christian groups). The psychiatrist consulted with Evadne's fellow church-members. To his astonishment, they said that Evadne's speech was not glossolalia, and that she was sick in the head. At this the psychiatrist decided that she might be psychiatrically ill, and offered medication. She co-operated willingly with treatment and improved, subsequently agreeing that she had had a breakdown.

Grady and Loewenthal (1997) discuss ways of distinguishing healthy from psychopathological glossolalia. In the same vein, Greenberg and Witztum (1994) discuss the difficult question of distinguishing "religious symptoms in a religious society". For instance, when does religious scrupulousness become obsessional-compulsive disorder (OCD)? And do religious scruples *foster* OCD (Lewis and Joseph, 1994)? Greenberg and Witztum (1994) think that religion merely provides a setting for the manifestation of OCD.

Many of these examples offer similar guidelines for good practice. As suggested above, the clinician requires information about religious beliefs and practices in the client's religious group, and access to reliable contacts in the group, who may be needed to help form judgment about psychiatric status. More detailed information on some common psychiatric dilemmas could be useful.

Spirit Possession, and Other Spiritual Causes of Illness

There are many mental health problems in the community involving religious issues, which are unlikely to come to professional attention. Witchcraft and spirit possession are often seen as causal factors in mental illness, especially among minority groups (Lefley and Bestman, 1977; Kua *et al.*, 1993; Dein, 1996; Millet *et al.*, 1996). There is often mistrust of medical and mental health professionals, particularly when religious issues are concerned. Apart from the fear of religious behaviour being misjudged, some people may feel that their sufferings are related to spiritual causal factors, and that medical remedies or psychological therapies are not as appropriate as religious help. Thus religious help may be sought first (Purdy *et al.*, 1983; Mollica *et al.*, 1986).

Several authors have reported that trust of mental health professionals has been improved when patients' religious interpretations of illness are acknowledged by mental health professionals. For example, when Margolin and Witztum (1989) suggested that impotence which had appeared several days after the death of a patient's father was the result of being "bound" by his vengeful deceased father as punishment for failing to observe the religious laws of mourning properly, the patient said that "this time he felt the therapist understood him". Witztum *et al.* (1990) offer a good example of co-operation between modern psychiatry and traditional religious healing resources in the case of a depressed man persecuted by a punishing angel.

Belief that illness may reflect personal failings, or is somehow wrong, can have implications for help-seeking and practice.

. . . Mrs Y has been very low since her last baby was born. She cries a lot when she is alone, and feels exhausted. She has five children under the age of six, and the family lives in a three-room flat on the third floor of a block occupied by other orthodox-Jewish families. Her husband is "very kind, but a bit short-tempered with the children", and he worries about his low earnings. Although the family is hard-up, the community is "very supportive", for instance recently providing a "new" dining-table and chairs. Mrs Y says she has so much to be thankful for, and is working on herself to improve her mood (I interviewed Mrs Y in 1993).

Mrs Y may believe that it is wrong to feel depressed, and is working on improving her mood by reminding herself how much she has to be thankful for. Provided that Mrs Y does not perceive a significant deterioration in her already difficult circumstances, she may stagger on indefinitely without seeking professional help.

. . . Mrs Z has been very low since her 20-year-old daughter left home to live in a bed-sitter by herself. Her daughter visits often and is on fairly good terms with her parents, but says she wants to live her own life and has no interest in an arranged marriage with a boy from Pakistan chosen by her parents. Mr Z says that their daughter's behaviour is because Mrs Z was not religious enough when their daughter was younger, and Mrs Z now fasts in Ramadan, prays regularly, is careful with her diet and is generally trying to be a better Muslim. Mr Z remarks that this may be too late (Khan, personal communication).

Mrs Z does not appear to be so concerned about her low state as with its cause: her daughter's social and religious defection, and the shame and stigma associated with this. She appears to have conceded her husband's point, that this is the result of her religious failings, and she is valiantly trying to improve herself. Although she has the symptoms of major depression she would see no point in going to a doctor.

Cinnirella and Loewenthal (1996) noted several important implications of these kinds of beliefs, that psychological illnesses may have religious causes. First, on the whole, most minority group members who are religious feel that professionals *from their own group* are more likely to understand their problems: "Because then they're on the same wavelength aren't they? If you start telling (an outsider) about the way you feel and they'll think you are little bit . . . ". However, own-group professionals may be avoided, especially if there is a shameful or stigmatising problem: " . . . a person might think, I don't want this to be known in my community". Second, there may be major efforts to engage in religiously endorsed (self-)help: prayers, thinking positive thoughts, enhanced religious behaviour, trusting that God will help, consulting the clergy. These acts are often seen as helpful, and indeed they may have therapeutic value. Outside professional help may be seen as a last resort when all else has failed, and viewed with some mistrust.

It has been suggested that somatisation – sometimes thought to be particularly likely in some minority groups – may be a result of religious and cultural factors (Jadhav, 1996; Witztum *et al.*, 1996; MacLachlan, 1997). One scenario is that a patient may not perceive him or herself as depressed, partly because this would imply that they are not a good religious person. Instead, stomach, back or other pains are presented for which no organic cause can be found. Cultural and linguistic factors can exacerbate such failure to perceive an association between the psychological and somatic elements of depression and anxiety.

Beneficial and Other Effects of Religion

There are many religiously influenced beliefs and practices with regard to mental health care which could be brought to professional attention, and which deserve closer scientific investigation.

These include prayer, meditation and related practices, the teaching and study of beliefs and ideas which may be helpful in coping with stress, and many forms of practical and social support. Some of these have already been studied (e.g. Shapiro, 1982; Finney and Maloney 1985; Loewenthal, 1995; Loewenthal and MacLeod, 1996) and beneficial physiological and emotional effects have been documented. Some are incorporated into practice in local culturally sensitive mental health help centres (Drew and King, 1995).

Several postures on multiculturalism have been outlined: most authors report that Western-trained professionals are pragmatically taking into account other ("non-Western") beliefs and, where indicated, are referring for treatment that is consistent with those beliefs (e.g. Lefley and Bestman, 1977; Richardson, 1991; Brent and Callwood, 1993).

Weiss (1997) and MacLachlan (1997) outline forms of interview to elicit:

- a description of all the things that are "wrong" with the patient (according to the patient), enabling understanding of culturally, linguistically and religiously shaped patterns of distress;
- what s/he thinks caused them;
- what s/he thinks other members of their social group/s think cause problems like this;
- what forms of help have been sought, could be sought and should be sought.

Patients may feel that religious forms of help are of no interest to the professional, who (it is felt) will be sceptical and possibly scornful of these "unscientific" and "superstitious" beliefs. Non-judgmental listening by the professional will at the very least improve trust, and will enable the professional to build an explanatory framework for the illness, enabling the clinician to draw up treatment goals in collaboration with the patient, and to draw on healing resources that are seen as appropriate, often using several different kinds of healing resource and cross-referring where necessary.

Future Developments

A number of **organisational improvements** could lead to improved access to those religious resources that patients have identified as potentially helpful:

- Creating opportunities for closer liaison between hospital chaplaincy services and the mental health team; Trusts and Health Authorities may set this as part of their quality assurance provision, and include such liaison in contracts for service specification.
- Trusts may encourage liaison brought about by the chaplaincy, between the mental health team and clergy or other leaders from the patient's own religious group. Often, patients are offered pastoral services from a chaplain seen as the "best match" for the patient's religious preference, and this match may be seen as inappropriate by the patient.
- Trusts may consider buying-in selected religious resources, where their efficacy is demonstrated.
- It may be helpful for The National Health Service Executive to support research on such efficacy.
- Allowing time and opportunity for psychiatrists and other personnel to carry out the practices described below.
- Trusts may consider funding accredited relevant continued education for psychiatrists, nurses and other professionals.

Improvements in clinical training and practice could include the following:

- Training in interview methods that enable the non-judgmental exploration of patients' ideas about religious factors related to their condition, including patients' ideas about possible forms of religious help that might be tried; such training could be available to (and sought by) general practitioners, psychiatrists, nurses, clinical psychologists and social workers.
- The development of treatment plans by individual professionals, which incorporate forms of religious help which the patient wishes to seek, disseminating these in the academic and professional press to encourage and develop models of good practice in this field, and monitoring suggested forms of religious help through (Trust or HA or NHSE-sponsored) clinical audit.
- The development by professional bodies and academic institutions of training in methods of gaining information about religious groups and their normative practices.
- Training in methods of developing contracts with religious groups when help is needed in deciding whether religious behaviour is psychopathological or not. Codes and models of practice might be developed by professional and academic institutions.

Finally, several **further specific issues and forms of action** are suggested as deserving attention:

- The preparation of published **guidelines on common forms of "religious psychopathology"** to enable professionals to avoid over-diagnosis, and to develop forms of help (where needed) which will not injure religious sensibilities: common scenarios for instance involve "religiously flavoured" African-Caribbean "psychosis"

(Littlewood and Lipsedge, 1981a, 1981b) and orthodox-Jewish OCD/ scrupulosity, again with a "religious flavour" (Greenberg, 1987; Greenberg and Witztum, 1994).

- **Suicide** is of much current concern. There is evidence that suicide is lower in religious groups that do not endorse suicide (e.g. Catholics, Jews, Muslims) and higher in groups that condone or encourage suicide in some circumstances (e.g. Protestants, Hindus; Loewenthal *et al.*, 1995; Ineichen, 1996; Williams, 1997), but there is scope for better understanding of these effects and how they are achieved, for example how the increase of suicide and parasuicide among young Asian women in the UK might be related to religious and cultural trends in UK Asian communities.

- **Somatisation**: many resources are expended fruitlessly on painful and debilitating symptoms which have no clear organic cause. There are indications that somatization is related both to stress and to cultural-religious factors, and a clearer picture of causal factors could lead to improvements in treatment.

- Better understanding is needed of whether, when and how **religious self-help** can be of use – beliefs in efficacy, actual use, and actual effects. This area of study must involve existing "culturally sensitive" therapy organisations, many of which endorse or encourage religious self-help. Careful descriptive and quantitative research is important. Psychiatry and religion do not need to co-exist uneasily in separate water-tight compartments. Adequate scientific methods do exist to investigate the claimed and actual impact of religion on mental health, and research will enable cross-cultural psychiatry to make informed and sensitive progress.

References

Allport, G.W. (1950) *The Individual and his Religion, a Psychological Interpretation*. New York: MacMillan.

Barker, E. (1996) New religions and mental health. In: Bhugra, D. (ed.) *Psychiatry and Religion*. London: Routledge.

Bergin, A.E. (1983) Religiosity and mental health: a critical re-evaluation and meta-analysis. *Professional Psychology: Research and Practice* **14**: 170–184.

Bhugra, D. (ed.) (1996) *Psychiatry and Religion*. London: Routledge.

Brent, J.E. and Callwood, G.B. (1993) Culturally relevant psychiatric care: the West Indian as a client. *Journal of Black Psychology* **19**: 290–302.

Capps, D. (1992) Religion and child abuse: perfect together. Presidential address of the Society for the Scientific Study of Religion 1991. Pittsburgh, Pennsylvania. *Journal for the Scientific Study of Religion* **31**: 1–14.

Cinnirella, M. and Loewenthal, K.M. (1996) Religious influences about mental illness in minority groups. Paper presented at a symposium on *Religious Issues in Mental Health among Minority Groups*, Royal Holloway, London University, November 1996.

Dein, S. (1996) Possession. Paper presented at a symposium "Religious Issues in Mental Health Among Minority Groups", Royal Holloway, London University.

Drew, T. and King, M. (1995) *The Mental Health Handbook*. London: Piatkus.

Evarts, A.B. (1914) Dementia praecox in the coloured race. *Psychoanalytical Review* **1**: 388–403.

Finney, J.R. and Maloney, H.N. (1985) An empirical study of contemplative prayer as an adjunct to psychotherapy. *Journal of Psychology and Theology* **13**: 284–290.

Grady, B. and Loewenthal, K.M. (1997) Features associated with speaking in tongues (glossolalia). *British Journal of Medical Psychology* **70**: 185–191.

Greenberg, D. (1987) The behavioural treatment of religious compulsions. *Journal of Psychology and Judaism* **11**: 41–47.

Greenberg, D. and Witztum, E. (1994) The influence of cultural factors on obsessive compulsive disorders: religious symptoms in a religious society. *Israeli Journal of Psychiatry* **31**: 211–220.

Ineichen, B. (1996) Suicide. Paper presented at a symposium on *Religious Issues in Mental Health among Minority Groups*, Royal Holloway, London University, November 1996.

Jacobsen, F.M. (1995) Can psychotropic medications change ethnoculturally determined behaviour? *Cultural Diversity and Mental Health* **1**: 67–72.

Jadhav, S. (1996) The cultural origins of Western depression. *International Journal of Social Psychiatry* **42**: 269–286.

Jung, C.G. (1958) *Psychology and Religion: West and East.* London: Routledge and Kegan Paul.

Kua, E.H., Chew, E.O. and Ko, S.M. (1993) Spirit possession and healing among Chinese psychiatric patients. *Acta Psychiatrica Scandinavica* **88**: 447–450.

Lefley, H.P. and Bestman, E.W. (1977) Psychotherapy in Caribbean cultures. Paper presented at the American Psychological Association, San Francisco.

Levin, J.S. (1994) Religion and health: Is there an association, is it valid, and is it causal? *Social Science and Medicine* **38**: 1475–1482.

Lewis, C.A. and Joseph, S. (1994) Religiosity: psychoticism and obsessionality in Northern University students. *Personality and Individual Differences* **17**: 685–687.

Littlewood, R. (1993) *Pathology and Identity: The Work of Mother Earth in Trinidad.* Cambridge: Cambridge University Press.

Littlewood, R. and Lipsedge, M. (1981a) Some social and phenomenological characteristics of psychotic immigrants. *Psychological Medicine* **11**: 289–302.

Littlewood, R. and Lipsedge, M. (1981b) Acute psychotic reactions in Caribbean-born patients. *Psychological Medicine* **11**: 303–318.

Littlewood, R. and Lipsedge, M. (1989) *Aliens and Alienists: Ethnic Minorities and Psychiatry,* 2nd edn. London: Unwin Hyman.

Loewenthal, K.M. (1995) *Mental Health and Religion.* London: Chapman and Hall.

Loewenthal, K.M. and MacLeod, A. (1996) Religion and cognitive aspects of coping. Paper given at the International Federation for the Psychology of Religion, International Congress of Psychology: Montreal, 1996.

Loewenthal, K.M., Goldblatt, V., Gorton, T. *et al.* (1995) Gender and depression in Anglo-Jewry. *Psychological Medicine* **25**: 1051–1063.

MacLachlan, M. (1997) *Culture and Health.* Chichester: Wiley.

Margolin, J. and Witztum, E. (1989) Supernatural impotence: historical review with anthropological and clinical implications. *British Journal of Medical Psychology* **62**: 339–342.

Millet, P.E., Sullivan, B.F., Schwebel, A.I. and Myers, L.J. (1996) Black Americans' and white Americans' views of the etiology and treatment of mental health problems. *Community Mental Health Journal* **32**: 235–242.

Mollica, R.F., Streets, F.J., Boscarino, J. and Redlich, F.C. (1986) A community study of formal pastoral counselling activities of the clergy. *American Journal of Psychiatry* **143**: 323–328.

Neeleman, J. and Persaud, R. (1995) Why do psychiatrists neglect religion? *British Journal of Medical Psychology* **68**: 169–178.

Purdy, B.A., Simari, C.G. and Colon, G. (1983) Religiosity, ethnicity and mental health: interface the 80s. *Counselling and Values* **27**: 112–121.

Redlener, I.E. and Scott, C.S. (1979) Incompatibilities of professional and religious ideology: problems of medical management and outcome in a case of paediatric meningitis. *Social Science and Medicine* **138**: 89–93.

Richardson, B.L. (ed.) (1991) *Multicultural Issues in Counselling: New Approaches to Diversity.* Alexandra, Virginia: American Association for Counselling and Development.

Schwieso, J.J. (1996) 'Religious fanaticism' and wrongful confinement in Victorian England: the affair of Louisa Nottidge. *Social History of Medicine* **9**: 158–174.

Shapiro, D. (1982) Overview: clinical and physiological comparison of meditation with other self-control strategies. *American Journal of Psychiatry* **139**: 267–274.

Turbott, J. (1996) Religion, spirituality and psychiatry: conceptual, cultural and personal challenges. *Australian and New Zealand Journal of Psychiatry* **30**: 720–727.

Weiss, M. (1997) Explanatory Model Illness Catalogue (EMIC): Framework for comparative study of illness. *Transcultural Psychiatry* **34**: 235–263.

Williams, M. (1997) *Cry of Pain: Understanding Suicide and Self-Harm*. Harmondsworth: Penguin.

Witztum, E., Buchbinder, J.T. and van der Hart, O. (1990) Summoning a punishing angel: treatment of a depressed patient with dissociative features. *Bulletin of the Menninger Clinic* **54**: 524–537.

Witztum, E., Grisaru, N. and Budowski, D. (1996) The 'Zar' possession syndrome among Ethiopian immigrants to Israel. *British Journal of Medical Psychology* **67**: 207–225.

Part III

New Directions in Service Provision

6

Psychiatry and Cultural Relativity

Dele Olajide and Kam Bhui

Introduction

To arrive at an objective understanding of himself, Descartes (1596–1650) sought to divest himself of any subjectivity and thus invented the mind–body dichotomy. In this mechanistic state he felt best able to contemplate the deeper meanings of life and the existence of God. This Cartesian dualism has dogged Western civilization ever since. In an attempt to gain respectability as an objective and a scientific pursuit, psychiatry has had to adopt objectivity as its principal tool of understanding human experiences. Jaspers (1913) took this a step further by using the "rigorous tool" of phenomenology in his inquiry of the patient's experiences. This consists of the enquirer recording as faithfully as possible the self-report of the patient's experiences. The phenomenological approach presupposes that the patient will report as faithfully as possible the events taking place in his/her internal world. If it is assumed that the internal world itself becomes destabilised by psychological distress, then *ipso facto*, self-reportage may not accurately reflect the subject's experiences. It is equally the case that the subject will only report experiences that s/he is capable of conceptualizing; in other words, culturally defined experiences. Can one therefore regard phenomenological examination as objective and culture-free?

These questions become relevant when one understands that non-Western philosophies do not recognize the Cartesian mind–body dualism. Most non-Western philosophies accept an integrated view of the mind and body as a continuum which has a diaphanous relationship with other worlds inhabited by ancestors and spirits benign and malign. There is thus a dynamic equilibrium between the known (here and now) and the unknown/unknowable world. The meaning of psychological distress is often sought in the interphase between these two worlds using an intermediary. In the traditional non-Western society, this intermediary could be the traditional healer, a herbalist or a religious leader. The doctor is the equivalent of the intermediary in Western medicine. To confound matters further, the non-Western world view consists of inter-related systems so that individuals are part of networks such as families and communities. An individual's role is defined within the context of these inter-related systems. Let us take the example of "A" from a non-Western culture: he can identify with his role as a spouse, a father, a son, and a member of the wider community without apparent contradictions. The influences that moulded his personality development combined to prepare him for these roles. Let us now take the example of "B" from a Western culture. He recognizes his roles as a spouse, father, son and his obligations within the wider community but has been conditioned to strive constantly to be an individual in his own right. This view of the self is pertinent to the interaction between the Western professional and the ethnic minority patient. Their mode of communication and interaction is shaped by their respective world views. The Western professional has the advantage that s/he comes from a culture which historically sees itself as superior to that of the patient. Neither the patient nor the professional may be consciously aware of this historical memory which dictates their pattern of communication. It may even be denied, if inappropriately raised, as a possible obstacle to a meaningful discourse between patient and the professional.

This chapter will aim to help both the professional and the care-seeker to acknowledge their respective cultural differences and show how such differences shape their patterns of communication. If not properly handled, these can lead to unsatisfactory encounters on both sides, which may lay the foundation for all future interactions. We shall also attempt to define the characteristics of a "culturally sensitive service" – an over-used terminology with no clearly defined meaning.

The Inherent Errors in the Current Classification Systems

The Western psychiatric nosological system is, in the main, based on categorisation of psychological disturbance with a possible aetiology, albeit as yet unknown. As indicated above, in its attempt at gaining scientific respectability, psychiatry has had to develop various psychometric schedules to ensure the reliability and validity of its categorisations. Numerous interview schedules (principally the Present State Examination – PSE; Wing *et al.*, 1974) are based on the phenomenological approach. Although given legitimization by its translation into several languages and its use in the World Health Organisation's International Pilot Study of Schizophrenia (WHO, 1973), it is nevertheless a Eurocentric instrument. The PSE places great reliance on **abnormal beliefs, experiences and behaviour** without cultural context. The fact that there is a significant reliability among its users (WHO, 1973) has been used to justify its sensitivity across the various cultures into whose languages it has been translated. This is a spurious argument, as the demonstrated reliability is a function of the initiation rites undertaken by its users in order to be competent in its use. There is hardly any individual competent in the use of the PSE who cannot trace his/her lineage to the inventors of the PSE. It is highly unlikely that such individuals, regardless of their cultural background, have not had to suspend cultural context at the altar of scientific objectivity.

The PSE appears to be highly successful in picking up cases of psychosis in ethnic minorities but has been singularly unsuccessful in identifying cases of depression and anxiety disorders in the same population. The question must therefore be asked as to its sensitivity in identifying the range of mental disorders for which it is designed when applied to non-Western populations.

Primary Care

Over 90 per cent of the general population are registered with a general practitioner (GP) although the figure for ethnic minorities is lower (Balarajan *et al.*, 1989; HEA, 1994; Koffman *et al.*, 1997; Chapter 13). The GP is in a unique and powerful position as a service provider, purchaser and "gate keeper" to specialist services. Furthermore, the recent NHS white paper advocates that primary care groups become responsible for purchasing health care through the establishment of trusts. The future of current mental health trusts providing community services is therefore uncertain. Yet another round of community care developments has been launched without due consideration of the impact on the health of ethnic minorities. Any serious attempt at understanding the pattern of service utilisation by ethnic minorities must therefore start at the primary care level.

There is a large body of evidence (Wilson and McCarthy, 1994; Jacob *et al.*, 1996) which suggests that there is a higher threshold for the recognition of mental illness in the ethnic minority population and that, even when there is adequate competence at recognizing mental ill-health, there appears to be a reluctance to refer to specialist services. This is more so with conditions such as anxiety, depression and personality disorders. Indeed, the diagnosis of personality disorder is seldom made in ethnic minority patients (DoH/HO, 1992). On the other hand psychotic conditions with significantly disturbed behaviour, when recognized, seem to access specialist services through emergency admissions following a crisis (Dunn and Fahy, 1990; Moodley and Perkins, 1991; Koffman *et al.*, 1997; Parkman *et al.*, 1997). The after-care of the severely mentally ill appears to be little different, judging by the frequency of relapse in the community (McGovern and Cope, 1987; Koffman *et al.*, 1997; Takei *et al.*, 1998). There is, therefore, a great need for GPs and other professionals to become competent in the basic skills of effective assessment of patients from ethnic minorities.

The Essential Ingredients of a Successful Consultation

It is incumbent on the professional to be cognizant of where the patient is coming from! By this we mean the totality of the patient's experience in the community. It is not uncommon for patients from ethnic minorities to have had problems with statutory agencies dealing with housing, employment, welfare benefits and, in some communities, "saturated policing". The sum total of these·experiences is to sensitise an individual coming into contact with psychiatry, especially for the first time, to expect further dehumaniz-ing experiences. Such an individual may approach a professional with displaced anger, there may be a reluctance to open up by discussing unpleasant or embarrassing personal experiences for fear that such dis-closure may be judged to be mental illness requiring hospitalisation. The professional who may be unaware of these psychosocial factors may attribute the patient's non-engagement or even hostility in personal terms and feel threatened and vulnerable. In some cases such professional vulner-ability may lead to over-reaction, necessitating the presence of other pro-fessionals or the police for "protection". There is a desire to conclude the encounter as quickly as possible whether or not the assessment is judged satisfactory. This cycle of mutual distrust can occur in the primary care setting, the patient's own home, the out-patient clinic and in the admission wards. The professional's discomfort may be blamed on the patient, using various stereotypical explanations usually related to the patient's culture.

The most intense contact that many psychiatrists and other professionals have with people from ethnic minorities occurs when the latter present in distress and seeking help or being compelled to receive treatment. Regard-less of cultural similarities or lack of these, patients in distress feel vulner-able when in the presence of a doctor. Straightaway, therefore, a patient from an ethnic minority background is disadvantaged because of the unequal nature of the relationship. It is the duty of the responsible doctor to handle the consultation with sensitivity.

We believe that observance of the following principles would go a long way to facilitating the consultation process with patients from ethnic mino-rities:

- Pay attention to the patient's name and if possible how to pronounce and spell it correctly; offence can be given if a patient feels that he or she is not seen as an individual but as a representative of an ethnic group with all the accompanying connotations.
- Pay attention to the age of the patient. Most cultures respect elders and a special effort should be made to avoid undue familiarity by calling elderly patients by their first names. Patronisation of an "elder" makes for a dissatisfied and possibly offended customer. This is not a good beginning for a therapeutic relationship.
- Show an interest in the unfamiliar such as dress style and current issues of cultural relevance.
- Give your undivided attention during consultation by not engaging in activities perceived by the patient as non-relevant to the consulta-tion, e.g. reading notes while talking to the patient.
- Realise that body language, such as gaze avoidance, may be cultu-rally patterned and invested with differing perceptions of intimacy, respect, confidentiality or fear. It would be presumptuous to apply psychopathological explanations for observed differences too readily. Appearing to be impatient while talking to the patient is a hazard to which all professionals are prone and which must be avoided. If a

patient is distressed and already anticipates that a professional will not understand his/her distress, impatience and urgency (especially if these contravene culturally accepted norms of mutual address) can very quickly result in the emotional unavailability of the patient and non-engagement with the professional.

● Be aware that most of what you know about patients from ethnic minorities derives from racial mythology, stereotyped images of immigrants provided by the media and images of their countries of origin both current and historical.

● Be aware of the public perception that psychiatry is a coercive agent of society with powers akin to those of the police and the criminal justice system.

● Be aware that many patients from the inner cities have had unpleasant experiences with statutory agencies such as housing, employment, welfare benefit, and the police.

● Realise that apparent aggression in body language may be a manifestation of fear of the unknown, based on hearsay account of the "power" of the psychiatrist.

● Put your patient at ease in any way you know how. If you do not know how, have the humility to learn from your patient.

To be able to achieve such cultural competence, given the pressure under which many professionals operate, it is essential to make conscious efforts to realise these aims. It is important, too, to acknowledge one's own feeling of vulnerability when confronted by an individual from an unfamiliar culture. It is only by so doing that one can conquer the fear of the unfamiliar that we all share – patient and professional alike.

Specialist Services

This is an area where ethnic minority communities believe that existing services have not taken on board local community views in service planning, development and evaluation. The Department of Health (1993) clearly stipulates that services must be local, sensitive, responsive, and accessible to the community which they serve. Ethnic minority communities perceive their service providers as not living upto these high ideals (Parkman *et al.*, 1997). The community's response has led to the development of the voluntary sector to provide for needs unmet by statutory agencies (see Chapter 9).

An even more drastic solution has been suggested by others – the development of a separate service that will cater solely for patients from ethnic minority populations. This is a serious indictment of the mainstream services.

We believe that these services would become more relevant and acceptable to the community which they serve if the following basic principles were observed in planning and developing services for a multi-cultural society:

- A commitment to ascertain the needs of the local community through consultation with the opinion leaders from youth organizations, churches, mosques and established voluntary service providers.
- Ensure that representatives of such organizations are appointed to various planning committees. This may require some training in how the health system works, and adequate remuneration as an incentive to attend meetings.
- Embark on as wide a publicity exercise as possible to allow the community to have a sense of ownership.
- Ensure that services provided have relevance to the daily experience of the local community with respect to the decor of the facilities.
- Provide a place of worship, even if this is only a room, as religion plays a significant role in the lives of many citizens from ethnic minority communities.
- Single-sex wards are desirable where religious cultures demand this.
- Make an effort to include ethnic food on the menu.
- The local hospital should be encouraged to stock specialist skin and hair care products for patients.
- Encourage collaboration with established voluntary agencies through participation in preparing pre-discharge care plans and after-care plans.
- Encourage the active participation of representatives from the community in setting quality standards as well as in-service evaluation.
- Establish an effective complaint forum that the community can access, and be ready to take on board legitimate grievances.
- Ensure that your service has a liaison officer between the service and the community to keep open a channel of communication.
- Ensure the rigorous monitoring and auditing of ethnic data collection in order to inform service planning and reconfiguration if necessary.
- Ensure that your Trust Board refelcts the demography of the local population.

The above principles can form the basis of local Trust objectives which will guide the business of the service provider.

The needs of ethnic minority communities are multifarious and require close inter-agency working in order to be able to provide a comprehensive and seamless service, cost-effectively. While health and social services have statutory responsibilities for providing community care for people suffering from mental illness, we recommend that strong alliances are forged with employment agencies, housing associations, adult education centres, local social security agency, the probation service and the local police. It is essential that these agencies are fully subscribed to the local service provider's objectives at the planning and development stages.

Treatment of Patients from Ethnic Minorities

The psychiatrist's roles in the treatment of patients include diagnostic assessment and management. These roles are increasingly being undertaken in conjunction with nurses, psychologists, social workers and a range of other professionals. The psychiatrist no longer practises in isolation; most care of the mentally ill is delivered through a multi-disciplinary team (MDT). This has significant advantages but also carries certain disadvantages, as we shall make clear presently.

If an assessment determines that a patient requires admission for further assessment and treatment, the patient's initial experience of the mental health service and its professionals can leave a lasting impression for good or bad. It is at this point that staff tolerance of inappropriate behaviour can determine the patient's treatment and subsequent passage through the system (Moodley and Thornicroft, 1988; Cope, 1989; Dunn and Fahy, 1990; Koffman *et al.*, 1997). Any disturbed patient generates anxiety in staff, but if he is "big and black" there may be a demand for the doctor to do "something". That something may be medication or permission to nurse the patient in an intensive unit in order to "protect others". The literature on aggression by in-patients both in the UK and the USA has not confirmed a higher level of aggression by "black" patients compared with whites, even though the former are more likely to receive acute treatment for aggression or to be secluded (Bond *et al.*, 1988; Noble and Roger, 1989; Koffman *et al.*, 1997).

The feeling of vulnerability by staff when confronted by patients from ethnic minorities also explains the use of physical restraint and potent medications, which occasionally result in sudden death (Institute of Race Relations, 1991; Jusic and Lader, 1994). It is the duty of the psychiatrist to be aware of the pressures being placed upon him/her in these situations and to be able to stand back sufficiently to take stock of a situation before taking drastic action. In our experience, such situations require leadership skills and courage. It is vital to reassure and support staff but it is also important to recognise our duty of care to the patient.

The care of patients from ethnic minorities is more likely to succeed if significant others are co-opted into treatment plans. The significant others should include family members when available, but members from the church, mosque or other local community groups to which the patient belongs can be a tower of strength. The identified supportive individual should be encouraged to attend MDT meetings, s.117 care plans and Care Programme Approach (CPA) meetings. It is the responsibility of the key worker to liaise with other agencies and ensure efficient communication in order to prevent the patient falling through the safety net, possibly into the criminal justice system or homelessness (see Chapter 7).

Care in the Community

The Community Care Act of 1990 (House of Commons, 1990) set the framework for community care provisions for the mentally ill. It made both health authorities and social services responsible for the care of the mentally ill in the community.

In theory, care in the community should lead to normalisation and improved quality of patients' lives. No longer will they exist in the margins of society, languishing in long-stay wards, toiling away at repetitive and childlike occupational therapy activities in day centres or sheltered workshops whose existence shamed society. The expectation of the Act was that individual patient's needs would be assessed and individualised care plans would be designed and with the help of the key worker/care manager, the patient will lead as normal a life as possible in the community. The CPA (DoH, 1989) was introduced to ensure co-ordinated care for the vulnerable severely mentally ill. This sounds too good to be true. But it could happen. A decade earlier, such a normal-isation programme saw the closure of the large institutions for patients with learning disability, with most of them relocated into purpose-built small accommodations in the community. Care in the community did not, unfortunately, lead to such structured decommissioning of the old hospi-tals and "community care" became a major social experiment with as yet undetermined outcome. A multi-cultural society with strong social net-works would have been an ideal foundation for community care. It is paradoxical that the political dogma of the day denied the existence of the community while at the same time embarking on a large-scale social experiment of relocation of asylum patients into the "community". The goodwill of the community that was a prerequisite of the success of the learning disability programme of the early 1980s had evaporated by the time that care in the community was introduced.

In spite of the above difficulties, there are places where community care seems to work well. What such centres seem to have in common is the ability to engage in effective partnerships, which includes a range of other agencies listed above. Additionally, such centres have successfully re-configured their services in order to provide a spectrum of services comprising:

- 24-hour nursing care for people with severe mental illness;
- crisis intervention service;
- respite care for users and support for their carers;
- employment schemes such as the Club House model;
- collaboration with housing associations;
- development of befriender schemes;
- provision of assertive outreach services;
- close collaboration with the police and close monitoring of the use of s.136.

While the above services are most likely to provide the most effective style of community care, and we are aware of the cost implications and the difficulties that many services experience in providing even a "tradi-tional" psychiatric service, it is our view that such service components can form the basis of service commissioning in a multi-cultural society. This is of the utmost importance in inner-city mental health service provision.

Physical Treatment

There is an on-going debate, both in academic and lay circles, with respect to the treatment of patients from ethnic minorities. This debate has been hindered by the paucity of empirical data and has led to some polarisation of the protagonists. Users and their carers have come to see medication as a form of "chemical restraint" akin to the other coercive tools in the psychiatrist's armamentarium. Psychiatrists argue the efficacy of pharmacological agents, quoting the wealth of randomised controlled trials as proof of their rational prescribing practice. Evidence-based medicine has now conferred legitimacy on rational prescribing. What are the central issues of the debate?

1. Are there pharmacogenetic differences across ethnic groups?
2. Are the side-effect profiles of psychotropics different across ethnic groups?
3. What factors influence compliance with medication across ethnic groups?

These are important and weighty matters that psychiatry has not begun to address and which we feel will be central to the debate surrounding patient management in the next millennium. Some readers may find this section rather technical but it is essential to explore some of the known facts with the implications for medication of patients from ethnic minorities. We shall attempt to answer these questions based on available research evidence.

The introduction of the various psychotropic medications such as antipsychotics, antidepressants, lithium and benzodiazepines led to a revolutionary change in the practice of psychiatry. Although these drugs were originally developed and tested in North America and Western Europe, they were introduced and used extensively for the treatment of psychiatric conditions in countries and societies with divergent cultural and ethnic backgrounds and socio-economic developments. Psychopharmacology has become the mainstay of psychiatric treatment worldwide (Lin *et al.*, 1993).

Ethnicity and Pharmacogenetics

The first recognition of ethnic differences in drug responses was noticed during the second world war when American soldiers were routinely given the anti-malarial, primaquine. A large number of African American soldiers suffered from severe haemolytic anaemia, the cause of which was discovered to be an in-born deficiency of an enzyme (biological catalyst), glucose-6-phosphate dehydrogenase (G6PD). In Africans, this same deficiency confers certain immunity to malaria in sickle cell disease carriers. The introduction of the anti-tuberculosis agent, isoniazid, in 1952 revealed that Asians developed obstructive jaundice when exposed to this agent whilst Caucasians developed peripheral neuropathy. Further investigations indicated that Asians are "slow acetylators" while Caucasians are "fast acetylators".

Acetylation represents an important metabolic pathway for a large number of psychoactive agents such as nitrazepam, caffeine and phenelzine. Weber (1987) has identified ethnospecific point mutations responsible for slow acetylation.

The well-recognized "flushing reaction" in East Asians (Chinese, Japanese, Koreans and Vietnamese) when exposed to alcohol has been found to be due to a genetically determined deficiency of aldehyde dehydrogenase which is accentuated in some individuals by an over-activity of alcohol dehydrogenase (Agarwal and Goedde, 1990; Yoshida, 1993).

With the exception of lithium, most psychotropics are lipophilic (fat soluble) and in order for these medications to be excreted from the body they must be made water soluble. There are two ways in which this can be achieved: oxidation or conjugation. It is now recognized that a group of enzymes (cytochrome P-450 mono oxygenases) are responsible for the metabolism and detoxification of the majority of chemotherapeutic agents through the process of oxidation (Gonzalez and Nebert, 1990; Shen and Lin, 1990; Karlow, 1993).

Pharmacogenetics is a relatively new area of academic pursuit but it is nevertheless capable of illuminating some of the differential responses to medication by various ethnic groups.

The following illustrate examples of differential drug metabolism of relevance to the care of ethnic minority patients.

Lithium
The sodium/lithium counter-transport system is less active in African Americans, thereby producing a higher red blood cell/serum concentration than in Caucasians. This predisposes African Americans to a greater risk of central nervous system toxicity.

Haloperidol
The pharmacokinetics and pharmacodynamics of haloperidol have been demonstrated to differ significantly between Asian and Caucasian patients suffering from schizophrenia. The plasma concentration of haloperidol was found to be 50 per cent higher in Asian than Caucasian patients (Potkin *et al.*, 1984). When the therapeutic doses of haloperidol were compared in four groups of patients, there were significant pharmacokinetic differences between Chinese and African Americans on the one hand, and Caucasians and Hispanics on the other (Jann *et al.*, 1993). There is anecdotal evidence that young male Africans and African Caribbeans are more prone to acute dystonic reaction when treated with haloperidol.

Clozapine
Clozapine-induced agranulocytosis has been found to be more prevalent in Ashkenazy Jews, especially among those possessing a particular cluster of human lymphocyte antigen (HLA) immunological typings that are found in this ethnic group (Lieberman *et al.*, 1990).

Tricyclic antidepressants

In contrast to neuroleptics, the results of ethnic differences in the pharma-cokinetics of the tricyclic antidepressants (TCAs) have been inconclusive although Asians appear to metabolize TCAs significantly more slowly than Caucasians (Kishimoto and Hollister, 1984). One study that compared the pharmacokinetics of imipramine among Asians, African Americans, Caucasians and Hispanics found elevated levels of desipramine in African Americans, but not in the other groups (Lin *et al.*, 1993).

Benzodiazepines

It has been found consistently that Asians metabolize diazepam more slowly than Caucasians (Rosenblat and Tang, 1987; Lin *et al.*, 1993). This suggests greater sensitivity to diazepam, with the risk of prolonged effect of its active metabolite (nordiazepam). Caution must be exercised in the long-term use of diazepam in this population.

Beta-blockers

Propranolol has been found to be relatively ineffective in treating hyperten-sion in African Americans (Moser and Lunn, 1981). By contrast, relatively smaller doses are effective in Asians compared with Caucasians. As pro-pranolol is sometimes used in anxiety disorders, it appears that propranolol is less likely to be efficacious in African Americans while relatively small doses should be used in Asians.

There is a compelling argument for research into the pharmacogenetics of antipsychotic drugs, as patients from ethnic minorities are often treated with large doses of them, with very little understanding of either their pharmacokinetics or pharmacodynamics in these populations. It is quite possible that pharmacogenetics holds the key to the understanding of the frequent unexplained sudden deaths of black Caribbeans, black Africans and Asians that have been reported in the literature (Institute of Race Relations, 1991; Jusic and Lader, 1994).

Ethnicity and Compliance with Medication

Non-compliance is a major problem in the treatment of any chronic condi-tion, and even more so in the treatment of chronic mental illness. The treatment of severe mental illness is complicated by poor compliance.

The following are possible causes of poor compliance with medication:

- Poor communication between doctor and patient with respect to treatment expectations and side-effects (full explanation of time of onset of action, when to discontinue, etc.).
- Acute- onset side-effects at the initiation of treatment which may be dose-dependent (e.g. acute dystonic reaction, dry mouth). Start at a smaller dose and gradually increase dose.
- Intermediate side-effects such as weight gain, sexual dysfunction, hair loss, craving for food, etc.

- Severe extrapyramidal side-effects that make the patient stand out and vulnerable to ridicule.
- Reluctance to accept a diagnosis of mental illness, with its associated social and economic implications.
- The rising tide of antimedication and the need to use alternative approaches to heal the emotionally wounded.

There are few studies of factors that predict compliance to medication, but good communication, rational prescribing and regular monitoring of the effect and continuing need are likely to enhance compliance.

Psychological Treatment

The origins of psychoanalytical psychotherapy in continental Europe condemned it, at its inception, to the middle class and the wealthy. It did not take root in the UK until after the second world war, in the wake of Jewish émigrés from the continent followed by a second wave of immigrants from across the Atlantic. Psychoanalysis typifies the myth that certain cultures are not "psychologically minded" and therefore incapable of introspection. Close scrutiny shows that of those excluded coincide with people who are more physically expressive in their music and life-style. This same group was spared the white man's burden in not suffering from depression or neuroses. Added to this group of outsiders are "insiders" who are working class and not given to introspection either. In order to remove any trace of elitism or racism, psychotherapists undergo an expensive initiation ceremony after which they can practise. As psychotherapy is traditionally provided in the private sector, only those with the economic wherewithal can afford it. Any accusation of elitism or racism can be countered by the argument that any one can gain access to the service at a price. Although psychotherapy is now available within the NHS to some extent, the selective process is still dictated by the historical myths about races upon which it was founded.

There are now other forms of psychological intervention that are based on pragmatic problem-solving approaches. There is no reason to believe that patients from ethnic minorities cannot benefit from interventions such as behaviour therapy, cognitive behaviour therapy, psycho-educational programmes for patients and their carers (Chapter 12). However, therapies that have not been developed with ethnic minorities as chief theorists or patients are subject to failures of theory, service delivery and economic or organizational availability. Delivery encompasses aspects of matching therapies and therapists for an optimal outcome (Bhugra and Bhui, 1998). Little reliable research exists into this complex yet crucial issue. (Chapters 2, 10, 12 and 19).

Conclusion

We have tried to provide some insight into the essential elements of a culturally sensitive service and the role of the psychiatrist within such a service. There is a movement towards separate service provision for ethnic minorities, but we believe this movement arose as a reaction to the insensitivity of mainstream psychiatry to the needs of this population. What we have come to recognise is that a culturally sensitive service is really one that is responsive to the population which it serves and which the local community feel comfortable with because they have a stake in it. The psychiatrist, as a member of a multi-professional team, has some insights that are complementary to those of other professionals. By working together, the MDT can deploy most efficiently their respective skills and insights in helping the user and the carer to overcome the awesome burden of mental illness so that the individual sufferer can take his/her place in society and feel worthwhile.

References

Agarwal, D.P. and Goedde, W. (1990) *Alcohol Metabolism, Alcohol Intolerance and Alcoholism.* Berlin: Springer.

Balarajan, R., Yuen, P. and Raleigh, V.S. (1989) Ethnic differences in general practitioner consultations. *British Medical Journal* **299**: 958–960.

Bhugra, D. and Bhui, K. (1998) Psychotherapy with ethnic minority clients. *British Journal of Psychotherapy* **14(3)**: 310–326.

Bond, C.F., DiCandia, C.G., MacKinnon, J.R. (1988) Responses to violence in a psychiatric setting: the role of the patient's. *Personality and Social Psychology Bulletin* **14**: 448–457.

Cope, R. (1989) The compulsory detention of Afro-Caribbeans under the Mental Health Act. *New Community* **15**: 343–356.

Department of Health (1989) *Caring for People with Mental Illness: The Care Programme Approach.* London: HMSO.

Department of Health and Home Office (1992) Services for people from black and ethnic minority groups: issues of race and culture. In: *Review of Health and Social Services for Mentally Disordered Offenders and Others Requiring Similar Services.* London: HMSO.

Department of Health (1993) *The Health of the Nation: Key Area Handbook – Mental Illness.* London: HMSO.

Dunn, J. and Fahy, T. (1990) Police admissions to a psychiatric hospital: demographic and clinical differences between ethnic groups. *British Journal of Psychiatry* **156**: 373–378.

Gonzalez, F.J. and Nebert, D.W. (1990) Evolution of the P-450 gene superfamily: animal–plant "warfare", molecular drive and human genetic differences in drug oxidation. *Trends in Genetics* **6**: 182–186.

HEA (1994) *Health and Lifestyles. Black and Ethnic Minority Groups in England.* London: Health Education Authority.

House of Commons (1990) *The National Health Service and Community Care Act.* London: HMSO.

Institute of Race Relations (1991) *Deadly Silence: Black Deaths in Custody.*

Jacob, K., Bhugra, D., Mann, A.H. *et al.* (1996) The use of the general practitioner by Indian females with psychiatric morbidity: recognition of the disorder and the role of social and cultural factors in help seeking. London: Institute of Psychiatry.

Jann, M.W., Lam, Y.W. and Chang, W.H. (1993) Haloperidol and reduced haloperidol plasma concentrations in different ethnic populations and inter individual variabilities in haloperidol metabolism. In: Lin, K.M., Poland, R.E. and Nakasaki, G. (eds) *Psychopharmacology and Psychobiology of Ethnicity*, pp. 133–152. Washington, DC: American Psychiatric Press.

Jaspers, K. (1913) *General Psychopathology.* Translated from the German by J. Hoenig and M.W. Hamilton. Manchester University Press (1963).

Jusic, N. and Lader, M. (1994) Post-mortem antipsychotic drug concentrations and unexplained deaths. *British Journal of Psychiatry* **165**: 787–791.

Karlow, W. (1993) Pharmacogenetics: its biologic roots and the medical challenge. *Clinical Pharmacology and Therapeutics* **54**: 235–241.

Kishimoto, A. and Hollister, L.E. (1984) Nortriptyline kinetics in Japanese and Americans (letter). *Journal of Clinical Psychopharmacology* **4**: 171–172.

Koffman, J., Fulop, N.J., Pashley, D. and Coleman, K. (1997) Ethnicity and use of acute beds: one day survey in North and South Thames Regions. *British Journal of Psychiatry* **171**: 238–241.

Lieberman, J.A., Yunis, J., Egea, E. *et al.* (1990) HLA-B38, DR4, Dqw3 and clozapine-induced agranulocytosis in Jewish patients with schizophrenia. *Archives of General Psychiatry* **47**: 945–948.

Lin, K.M., Poland, R.E. and Nakasaki, G. (eds) (1993) *Psychopharmacology and Psychobiology of Ethnicity.* Washington, DC: American Psychiatric Press.

McGovern, B. and Cope, R. (1987) The compulsory detention of males of different ethnic groups with special reference to offender patients. *British Journal of Psychiatry* **150**: 505–512.

Moodley, P. and Perkins, R.E. (1991) Routes to psychiatric inpatient care in an inner London borough. *Social Psychiatry and Psychiatric Epidemiology* **26**: 47–51.

Moodley, P. and Thornicroft, G. (1988) Ethnic group and compulsory detention. *Medical Science Law* **28**: 324–328.

Moser, M. and Lunn, J. (1981) Comparative effects of pindolol and hydrochlorothiazide in black hypertensive patients. *Angiology* **32**: 561–566.

Noble, P. and Roger, S. (1989) Violence by psychiatric inpatients. *British Journal of Psychiatry* **155**: 384–390.

Parkman, S., Davis, S., Leese, M., Phelan, M. and Thornicroft, G. (1997) Ethnic differences in satisfaction with mental health services among representative people with psychosis in South London: PRiM Study 4. *British Journal of Psychiatry* **171**: 260–264.

Potkin, S.G., Shen, Y., Pardes, H. *et al.* (1984) Haloperidol concentrations elevated in Chinese patients. *Psychiatry Research* **12**: 167–172.

Rosenblat, R. and Tang, S.W. (1987) Do oriental psychiatric patients receive different dosages of psychotropic medication when compared with Occidentals? *Canadian Journal of Psychiatry* **32**: 270–274.

Shen, W.W. and Lin, K.M. (1990) Cytochrome P-450 monooxygenases and interactions of psychotropic drugs. *International Journal of Psychiatry in Medicine* **21**: 21–30.

Takei, N., Persaud, R., Woodruff, P., Brockington, I. and Murray, R.M. (1998) First episodes of psychosis in Afro-Caribbean and White people: an 18 year follow-up population based study. *British Journal of Psychiatry* **172**: 147–153.

Weber, W.W. (1987) *The Acetylator Genes and Drug Responses.* New York: Oxford University Press.

WHO (1973) *International Pilot Study of Schizophrenia.* Geneva: World Health Organisation.

Wilson, M. and McCarthy, E. (1994) GP consultation as a factor in the low rate of mental health service use by Asians. *Psychological Medicine* **24**: 113–119.

Wing, J.K., Cooper, J.E. and Sartorius, N. (1974) *The Measurement and Classification of Psychiatric Symptoms.* London: Cambridge University Press.

Yoshida, A. (1993) Genetic polymorphisms of alcohol-metabolizing enzymes related to alcohol sensitivity and alcohol diseases. In: Lin, K.M., Poland, R.E. and Nakasaki, G. (eds) *Psychopharmacology and Psychobiology of Ethnicity,* pp. 169–186. Washington, DC: American Psychiatric Press.

7

The Probation Service

Hindpal Singh Bhui

Introduction

Using a broad definition of a mentally disordered offender (MDO), which includes those who experience significant mental distress but do not necessarily fit the criteria of the Mental Health Act 1983, most statistics indicate that MDOs constitute around 15–20 per cent of the average probation caseload (e.g. Pritchard *et al.*, 1992; ILPS, 1997). At 11 per cent, the proportion of MDOs from minority ethnic groups closely resembles that of minority ethnic offenders on the national probation caseload (Hudson *et al.*, 1993).

Probation officers occupy a pivotal position in the criminal justice system, have a major role in the assessment, diversion, management and, perhaps most controversially, treatment of such offenders, and consequently are in a position either to reinforce or redress the discrimination which exists in that system. Despite this, many professionals in both the mental health and criminal justice fields often appear to have a minimal understanding of the probation role in work with MDOs. This is partly due to the low public profile traditionally maintained by the Probation Service, a position reinforced during recent years when its often complex and unpopulist work has, notwithstanding its many proven merits (e.g. Oldfield, 1997), been undervalued and undermined by both the media and politicians.

When the Service does receive positive publicity, it usually focuses on its controlling function; the value of the probation officer's role as a caring professional is rarely highlighted. However, until recently, the Probation Service itself has given limited attention to working creatively with MDOs and building closer links with the mental health services. The result has, unsurprisingly, been an inconsistency of service, with pockets of highly competent and sometimes inspired work by individual probation officers and certain probation areas, often co-existing with practice which meets the needs of neither the client nor the wider community. Clearly, a crucial prerequisite to culturally sensitive work with ethnic minority MDOs is improved probation practice with MDOs in general. Consequently, this chapter ranges widely across issues that affect work with all such offenders, making it impossible to avoid treating some complex issues with excess brevity. One can only hope that this does not detract from the overall usefulness of the analysis. This chapter has four fundamental aims:

1. To present an accessible account of the probation officer's role in work with MDOs and in particular to outline the distinctive influence which the Probation Service can bring to bear in the achievement of an effective anti-discriminatory and culturally sensitive service.
2. To offer a critical analysis of some of the most important issues facing the Probation Service in its work with MDOs.
3. To explore ideal models of organisation and practice.
4. To offer a probation practitioner's perspective on other services in the multi-agency environment.

The chapter cannot claim to be the final word on the Probation Service, MDOs and cultural differences, and is certainly not all-encompassing, drawing as it does largely on the work of the Inner London Probation Service (ILPS). The ILPS is, however, the largest and most cosmopolitan of the 54 probation areas in England and Wales. It employs around 10 per cent of all probation officers, and one third of their caseloads are comprised of offenders who describe themselves as black.

The Probation Service and MDOs

Statutory Contact with MDOs in the Community and Prisons

1. **Psychiatric and standard probation orders**. A probation order can be imposed if it is deemed to be in the interests of the rehabilitation of the offender or the protection of the public from harm or reoffending. Probationers must attend regular compulsory probation sessions for between six months and three years. Mental Health Act criteria for treatability do not have to be met for a psychiatric probation order to be imposed and, if the psychiatrist and probation officer consider it appropriate, personality – disordered offenders (whose conditions could include elements of mental illness and who may well have differing diagnoses over time; see, for example, Davis, 1990, pp. 41–45) can be dealt with using this disposal (HMIP, 1993; Stone, 1995).
2. **Psychiatric supervision orders**. These apply to young offenders under 18 years old and are in most respects similar to probation orders (Stone, 1995).
3. **Guardianship orders**. These are undoubtedly underused; they ought to be considered when an individual's offending behaviour can be attributed to a psychiatric condition which could be controlled through medication and access to appropriate health and social care resources.
4. **Supervision and treatment orders**. These are normally supervised by social workers; only one is being supervised by an ILPS probation officer at time of writing. They are very similar in nature to psychiatric probation orders, but, as is the case with guardianship

orders, there is no power of breach (see Stone, 1995, for other differences).

5. **Throughcare, parole and licence supervision**. Any offenders who receive custodial sentences of more than 12 months will be allocated a probation officer whose role it is to assist the offender's rehabilitation in the community and take all reasonable steps to minimise the chances of reoffending. On release, they are subject to a period of compulsory supervision by a probation officer. Young offenders will be on licence regardless of the length of sentence.

6. **Social supervision of restricted patients conditionally discharged from hospitals**. At the end of 1996, 138 conditionally discharged patients were being supervised by probation officers (Home Office, 1997). There are currently about 50 restricted patients on probation caseloads in the Inner London area. In-house training has recently been instituted to ensure that each one of these potentially high-risk offenders is supervised by specially trained officers.

7. **Prisons**. Probation officers seconded to work in prisons, whose numbers have been drastically reduced in the wake of funding cuts to the prisons, are ideally placed to act as links between the prison and community mental health services, maximising communication between agencies. They are also likely to be prominent in identifying mental disorder in prisoners, an important role given that the results of a major research study concluded that about one third of male adult sentenced prisoners had some form of mental disorder (Gunn *et al.*, 1991).

Probation Officers in the Court Setting – Diversion and Custodial Remands

The Probation Service, through its links with the criminal justice system and with outside agencies, is well placed to organise diversion schemes and is the body most likely to do so (Blumenthal and Wessely, 1992; unpublished study quoted in Hudson *et al.*, 1993). In some areas a full multi-disciplinary panel, usually co-ordinated by a probation officer, will assess the options (for a more detailed discussion see Wickham, 1994). As Smith (1993) points out, the presence of a psychiatrist means that probation officers are more likely to take "risks" with bail hostel referrals and that sentencers are less likely to feel obliged to incarcerate MDOs because of a fear of violence to the community. However, Browne (1995), who conducted a series of interviews with criminal justice officials, including probation officers and magistrates, found that they are "more likely to err on the side of caution with black mentally vulnerable defendants and to be affected by a heightened perception of dangerousness with regard to this group" (1995, pp. 70–71). As the decision to remand in custody appears in many cases to be "largely intuitive" (Browne, 1995, p. 70), there is a need for probation officers and others in a position to influence decision-makers, not only to be aware of their own prejudices, but also to be pro-active in challenging discriminatory attitudes in the court setting and at court staff liaison meetings. The Bail Act 1976 requires sentencers to state clearly the reasons for a refusal to grant bail. A 1994 survey commissioned by ILPS from the "Revolving Doors" agency found that, in addition to the common criteria of lack of community ties and likelihood of reoffending, courts offered reasons distinct from the legal requirements of the Bail Act such as the "defendant's demeanour in court" (Browne, 1995, p. 24). This latter criterion clearly demands particular vigilance and concern, given evidence that the body language and statements of people from minority ethnic backgrounds can be misinterpreted and lead to racist stereotyping and discriminatory decisions (Littlewood and Lipsedge, 1997).

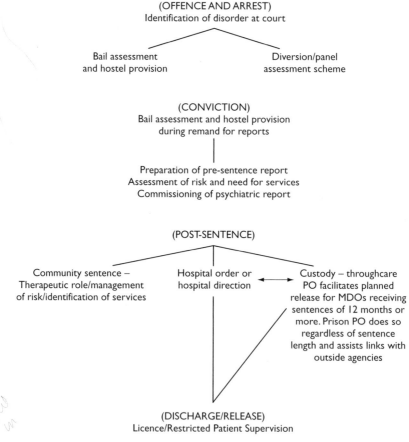

Figure 7.1 Probation involvement with mentally disordered offenders. PO, probation officer.

Probation Officers' Assessment as a Complement to the Medical Model

If one accepts to any degree Fernando's argument that the medical approach to mentally distressed people generally minimises the importance of racial and cultural issues in what is seen as a question of "illness identification" (1995, p. 35), the value of a broader non-medical assessment in ensuring that black and other minority ethnic people are neither held more starkly responsible for their offending than is justifiable by the facts, nor deprived of appropriate assistance, becomes apparent. Probation officers need to be aware of the importance of their role in the context of a system of psychiatric classification which is based on limited knowledge and understanding of distressing conditions, which in turn vastly increases the scope for discretion and discrimination.

A fascinating study of forensic psychiatric assessments in Sweden (Belfrage and Lidberg, 1996) illustrates this powerfully: it found a "remarkable degree of discrepancy in decision-making" among senior forensic psychiatrists. In some cases there were even "negative correlations" between assessments, "that is, if one psychiatrist assessed an offender as in need of treatment, another one assessed him as not in need of treatment" (p. 331). Pre-sentence report (PSR) authors are trained to present a criminological analysis of offending which addresses the contribution of socio-economic and environmental considerations, and to give an opinion on their relevance to the sentencing decision. Consequently, the fact that a black MDO's psychiatric condition, behaviour and personality may have been profoundly influenced by racism and the resultant disadvantage should be explicitly recognised.

The Probation Officer's Role in the Context of Community Care

The closure of residential facilities for psychiatric patients has not been matched by a proportionate increase in community care facilities; consequently the Probation Service has become increasingly important in the care of MDOs in the community. Although the lack both of systematic monitoring and a standard definition of mental disorder in probation areas makes it difficult to measure changes in numbers (Vaughan and Badger, 1995, pp. 8–12), there is little doubt that there is a far greater awareness of such offenders on probation caseloads.

A number of these offenders will be classed as having a psychopathic or other form of personality disorder and be considered by psychiatrists not to warrant a significant commitment of time and resources because they are not thought to be treatable. As addressing offending behaviour and managing risk are the overriding responsibilities of the Probation Service, regardless of any measure of treatability, probation officers do not have the option of avoiding responsibility for these offenders. It appears to be a common perception amongst probation officers that over-stretched psychiatric and social services tend to limit their own involvement if they know that a probation officer is involved. In some cases this may well be justified; but if the disengagement is due more to a lack of resources than to a consideration of the needs of the individual, then the probation officer's role becomes problematic, even dangerous, when more appropriate services are withdrawn.

Clients with a dual diagnosis, that is with both a psychiatric condition and problematic drug or alcohol use – who form a large, vulnerable, often high-risk group – are more likely to be excluded or to receive inadequate treatment from mainstream treatment services. Like those people given a vague label of personality disorder, they are liable to end up as long-term clients of the Probation Service because their offending remains a constant problem. The probation officer has a particularly crucial role as an advocate for appropriate services, a conduit for effective communication between the different agencies and as provider of up-to-date assessments, facilitating specialist intervention at the time when it is likely to be most successful (for a more detailed consideration of the implications of the social care market for the Probation Service, see Haynes and Henfrey, 1995).

Probation Officers as Therapists

All currently practising probation officers are trained social workers, versed in casework methods that can reduce reoffending. One, albeit small, study (Mendelson, 1992; quoted in Hudson *et al.*, 1993, p. 38), estimated that probation officers took a therapeutic role with 30 per cent of psychiatric out-patient cases, more than any other professional group, bar psychiatrists. Addressing offending behaviour and managing risk, the central functions of the modern probation officer, may often involve substantial use of counselling skills and "supportive psychotherapy" (Pringle and Thompson, 1986, pp. 113–114) to promote emotional calm, increase a client's ability to cope, and minimise the chances of psychiatric relapse and reoffending. Although the probation officer's role inevitably involves appropriate use of authority, this is not akin to driving a wedge between worker and client. Many clients respond very positively to the boundaries which are in themselves an integral part of the therapeutic process in any setting (Buchanan and Millar, 1997). As people who have some form of mental disorder and/or abuse drugs or alcohol frequently lead chaotic lives in which appointments are likely to be missed, perhaps more out of habit than design, the threat of court action can frequently facilitate progress.

With regard to black MDOs, a particularly important point, which should not be underestimated, is that the Probation Service is the only criminal justice agency which has succeeded in attracting black staff in numbers at least proportionate to their representation in the general population. At the end of 1996, 8.4 per cent of all probation officers were from minority ethnic backgrounds, compared to 6.1 per cent of the general population. There were proportionately three times as many black African-Caribbean staff as in the general population, although only half as many South Asians (Home Office, 1997). Whilst the presence of black staff does not guarantee a culturally sensitive service, it can inspire a greater sense of identification and confidence, and often encourages therapeutic engagement amongst black offenders (Jeffers, 1995, p. 19). Support and campaigning organisations such as the Association of Black Probation Officers and the National Association of Asian Probation Staff have also become well established within the Probation Service.

Partnerships Between the Probation Service, the Voluntary Sector and other Community Organisations

The Probation Service has been encouraged by the government to set aside about 5 per cent of its budget (at the time of writing, ILPS is spending about 7 per cent) for funding partnership workers and agencies (Home Office, 1992). ILPS has developed eight MDO partnerships, two of which are targeted specifically at black MDOs. They have proven to be an invaluable aid to working with those MDOs who either have a condition which the mainstream mental health services have not considered serious enough to warrant allocation of resources, or who are unwilling or unable to engage with those services. Given the publicity surrounding black people's deaths while in custody or psychiatric care, black people may have a quite legitimate fear of consenting to psychiatric or probation assessment. Such apprehension may be exacerbated by a pre-existing paranoid belief system, or be dismissed by mental health professionals as something with no rational basis. The following case study illustrates how black partnerships can play a vital role:

TH is a black man in his twenties who was exhibiting psychotic symptoms. He had refused to see a psychiatrist or co-operate in the assessment process because he was convinced that his life would be in danger, particularly as a mentally ill friend had recently died in a psychiatric hospital. He was eventually remanded in custody, and was still refusing to co-operate until one of the ILPS black partnership workers visited him, and gradually managed to gain his trust. It seems that one of the main reasons that she succeeded where others had failed was because she was a member of an independent organisation and not identified as part of an oppressive system. She and the involved probation officer subsequently persuaded the court that TH needed to be bailed so that he could visit the partnership project itself, where a black psychiatrist was eventually able to complete the assessment.

Similarly, black voluntary organisations can also enhance the responsiveness of black MDOs to probation intervention by giving assistance which is neither available nor acceptable from a criminal justice agency or from predominantly white organisations. One of their most important contributions is the perspective they can offer to a Probation Service often bogged down with the imperatives of government criminal justice policy. In order to provide a service to minority ethnic clients which is both just and effective in reducing crime, the Probation Service needs to hear and respond to the voices of groups that evolve out of local communities.

Provision of a High-quality, Anti-discriminatory and Culturally Sensitive Service

Probation Officer Training

All probation officers should have sufficient knowledge to ask informed questions of mental health professionals and be able to challenge their decisions constructively when appropriate. They should also have enough knowledge of psychiatric symptomatology to make reasoned and non-discriminatory preliminary assessments of clients presenting with mental health problems. Hudson *et al.*'s (1993) study into probation officer training for work with MDOs covered 25 per cent of officers in eight probation services, which employed 20 per cent of all probation officers in England and Wales. It elicited 193 responses (73 per cent), and provides one of the best available guides to the state of probation knowledge with regard to this client group. The lack of specific mental health training and consequent lack of ease amongst many probation officers working with MDOs figured strongly in the questionnaire responses, with the vast majority expressing "considerable professional concern about work with mentally disordered offenders and their awareness of key issues" (p. 39). Of those who had trained in the preceding four years, 50 per cent reported training on ethnic differences and mental disorder during their courses, but of those trained between five and nine years before the survey, only 22 per cent had received such training. Only 4 per cent of those trained more than ten years before completing the questionnaire reported having had this training either in college or while in post (p. 34). While all of the ten "specialist" workers interviewed (including three probation officers working in mental health settings) agreed that probation officers were sensitive to issues of discrimination and racism, "more problematic was whether their training had been sufficiently thorough in dealing with the complex and subtle interaction among racial identity, culture, the experience of discrimination and oppression and mental disorder . . ." (p. 17).

The inevitable result of such shortcomings is imbalanced and inappropriate assessment, a concern expressed by several respondents in the survey, and one of the most worrying consequences of this is the potential for flawed risk assessments. Probation officers, anxious not to label inappropriately or discriminate, may easily underestimate an offender's dangerousness in their eagerness to avoid stereotyping and reluctance to increase distress. Yet, if they are paralysed by fear of being racist or discriminatory, this in itself leads to discrimination which neither helps the offender nor protects the public. The Christopher Clunis case is a particularly high profile example of how the desire to prevent stigmatisation of a black person may have contributed to the underestimation of his dangerousness and the tragedy that subsequently occurred (Ritchie *et al.*, 1994, para. 9.3.3).

The reputation of training courses in actually promoting – as opposed to merely stating a commitment to – general anti-racist practice has not been particularly good. Dominelli *et al.* (1995, pp. 58–62) refer to several studies carried out between 1988 and 1991 which paint a picture of poor anti-racist content in training courses. One of those studies, by Davies and Wright (1989), reported that 61 per cent of their respondents considered "race awareness to be minor or marginal on their courses", with 13 per cent saying it was altogether absent. It is not surprising then that Denney's research led him to conclude that probation officers writing PSRs on black people often "combine familiar conventional accounts based on such factors as traumatic family background and alcohol dependence with less familiar and unconventional explanations like 'anti-authoritarianism' and 'irresponsibility'" (1992; quoted from Denney, 1996, p. 62) – explanations which clearly portray the offender as being more intractable and culpable. In a brief review of anti-discriminatory practice and anti-racism in the Probation Service, Jeffers refers to the dangers of "reducing black people's experience to solely their experience of racism or of transforming anti-racism into a de-politicised bureaucratic exercise . . ." (1995, p. 7). The fact that even "bureaucratic exercises" such as ethnic monitoring appear to have been haphazardly conducted by probation officers (RDA, 1994; Jeffers, 1995; Home Office, 1997) suggests that, in spite of a relatively high level of organisational commitment to anti-discriminatory practice, it has not made the transition from an attractive theory to a legitimate and important part of probation officers' daily practice.

The Central Council for Education and Training in Social Work (CCETSW), which was, until very recently, responsible for probation officer training, made anti-racist training and practice a requirement for would-be probation officers who wished to attain their Diploma in Social Work (CCETSW, 1991). However, the opposition to this move from politicians, the media and from within the CCETSW itself was tremendous, the main objection being that CCETSW was overstating the need for a strong anti-racist perspective and consequently "alienating" people through its "extremism" (Denney, 1996; Dominelli *et al.*, 1995). A telling indication of the former Conservative government's attitude towards the Probation Service's ethos was the Dews Report into probation officer training, a document widely condemned as one of the most appalling and clearly politically driven reports ever to be produced by the Home Office. A central, clearly racist and sexist "criticism" was that the Service had too many black and female entrants, portraying this as a reflection of in-appropriate political correctness rather than a successful recruitment policy (Dews and Watts, 1995). The signs are that the current Labour govern-ment's approach to the Service is more rational and sympathetic, but it is too early to offer a considered opinion.

Probation Commitment to Working with MDOs

In London and other areas, a great deal of excellent, innovative work is being done with MDOs. However, such work appears in many cases to rely on a small number of committed officers. Smith goes as far as to argue that since the Mental Health Act 1983 placed primary responsibility for dealing with mentally ill people onto the social services, many probation services appear "almost, it seems, with a sigh of relief" to have decided that it is legitimate to pass virtually all of the responsibility for working with MDOs who have "serious" mental illnesses such as the schizophrenias to other services (1993, p. 119). The combination of a lack of confidence with the perception that psychiatric support is inadequate appears to be the main reason that probation practitioners may avoid responsibility for MDO work. A frequent complaint is that officers are left unsupported in their work with those offenders who are given the label of "personality disorder" by psychiatrists. While recognising that the notion of "treatability" is a legitimate criterion for any substantial psychiatric involvement, probation officers seem to retain an enduring suspicion that, as Davis puts it, the "subjectivity and ambiguity which surrounds the diagnosis of personality disorder . . . enables medical professionals to exclude disliked, problematic patients . . . " (1990, p. 41). She goes on to argue that "in all but the most serious and acute cases, psychiatrists prefer to offer medical assistance on a voluntary basis thereby enabling a 'therapeutic relationship' with the patient" (Davis, 1990, p. 58). In practice this means absolutely nothing for the many MDOs who do not have the motivation to attend psychiatric appointments, leaving the probation officer to manage the case alone.

While the evidence for the effectiveness of psychiatric conditions attached to court orders is inconclusive (Stone, 1995, p. 85), one of the most telling results of Hudson *et al.*'s research was the high correlation between reports of formal psychiatric advice arrangements, which meant that probation officers did not feel isolated in their attempts to work with MDOs, and good ratings of probation/psychiatric relationships (1993, p. 26). In any event, probation officers should not consider that they do not have the skills or moral/professional responsibility to work with such clients. Indeed, they should be taking the opportunity to tackle seemingly intractable offenders from the perspective that their training gives them, not only because it is the most conscientious and professional approach, but also because they cannot avoid having such people on their caseloads. The following case study illustrates what committed probation work can achieve with personality disordered offenders.

MS is a black man in his early twenties with a diagnosis of personality disorder. He appeared to his white male probation officer to fit almost every conceivable negative and racist stereotype of young black men, being a drug-user, seemingly alienated from society, aggressive and sexually intimidating. Other agencies had withdrawn their assistance as a result of MS's behaviour and a lack of progress. It was with some difficulty that the probation officer had persuaded the courts to allow him the chance to work with MS and a large part of his early involvement with this man consisted of negotiations with sentencers, who were generally minded to imprison him for short periods. Although MS was not considered to be treatable by assessing psychiatrists, the officer sought psychiatric opinion on a number of occasions, if only to give him the chance to discuss his concerns and to reflect on his method of working. He was often uncertain about exactly what he was achieving and admits that he considered applying for revocation of MS's several concurrent probation orders as his behaviour did not appear to be improving. However, against expectations, MS became one of the officer's most reliable attenders and over a period of five years he established a stable, trusting and frank relationship with the officer who relentlessly and firmly challenged his behaviour, without ever rejecting involvement with him.

A vital function of the probation officer in this case, the importance of which is often underestimated, was "holding" MS by providing support and contact at times of crisis which was in excess of that made available by other services. Eventually, MS was able to talk about his tragic past, characterised by familial instability, bereavement and isolation, and, once more contrary to expectations, his offending reduced in frequency and in seriousness and his general behaviour improved. The probation officer had put into practice principles which Prins considers to encapsulate all work with apparently intractable personality disordered offenders, namely *"consistence, persistence and insistence"* (1986, p. 161). Unlike those cases where the personality disordered offender is offered no opportunity for probation involvement, almost everything that could have been done, to address both the risks posed and the distress MS was experiencing, was done. It is, of course, only by offering positive treatment and action packages in court reports that probation officers can prevent the imprisonment of such offenders – often for short periods which would not lead to a period of licence supervision – without any of the criminogenic factors they present being tackled effectively.

While probation practitioners commonly complain that ignorance of their role amongst other agencies leads to exclusion from case conferences and a failure to consult them about care plans, there is as yet little widespread ownership of the role which they themselves could play. Probation officers harm their cause by continuing to perceive themselves as outsiders in a process that should be a routine part of their own practice. For instance, the institution, or lack of it, of the CPA should be part of every officer's checklist when s/he begins supervision of an MDO. It represents a great opportunity for probation officers to obtain as well as give advice on risk assessment and most effective practice, to build the all-important inter-agency links which every major mental health inquiry has identified as crucial, and to hold other agencies to account for provision of services, particularly to the so-called "untreatable" MDOs with personality disorders.

The Probation Service Role in Multi-agency Working

Although the Probation Service role in the multi-agency context is a major theme of this chapter, the following points need to be highlighted. The Reed Report (DoH and HO, 1992), Home Office circular 66/90 and most recently Home Office circular 12/95 have all emphasised the Probation Service's role in facilitating effective inter-agency work. While multi-agency communication has greatly improved in recent years, much has yet to be done to actualise the role envisaged for the Probation Service. Despite evidence of otherwise positive developments in all of the study areas, a recently published report on the development of multi-agency working in the provision of services for MDOs (SSI, 1996) concludes that the omission of probation staff "in strategic or locality planning" is a common problem (p. 16) and that in some cases the "criminal justice dimension [is] excluded or underdeveloped" (p. iv). Interestingly, practitioners from different agencies expressed concern about risk assessment and management (p. 23), areas in which the Probation Service has considerable but obviously unexploited experience and expertise. In a number of the London boroughs, ILPS, with varying success, has taken a lead in organising multi-agency meetings both at a management and, to a lesser extent, practitioner level. However, the lack of practitioner involvement in *existing* local non-MDO forums remains a major problem. One of the probation officer's main roles should surely be to offer a Probation Service perspective and to bring into the consciousness of other agencies the criminogenic and other needs of MDOs by being an effective presence on such bodies.

Diversion and Hostels

In spite of concerted attempts by probation and bail hostel management to encourage referrals on high-risk offenders, there is a widespread suspicion amongst referring probation officers that hostels are reluctant to accept MDOs. The authors of the Revolving Doors Agency (1994) report on psychiatric bail hostel provision certainly gained the impression that the often "stressful environment" in probation and bail hostels was not considered to be suitable for vulnerable people (p. 26). A commonly heard theory amongst field probation officers is that prejudices associated with mental disorder lead both court officers and hostel workers to exaggerate the importance of past violent and dangerous offences, which may actually be no worse than those committed by other offenders. This clearly has implications for black MDOs who are in any case more likely to be considered dangerous (Browne, 1995, pp. 70–71). A central message of the Revolving Doors Agency report was that existing bail hostels need to develop closer links with psychiatric support services so that courts will have greater confidence in bailing MDOs and hostel staff will have more confidence in accepting referrals. During the last three years at least two London hostels have indeed developed formal links with psychiatric services and *ad hoc* arrangements exist with others. However, MDOs remain as difficult as ever to place and there is still no clear understanding of why this is so. Meanwhile, bail information probation officers reported in 1994 that they were less confident of assessing people as having a mental health problem than they were of identifying an alcohol or drug problem. This can clearly lead to the former being obscured (Browne, 1995, p. 20) and again demands a greater emphasis on training.

The Way Forward

Probation Officers' Training

In spite of Home Office and Department of Health urgings (e.g. HO and DoH, 1995), there is as yet no common anti-discriminatory practice and little sign of a common policy for MDOs amongst agencies. A co-ordinated approach to training, in which each agency is given the opportunity to become familiar with the workings of others, can clearly help to break down destructive professional barriers and tackle the potential discrimination that may arise in the treatment of MDOs. As Fernando puts it, "a common frame of reference, at least on basic issues, must evolve (or be created) and for this to happen a common text is essential" (Fernando, 1995, p. 3).

The Probation Service's pivotal role in the management of MDOs, high stated commitment to anti-discriminatory practice and experience in risk assessment – identified as a training priority in a number of areas (SSI, 1996, p. v) – suggests that it is perhaps the best placed agency to take a lead role in the co-ordination of joint training and policy, something that has not yet occurred on a wide scale. One reason for this may be the negative attitude of staff in other criminal justice agencies to the Probation Service's stance on anti-discriminatory issues; probation officers responding to one wide-scale survey considered them to be unhelpful and disinterested (Holdaway and Allaker, 1990). This is perhaps a reflection of a general lack of ground level commitment, certainly in the criminal justice system.

Where the Service itself has been lacking in imagination and commitment, two important explanatory factors (but not excuses) might be cited: first, there has been an unprecedented proliferation of criminal justice legislation during the 1990s, which has generally swallowed probation training resources. Second, and more fundamentally, the Probation Service has been understandably preoccupied with preserving its own identity and training base in the wake of government attacks. In 1996 the Conservative Home Secretary removed the requirement of the two-year full-time university Diploma in Social Work for probation officers despite enormous opposition from all areas of the criminal justice system. Although at the time of writing no replacement system has been implemented, it was with some relief that probation officers received the current Home Secretary's announcement that future probation officers would be required to complete a professional diploma located in higher education (House of Commons announcement, 29.7.97).

One of the positive outcomes of the removal of the old arrangements is that it represents a great opportunity to make long-needed improvements in mental health training, provided the profession is both allowed to and has the will to take it. There is a pressing need for courses not only to provide training that relates specifically to the issues faced by minority ethnic MDOs, but also for student probation officers to gain experience of specialist areas of practice. Hudson *et al.*, for example, recommended that all trainee probation officers be required to "spend at least a short and preferably a long placement in a forensic mental health setting" (1993, p. 45), thus ensuring a degree of pre-qualifying experience which would probably surpass that of most experienced probation officers currently practising.

Policy and Partnerships

One of the ways in which minority ethnic MDOs' voices can be more clearly heard in the Probation Service is through both formal and informal partnerships with relevant organisations. It is important that this is explicitly a two-way deal. Probation services cannot expect to take the benefits offered by such agencies in helping to reduce reoffending, without giving far greater attention to their campaigning role. Broad (1991) talks of the profound disappointment of voluntary organisations at the time of the inner-city riots of the early 1980s, at the Probation Service's silence about important issues such as poverty and discrimination. The increasing pull which the Probation Service is experiencing towards being an integrated criminal justice agency, illustrated by the punitive thrust of recent probation policy and the loss of the social work basis of probation training, may well undermine the Service's commitment to confronting the social disadvantage, oppression and victimisation which many of its clients themselves experience. Community partnerships can provide a valuable balance and increase the responsiveness of the Service to local communities.

Although this chapter has focused on the difficulties experienced by African-Caribbean MDOs, who are most obviously discriminated against, it is important to acknowledge the needs of other minority ethnic MDOs. Irish people, for example, experience substantial discrimination and hardship, and probation services need similarly to involve their community organisations in the local policy-making process. Partnerships should, in short, be seen as integral to the development of sensitive and inclusive probation MDO policy.

The ILPS partnership plan and the strategy document on black offenders recognises the value of developing such links, and ILPS assists smaller initiatives to survive and develop by offering organisational support, financial know-how and in some cases limited funding. However, the specialist mental health partnership resources for black people which have existed in ILPS have suffered from a shortage of referrals. This appears to be because of limited awareness and acknowledgement of their value amongst probation officers, a problem which to some extent can be tackled by local managers, who should explicitly encourage appropriate referrals and take a lead in supporting MDO initiatives in their areas.

Competent and knowledgeable local supervisors can be tremendously important in encouraging greater practitioner confidence in working with mentally disordered clients, who are, of course, particularly likely to evoke high amounts of stress and negative emotion. However, local managers in turn depend on a clear vision from the centre. While in a large and diverse probation area such as Inner London, there must obviously be some flexibility in the creation and implementation of local strategies, the commonly heard argument, that the existence of diversity and the need to respect local autonomy means that it would be pointless to "impose" a London-wide policy, seems to miss the point. Certainly, there is a limit to what can be done from the centre, but this does not justify a lack of *purpose* and *expectation* emanating from the centre.

The ILPS Policy Statement on MDOs and the Black Offender Strategy are in many respects admirable documents, but it is noticeable that neither makes substantial reference to the needs of minority ethnic MDOs. A more extensive and focused statement of intent is needed in all areas. Greater engagement of probation officers in the multi-agency environment would increase the Probation Service's profile and should lead to a greater appreciation of the probation perspective. This in turn is likely to help probation management to make its influence felt more keenly in joint commissioning arrangements; realistically, it is only through joint funding that smaller organisations, such as those that provide services for minority ethnic MDOs, will survive.

The Case for MDO Specialisms in Probation

Many of the major problems described above could be alleviated through the wider development of "special responsibility MDO posts" within the Probation Service. In the context of the modern and rapidly changing multi-agency environment, effective work (and by implication anti-discriminatory practice) can only be facilitated through officers having the time and the encouragement to develop a sophisticated awareness of their potential role and that of the health and social services. The oft-heard argument, that specialisms encourage abdication of responsibility by the majority of officers for working creatively with demanding client groups, does not acknowledge the crucial point that without them probation practice has in any case been inconsistent. While the specific model to be applied would vary according to local conditions, it is necessary for at least one probation officer in each area to take a lead role in the development of practice. In some localities this may result in the creation of semi-specialist caseworker posts; these are, for example, evolving in Lambeth, a London borough with higher than average numbers of black MDOs subject to compulsory detention in hospital and to section 41 MHA restrictions.

A model of practice which may suit many other areas is the "focus group" model which has been successful in the borough of Hackney. In Hammersmith and Fulham the model being developed focuses on the functions and needs of probation practitioners. An officer with special responsibility for MDO work co-ordinates a working group consisting of probation officer representatives from each of the four borough teams, a probation manager and the mental health partnership workers. Although other agencies are invited to meetings and kept informed of the Probation Service's activities, the group convenes regardless of their attendance. This "two-tier" approach, with the emphasis on the development of probation practice, means that a lack of commitment from other agencies will not undermine the essential purpose of the group. Members discuss specific cases, the main issues with regard to MDO work in the borough and the degree of progress that has been made in meeting policy objectives. Each member of the group feeds back to individual teams while the co-ordinator carries out the functions of the lead worker or semi-specialist as described below. In accordance with the lessons of some major reports (e.g. Woodley, 1995), one of the permanent agenda items for each meeting is anti-discriminatory practice, the different understandings of this concept within agencies and the responsiveness of probation officers and others to local needs. It is too soon objectively to evaluate the success of this initiative, but it promises to enhance the standard of MDO work in ILPS.

The main benefits of MDO lead workers or semi-specialists within the Probation Service can be summarised as follows:

- Greater knowledge and experience, leading to more *balanced and confident* assessment and supervisory practice. For example, the fact that conditionally discharged patients are very few in number means that without a specialist system it is unlikely that a probation officer could develop much experience in working with offenders who are liable to be among the most demanding of all clients.

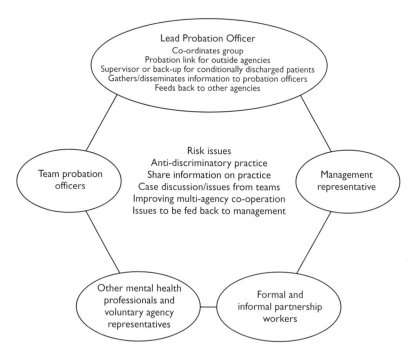

Figure 7.2   Hammersmith and Fulham Mentally Disordered Offender Practitioner Forum.

- An enhanced awareness of research and the major debates with regard to MDOs which would increase the worker's ability to identify gaps in competence. For example, it is only if a probation officer appreciates the competing explanations of why black people are overrepresented in the system that s/he will be better able to minimise unintentional discrimination and provide a higher quality service.
- Improved inter-agency communication. The existence of a named link officer facilitates a more personal relationship which is likely to encourage and enhance professional co-operation and allow a sharing of knowledge and experience. Other professionals should be able to call upon the lead worker's advice whether or not the MDO in question is a current probation client. S/he would also be a more effective presence at local multi-agency practitioner meetings, generating greater awareness of the probation role and the principles of anti-discriminatory practice underpinning probation policy.
- Greater experience and the support of other probation officers in similar posts should have the effect of increasing the individual officer's ability to cope with the stress of working with offenders who often present very complex needs and are more likely to pose a high risk of harm to themselves or others. It should also help to counter the kind of over-reaction which black MDOs in particular might excite.
- The provision of an office resource, advising and assisting other staff, leading to higher quality reports and improved supervisory practice across the board. This would also raise the awareness and use of local resources amongst other probation officers.
- An enhanced reputation amongst sentencers of probation officers' skills in working with MDOs, a logical consequence of which would be more community orders being imposed, better use of psychiatric treatment conditions and more appropriate use of Mental Health Act powers by courts properly informed by probation reports.
- Lead workers and/or focus groups provide a pool of informed probation officers who can be consulted by management about practice issues and give advice on the need for specific resources.

Conclusion

Black and other minority ethnic MDOs face additional discrimination because of their ethnicity and/or colour in a system which scarcely delivers justice for white English MDOs. They start from a position of double disadvantage and are particularly in need of the kind of improvements in policy and practice suggested above. There is no doubt that, albeit slowly, a culture of co-operation in the field of MDO work is evolving. Probation officers have an opportunity to be central to that work and in some areas specialist posts are already well established. More sophisticated models which can facilitate the translation of theory into practice will only develop with committed managerial level action and, crucially, practitioner involvement sanctioned and encouraged by management. No amount of training will help if probation officers are not given the opportunities to put what they have learned into practice. The principles of anti-discriminatory practice must be central to any strategy, not only because this is the most just way to proceed, but also because a model of practice that recognises difference and promotes equality is far more likely to be effective in achieving its ends.

Acknowledgements

Thanks are due to Gwyneth Boswell, Liz Dixon, Tony Hearne, Herschel Prins, Stephen Parvez Rashid and, in particular, Angus Cameron, for their invaluable advice.

References

Belfrage, H. and Lidberg, L. (1996) Forensic psychiatric assessments in practice: a blind study of different forensic psychiatrists' assessments of the same cases. *Criminal Behaviour and Mental Health* **6**(4): 331–337.

Blumenthal, S. and Wessely, S. (1992) The extent of local arrangements for the diversion of the mentally abnormal offender from custody. Unpublished report quoted in Hudson *et al.* (1993) *Training for Work with Mentally Disordered Offenders*. London: Central Council for Education and Training in Social Work.

Broad, B. (1991) *Punishment Under Pressure: The Probation Service in the Inner City*. London: Jessica Kingsley.

Browne, D. (1995) Sectioning: the black experience. In: Fernando, S. (ed.) *Mental Health in a Multi-ethnic Society*. London: Routledge.

Buchanan, J. and Millar, M. (1995) Probation: reclaiming a social work identity. *Probation Journal* **44**(1): 32–36.

CCETSW (1991) *Requirements for the Diploma in Social Work, Paper 30*. London: Central Council for Education and Training in Social Work.

Davies, M. and Wright, A. (1989) *The Changing Face of Probation*. Norwich: University of East Anglia Social Work Monographs.

Davis, J.L. (1990) *Personality Disorder: A Suitable Case for Probation?* University of West London: Brunel Socio-Legal Working Papers.

Denney, D. (1992) *Racism and Anti-Racism in Probation*. London: Routledge.

Denney, D. (1996) Discrimination and anti-discrimination in probation. In: May, T. and Vass, A. (eds) *Working With Offenders: Issues, Contexts and Outcomes*. London: Sage Publications.

Department of Health and Home Office (1992) *(The Reed Report) Review of Health and Social Services for Mentally Disordered Offenders and Others Requiring Similar Services*, Final Summary Report, Cmnd 2088. London: HMSO.

Dews, V. and Watts, J. (1995) *Review of Probation Officer Recruitment and Qualifying Training*. London: The Stationery Office Ltd.

Dominelli, L., Jeffers, L., Jones, G., Sibanda, S. and Williams, B. (1995) *Anti-racist Probation Practice*. Aldershot: Arena.

Fernando, S. (1991) *Mental Health, Race and Culture*. London: Macmillan/MIND.

Fernando, S. (1995) *Mental Health in a Multi-Ethnic Society – A Multi-Disciplinary Handbook*. London: Routledge.

Gunn, J., Madden, J. and Swinton, M. (1991) *Mentally Disordered Prisoners*, Report to the Home Office. London: HMSO.

Haynes, P. and Henfrey, B. (1995) Making a reality of Reed? *Probation Journal* **42**(2): 83–87.

HM Inspectorate of Probation (1993) *Probation Orders With Requirements for Psychiatric Treatment*. London: HMSO

Holdaway, S. and Allaker, J. (1990) *Race Issues in the Probation Service: A Review of Policy*. London: Association of Chief Officers of Probation.

Home Office (1990) *Provision for Mentally Disordered Offenders*, Home Office Circular No. 66/90. London: HMSO.

Home Office (1992) *Partnership in Dealing with Offenders in the Community*. London: HMSO.

Home Office (1995) *Mentally Disordered Offenders: Inter Agency Working*, Home Office Circular 12/95. London: HMSO.

Home Office (1997) *Probation Statistics for England and Wales, 1996*. London: HMSO.

Home Office and Department of Health (1995) *Mentally Disordered Offenders: Inter Agency Working*. London: Home Office.

Hudson, B., Cullen, R. and Roberts, C. (1993) *Training for Work with Mentally Disordered Offenders: Report of a Study of the Training Needs of Probation Officers and Social Workers*. London: CCETSW.

ILPS (1995) *Partnership Plan*. London: Inner London Probation Service.

ILPS (1997) *Professional Guidance on Work with Mentally Disordered Offenders*. London: Inner London Probation Service.

Jeffers, S. (1995) *Black and Ethnic Minority Offenders' Experience of the Probation Service*. London: Inner London Probation Service.

Littlewood, R. and Lipsedge, M. (1997) *Aliens and Alienists: Ethnic Minorities and Psychiatry*, 3rd edn. London: Routledge.

Oldfield, M. (1997) What worked? A five year study of reconvictions amongst probationers. *Probation Journal* **44**(1): 2–10.

Pringle, N.N. and Thompson, P.J. (1986) *Social Work, Psychiatry and the Law*. London: Heinemann Medical.

Prins, H. (1986) *Dangerous Behaviour: The Law and Mental Disorder*. London: Tavistock.

Pritchard, C. *et al.* (1992) Mental illness, drug and alcohol abuse and HIV risk behaviour in 214 young adult probation clients. *Social Work and Social Sciences Review* **3**(3): 227–242.

RDA (1994) *The Need for Psychiatric Bail Provision in Inner London*. A Report to the Inner London Probation Service. London: Revolving Doors Agency.

Ritchie, J.H., Dick, D. and Lingham, R. (1994) *The Report of the Inquiry into the Care and Treatment of Christopher Clunis*. London: HMSO.

Smith, G.W. (1993) A view from the Probation Service. In: Watson, W. and Grounds, A. (eds) *The Mentally Disordered Offender in an Era of Community Care: New Directions in Provision*. Cambridge: Cambridge University Press.

SSI (1996) *Mentally Disordered Offenders: Improving Services*. London: Social Services Inspectorate/Department of Health.

Stone, N. (1995) *A Companion Guide to Mentally Disordered Offenders*. Ilkley: Owen Wells.

Vaughan, P.J. and Badger, D. (1995) *Working with the Mentally Disordered Offender in the Community*. London: Chapman and Hall.

Wickham, T. (1994) *A Psychiatric Liaison Service for the Criminal Courts*. Norwich: University of East Anglia Social Work Monographs.

Woodley, L. (1995) *Report to the Independent Review Panel to East London and The City Health Authority and Newham Council*. London: East London and the City Health Authority.

8

Cultural Competence and the Law of Mental Health

Satvinder S. Juss

Introduction

Lawyers in Britain have much to answer for regarding the benign neglect of the rights of mentally disordered people. The American "legal rights movement" of the 1960s and 1970s which ran contemporaneously with anti-psychiatry and de-institutionalisation movements appears to have passed Britain by. As a result, "despite the much-vaunted concern of the common lawyer for individual freedom, lawyers in this country played little part in all this ferment" (Hoggett, 1990, p. 3). This neglect has meant not only a failure by lawyers in Britain to protect the basic rights of mentally disordered persons but has also meant a failure by them to assist in the establishment of a comprehensive framework of mental health legislation. The Mental Health Act 1983 stands as a paradigm example of this failure. In 1993, the Mental Health Act Commission, set up under the Act of 1983, called for a comprehensive review of the Act (see Mental Health Act Commission, 1993). The House of Commons Select Committee on Health has described the Act as "obsolescent though far from obsolete" (Health Committee, 1993, para 87). Even at the time of its passage, one commentator (now a High Court Judge) wondered whether anyone would actually gain from the provisions of the 1983 Act (Hoggett, 1983). Another High Court Judge has recently written that "apart from a weak obligation on the Health and Social Services Authorities to provide 'after-care' for patients discharged from long-term detention . . . there was nothing in the legislation to develop the rights of patients to receive services in the community, or to encourage a genuine community concern for the mentally afflicted. Now that since 1991 we have been pitchforked into care in the community, where is the legislative response to the protection of incapacitated and vulnerable people living in the community?" In his view, "the 1983 Act is not just out of date and out of step with the times; it presents entirely the wrong image to practitioners in the mental health system. Any legislation in this field must, of course, provide for safeguarding the rights of patients detained for treatment for psychotic disorders. But if the shift of care and treatment from hospital to community is to be a reality, the legal framework must reflect the primacy of rights and duties of community care, with infringements of liberty taking on a supportive, hospitalising role. Society's values relating to mental health cannot go legislatively unacknowledged" (Blom-Cooper QC, 1996). These cumulative failures have a direct impact on the rights of mentally disordered persons from ethnic minority and culturally diverse backgrounds.

Let us first consider the operation of the 1983 Act itself. There is a cultural gap here between consumers and providers which leads to a misdiagnosis of consumers by providers. The blame for misdiagnosis rests heavily on cultural insensitivity. Unlike other fields of medicine, where diagnosis may be dependent on aetiology or malfunction, psychiatry relies on symptoms and signs. This cultural distance between the therapist and the patient has been accepted as "a major drawback" because "symptoms and behaviours may be culturally related and thus differ from one ethnic group to another" (Jones and Gray, 1986). Consequently, the compulsory admission of African-Caribbeans under section 2 or section 3 of the Mental Health Act 1983 into the Mental Health Services is far greater than for the general population. It has been found that while, during the 1980s, fewer than 10 per cent of all admissions were compulsory, for African-Caribbeans the figure lies between 20 and 30 per cent (Cope, 1989). These disparities are evident also in the use of section 136 of the Act where the police have specific powers to detain persons for up to 72 hours in a "place of safety" should they be regarded as a danger to themselves or to others. Once again studies indicate that African-Caribbeans are particularly likely to be detained under this section (Littlewood and Lipsedge, 1989). Young African-Caribbean males, between the ages of 16 and 30 years, are up to seventeen times more likely than white males to be compulsorily admitted (Cope, 1989). Another recent study has found that, for African-Caribbeans, "nearly half of all admissions were compulsory, compared with only one fifth for whites" (Bebbington *et al.*, 1994, p. 747). In addition, whereas African-Caribbean males are considered to be susceptible to schizophrenia, although this has been strongly contested (Fernando, 1988, pp. 138, 140), other patients, particularly women, are considered to suffer more from depression and suicidal tendencies (a newspaper article went so far as to speak in terms of a "suicide epidemic among young Asian women": *Observer*, 29 August 1993). Studies show that a popular representation of people in a particular manner influences diagnosis (Hellman, 1990, p. 225).

Let us next take the movement towards de-institutionalisation and the concept of care in the community. As we have seen, the Mental Health Act 1983 does not cater for these developments and an appropriate legislative response is still awaited. However, the high rates of compulsory admissions that we have referred to above surely point to the conclusion that black people on the whole are not accessing Mental Health Services through "voluntary" admissions. They are not using the process of referral from a GP to a psychiatrist or another mental team. Indeed, there is no evidence that Asian people are any more prone to using the services at primary health care level. Before any legislative initiative is taken on board the rate of utilisation of existing services must be thoughtfully considered. It is here that lawyers and advocacy groups have an important role to play in Britain as they have done in the United States. Lawyers in the United States have used the "legal rights movement" to oppose the interests of psychiatry and of medical paternalists. They have opposed medical autonomy and applied the perspective of a modestly egalitarian social contract. Under this, society as a whole, including patients, physicians and other providers, has legitimate rights and interests in the health care system. The role of the law is seen as a device to achieve a fair resolution of those interests in the face of often highly unequal relationships. A major component of this approach is the realisation that fair individual relationships are often not possible between unequally situated parties so that the law must enforce a "social contract" to achieve equitable relationships (Law *et al.*, 1997). This directly challenges the principle of medical autonomy and lawyers have a public duty, where it is appropriate, to make this challenge. One such area is the psychiatric profession's persistent "clinging to outmoded theories and practices" (Kleinman and Cohen, 1997). Recently, researchers at the Harvard Medical School have argued for a better understanding of the links between culture and mental disorders, as a way of reaching fairer and more equitable results. Kleinman and Cohen (1997) point to the persistence of myths in psychiatry:

> The first is that the forms of mental illness everywhere display similar degrees of prevalence. Myth number two can be described as an excessive adherence to a principle known as the pathogenetic/pathoplastic dichotomy, which holds that biology is responsible for the underlying structure of a malaise, whereas cultural beliefs shape the specific ways in which a person experiences it. The third myth maintains that various unusual, culture-specific disorders whose biological bases are uncertain occur only in exotic places outside the west. The fourth, held by many international health experts who discount mental health problems to begin with, holds that not much can be done to treat mental illness.

Certainly, cultural distance is proven to be largely responsible for problems of miscommunication, misdiagnosis and mistreatment of persons from diverse minority cultural and ethnic backgrounds. But is the answer to increase the number of minority social workers, psychologists, psychiatrists, mental health service administrators and advocates in the health system? Whereas non-minority providers may be culturally sensitive, there is evidence to suggest that they cannot replace the direct perspective of providers who are themselves members of the same minorities in every case (Williams *et al.*, 1978) and in some cases only a minority provider can establish the trust necessary for effective health care (Terrell and Terrell, 1984). However, it is a mistake to assume that a minority provider will always be effective. To allow only black staff to "care for their own" not only denies black consumers access to all sectors of the mental health profession (Carter, 1982) but there is evidence to suggest that middle class black psychiatrists do misdiagnose low income patients even where they come from the same racial or ethnic background (Mukherjee *et al.*, 1983; Grevious, 1985).

What is required, therefore, is a programme of culturally appropriate services at the heart of the health care system. Culturally appropriate service means recognising race and culture as a factor, while still treating the consumer as an individual (Rosen and Frank, 1962; Rogler *et al.*, 1987). The recognition and servicing of cultural attributes in the health care system will create a corresponding cultural imperative in legal rights protection and advocacy for lawyers. At present, little work has been done to define the advocacy issues or to develop strategies for resolving problems of culture. This chapter concentrates on the main advocacy issues for lawyers. These advocacy issues are not, on the whole, any different for lawyers than for other professionals. Nevertheless, they are worth outlining. The very same cultural distance exists between low income minority mental health consumers and predominantly white middle class lawyers, as exists between these consumers and medical health providers, thus creating barriers to appropriate protection and advocacy. The legal system is as intimidating as is the psychiatric world to most minority health consumers. As a result, the very concept of patients' rights is simply unknown to people from diverse ethnic minority backgrounds.

Culturally Competent Mental Health Care

How is it Achieved?

Culturally competent mental health care policies are brought into focus by considering the following six questions to which particular thought has been given in the United States.

1. How and by whom is mental health and illness defined?

The definitions of mental health and illness are critical in the proper development of services for ethnic minority populations. Lawyers should ensure that psychiatrists properly substantiate their medical opinions and not merely reach medical conclusions so that their psychiatric diagnostic and predictive skills are fully scrutinized to ensure that cultural aspects are not ignored. The approach does not have to be combative. Ideally, it should be collaborative. But this does not mean that a patient-centred, rights-driven, and culturally competent approach should be sacrificed. At present, the diagnostic classification scheme uses traditional Western definitions focusing on inherent personality, genetic or biological differences within the individual. Lawyers advocating on their client's behalf can couch their arguments in cultural, rather than medical, terms. Few diagnostic classifications addresses the impact of race, ethnicity or culture on the manifestation of symptoms and behaviours. Yet, the definition of mental health for ethnic minorities may be broader because of the impact of discrimination, poor housing, poor education, poverty, lack of employment, and social isolation leading to increased psychological and emotional difficulties.

2. What are the factors used to address a mental health problem?

There is evidence to suggest that when traditional assessment instruments are used the normative differences between black and white respondents are large enough to result in a misdiagnosis of a significant proportion of black respondents as psychotic (Gynther, 1972). But traditional assessment instruments do not take into account questions of ethnic identity (Bernal *et al.*, 1990). Lefley has concluded that "there is considerable evidence that, lacking normative data on non-psychiatric community populations, the scores of non-white, non-English speaking patients on diagnostic screening instruments may be of dubious validity, and in some cases, seriously mis-leading" (Lefley, 1986, p. 12). Assessment instruments should take into account the level of acculturation and assimilation; the migration experi-ence; the language spoken in the home; race and country of origin; family's place of residence; socio-economic status, educational achievement, and upward mobility of family members; the emotional process in the family; the political and religious ties to the ethnic group; the family lifecycle; value orientations; and strengths and positive coping strategies (McGoldrick *et al.*, 1982). Lawyers know only too well themselves that nothing is more vague, elastic and indeterminate than the concept of "dangerousness" in mental health law. A failure to recognise the factors outlined above medi-cally only promotes avoidable litigation.

3. How are mental health services offered and made accessible to the ethnic minority population?

Ethnic minority groups under-utilise and prematurely terminate mental health services, yet little attention has been paid to the biased referral processes whereby ethnic minority groups have ended up in the correc-tional system rather than the mental health system. Similarly, little attention has been paid to the cultural factors that may play a role in under-utilisation or premature termination. The geographical location of the services, hours of operation, and community perception of the facility's function are important considerations for increasing access and use of mental health services by minority ethnic groups. More positive interac-tions between the community and the programme are required to increase access (Wong, 1980).

As a result of the Mental Health Act's failure to provide for patients in the community, and not just in hospitals, the Government has introduced a new statutory procedure for "supervised discharge", which came into effect in April 1996, but this does not fully address the cultural difficulties of minority groups that could militate against the proper utilisation of available services. Even before utilisation in the community, the whole question of conditional release needs to have the cultural dimension incor-porated into the legal decision-making process if the minority patient's interests are to be well served. We know, for example, from health care psychology that a patient's compliance with medical advice, to take regular medication for instance, will be greater if the patient gives a public com-mitment and family members are made aware of the terms of the release. Lawyers need to ensure that the cultural support mechanisms of extended family networks are woven into the legal release decision-making process.

4. What methods/interventions are chosen to alleviate and solve mental health problems?

The methods of interventions used to address mental health problems depend upon the understanding of their causes and consequences. Certain types of interventions are more effective with ethnic minority populations, such as recognition of an intervention in social problems, group therapy, family-focus therapies, in home services, crisis intervention and problem-solving services, case management and brokering services, didactic and educational approaches, community level interventions, and appreciation and recognition of cultural issues or problems (Szapocznik *et al.*, 1990). Let us consider for a moment the most serious scenario. When Mental Health Review Tribunals decide (under the MHA 1983, Part V) whether detained patients should be released from hospital or not, they may make recommendations so that the Parole Board can order the release of discretionary life-sentence prisoners. The patient may be discharged into the community from a hospital or a prison. This is a large step to contemplate. Yet, without a willingness to consider all the substantive factors of the case, and not just the procedure, the decision-making process does not lead to "high-quality" decisions.

The result is that the Parole Board does not make bold, forward-looking decisions where it needs to. A challenge in the Court of Appeal to the diffident approach of the discretionary lifers panel (in R v. Parole Board, ex parte Telling, unreported, Lexis, 6 May 1993) was rejected when the Court applied traditional medical assessment techniques to concepts of "dangerousness" and "reasonableness". Lawyers need to ensure, in conjunction with other mental health professionals, that the emphasis is on qualitative decision-making. This is an almost impossible test to verify objectively. An emphasis on quality decision-making, in collaboration with other professionals, can mean that both may be involved in the development and positive monitoring of risk-taking policies to facilitate early release. Thus, clinicians can use this opportunity incrementally to give more freedom and responsibility to patients. Lawyers can use the opportunity to analyse forensically whether an appropriate programme of risk-taking, which is avowedly designed to facilitate the patient's competence and eventual release, is being applied practically and meaningfully.

5. Who should administer/provide the intervention?

The issue of ethnic staffing for programmes and services is one of the most intensely controversial whenever cultural competence is discussed. Studies in the United States indicate that the higher the number of staff from the minority group, the higher the rate of utilisation of services by ethnic minority groups (Wu and Windle, 1980; Snowden *et al.*, 1989). The staffing dilemma has to do with problems with and the lack of creativity around identifying, recruiting and retaining minority professionals. Two approaches may be used to overcome these problems. One is to utilise paraprofessionals, who are unfortunately considered merely to be substitutes for culturally unskilled professional therapists and practitioners, but are rarely recognised as skilled and trained ethnic minority professionals in their own right.

Another way of resolving staff dilemmas is to train majority staff to understand and work more effectively with different ethnic minority populations, thereby making them a more culturally competent workforce. Such training should ideally be given during undergraduate or graduate studies but in-service courses can also be run. As Pedersen and Lefley (1986) observe, "adequately trained mental health professionals will have an awareness of their own cultural biases, knowledge about the research literature relating culture to mental health, and skills to implement the insights resulting from knowledge and awareness in a culturally appropriate format . . . The goal of cross-cultural training is to increase a counsellor's intentionality through increasing the person's purposive control over the assumptions which guide his or her behaviour, attitudes, and insights."

A very good example of current topicality is the present Law Commission's approach to the decision-making rights and powers of mentally incapable adults. Their capacity to make personal, ethical, ethnic, sexual, private, medical and financial decisions is approached by the Law Commission as a technical legal question only, with the aim being simply to develop a framework within which a consensus can be reached. However, the consensus is just a legal consensus. What it should really do is approach the matter as if the persons in question were not incapacitated, but incapable at present, with the aim being to teach them skills designed to enable them eventually to make those decisions. Cultural beliefs and attributes, which would be lost in a consensus-seeking legal framework, would now be protected and preserved. Only lawyers can bring these pressures to bear on the other professionals in this field.

6. What are the expected or anticipated outcomes?

The measuring of client outcomes and the effectiveness of treatment programmes has always been difficult in the field of mental health. There is little research here. However, there is some evidence to suggest that ethnic matching between clients and therapists leads to higher utilisation and length of stay in treatment than when clients are matched with ethnically dissimilar therapists (see Snowden *et al.*, 1989). There is also evidence to suggest that culturally tailored programmes are effective in reaching and engaging hard to reach ethnic minority populations (see Neighbors, 1990).

The basic problem is that the cultural values and orientation of ethnic minorities are different from those of mainstream British society. Table 8.1 identifies some of the differences in cultural values and orientations.

It can be seen from the discussion above that cultural competence is a set of congruent behaviours, attitudes and policies that come together in a system, agency, or among professionals and enable that system, agency or professionals to work effectively in cross-cultural situations. The word

Table 8.1 Comparison of common values.

Western cultures	Harmony with nature
Mastery over nature	Fate
Doing-activity	Being
Time dominates	Personal interaction dominates
Human equality	Hierarchy/rank/status
Individualism/privacy	Group welfare
Youth	Elders
Self-help	Birthright inheritance
Competition	Co-operation
Future orientation	Past or present orientation
Informality	Formality
Directness/openness/honesty	Indirectness/ritual/"face"
Practicality/efficiency	Idealism
Materialism	Spiritualism

"cross-culture" means an integrated pattern of human behaviour that includes thoughts, communications, actions, customs, beliefs, values and institutions of a racial, ethnic, religious or social group. The word "competence" implies having the capacity to function effectively. By following the above precepts lawyers can help to bring about a more culturally competent delivery of mental health care services. The relationship between lawyers and clinicians has always been antagonistic. Measures such as the ones outlined above can help all professionals seek synergies in what they do. The point about cultural competence in medical care (unlike medical competence) is that it advocates an interdisciplinary co-operation without requiring that either lawyers or clinicians give up their core competences. Lawyers undoubtedly benefit themselves very greatly in this because they will have a lens through which to look at their client's broader interests.

Becoming Culturally Competent

In order to understand fully where one is in the process of becoming culturally competent, one can imagine a continuum that ranges from cultural destructiveness to cultural proficiency. There are at least six different positions between these two extremes.

1. Cultural destructiveness

The most negative end of this continuum is represented by attitudes, policies and practices that are destructive to cultures (Hune, 1977) and consequently to individuals within that culture. The most extreme example of this is an immigration policy that has prohibited Asians from bringing in their spouses from the Indian subcontinent following the Immigration Act 1971 (Juss, 1997).

2. Cultural incapacity

The next position on the continuum is where a system or agency does not intend to be culturally destructive but rather lacks the capacity to help minority clients or communities. The system may disproportionately apply resources, discriminate against people of colour on the basis of whether they "know their place", and believe in the supremacy of the dominant culture helpers. The characteristics of cultural incapacity here include discriminatory hiring practices, subtle messages to people of colour that they are not valued or welcomed, and generally lower expectations of minority clients.

3. Cultural blindness

Halfway along the continuum, the system and its agencies provide services with the express philosophy of being unbiased. Culturally blind agencies are characterised by the belief that helping approaches traditionally used by the dominant culture are universally applicable. If the system worked as it should then all people, regardless of race or culture, would be served with equal effectiveness. This view is the product of a well-intentioned liberal philosophy. It results, however, in services becoming ethnocentric, and consequently virtually useless to all but the most assimilated minority people. A philosophy of cultural blindness ignores cultural strengths, encourages assimilation, and blames the victim for their problems.

4. Cultural pre-competence

A system or agency that moves towards the upper end of the scale is pre-competent because it realises its weaknesses in serving minorities and attempts to improve some aspect of its services to a specific population. Such agencies hire minority staff, explore how to reach minority people in their service area, initiate training for their workers on cultural sensitivity, enter into needs assessments concerning minority communities, and recruit minority individuals for their boards of directors or advisory committees. Pre-competent agencies respond to minority communities' cries for improved services by asking, "What can we do?". There are two dangers to avoid here, however. One is a feeling of a false sense of accomplishment or of failure that prevents the agency from moving forward along the continuum. The other is the danger of tokenism. An agency will usually hire one or more assimilated minority workers and feel that they are then equipped to meet the need. Since the minority professional is trained in the dominant society's frame of reference, such a professional may be little more competent in cross-cultural practice than his/her co-workers.

5. Cultural competence

Culturally competent agencies are characterised by acceptance and respect for difference, continuing self-assessment regarding culture, careful attention to the dynamics of difference, continuous expansion of cultural knowledge and resources, and a variety of adaptations to service models in order to meet the needs of minority populations better. Such agencies view minority groups as being distinctly different from one another and as having numerous subgroups, each with important cultural characteristics. Culturally competent agencies work to hire unbiased employees, seek advice and consultation from the minority community, and actively decide what they are and are not capable of providing to minority clients.

6. Cultural proficiency

The most positive end of the scale is advanced cultural competence or proficiency. A culturally proficient agency seeks to add to the knowledge base of culturally competent practice by conducting research, developing new therapeutic approaches based on culture, and publishing and disseminating the results of demonstration projects. Culturally proficient agencies hire staff who are specialists in culturally competent practice.

To summarise, a culturally competent system of care is made up of culturally competent institutions, agencies and professionals. Lawyers and the legal system have to become as culturally competent as clinicians and medicine must be. There are five essential elements which go to contributing to a system's, institution's or agency's ability to become more culturally competent. A culturally competent system has the following characteristics:

- It values diversity – because a system of care is strengthened when it accepts that the people it serves are from very different backgrounds and will make different choices based on culture.
- It has the capacity for self-assessment – because planners and administrators who understand that a system of care is shaped by culture, know that it must be able to assess itself and have a sense of its own culture.
- It is conscious of the dynamics inherent when cultures interact – because when a system of one culture interacts with a population from another, both may misjudge the other's actions based on learned expectations.
- It has institutionalised cultural knowledge – because the system of care must sanction and in some cases mandate the incorporation of cultural knowledge into the service delivery framework since every level of the system needs accurate information or access to it.
- It has developed adaptations to diversity – because adaptations allow for a better fit in the system's approach between the needs of minority groups and the services available.

Each of these five elements must function at every level of the system and the attitudes, policies and practices must be congruent within all levels of the system. The practice must be based on accurate perceptions of behaviour, policies must be impartial, and attitudes must be unbiased. Unbiased does not mean colour blind; unbiased means acceptance of the difference of another. In this way, all professionals, including lawyers, can become equipped to deal with minority clients from the mentally ill population.

Implementation of Policy

Finally, we need to say something about how these ideas can be implemented at a policy level. Systems do not start out by being culturally competent. Cultural competence is developed over time, through training, experience, guidance and self-evaluation just like any other type of competence. Attitudes have to be cultivated through training, modelling and experience. Policy evolves through research, goal setting and advocacy. Practice grows with information, training and the development of new alternatives. The system or agency has to develop and create cultural attributes at policy-making, administrative, practice and consumer levels. Let us consider each of these.

Policy-making level

The policy-makers may be board members of private agencies, public agency officials, legislators and commissioners, or Advisory Committee members. A number of actions must be undertaken at this level. First, there has to be community involvement (Higginbotham, 1984; VanDenberg and Minton, 1987). Minority community persons can be recruited and asked to serve on Boards, Advisory Committees and Commissions that already exist in the agency or system. Special task forces or advisory groups can be created using the representatives of minority communities to study and address issues of that particular community. Further, an agency might create an evaluation committee and submit its cross-cultural performance to minority community review. Policy-makers can set standards for cross-cultural services and an agency may develop standards that it expects its employees to follow. Planners should commit the resources to implement such policies (Zane *et al.*, 1982; Meinhardt and Vega, 1987). Policy-makers should use research findings to guide their decision-making. A decision-making structure in a system that is flexible and empowers less powerful segments of the community contributes to the minority voice being heard (McDiarmid, 1983). At the legislative level, policy can be integrated into existing laws and be formulated into new laws. Funding can be used as an incentive for developing cultural competence. Programmes at the policy level might take the form of a written mission statement and a comprehensive plan to develop culturally competent services (Hawkins and Salisbury, 1983). An agency or government department may enter into arrangements such as resource development and programme fostering. None of these ideas are new concepts and they are not the only possibilities. However, what is new is the idea that these actions can come together in an agency's policy-making body so that the agency becomes more competent to make policy for services to minority populations.

Administrative level

The administrative level of service delivery is made up of agency directors, managers, department heads, and a variety of other people in the organisation. It is this level that interprets and implements policy. This power can be used to move the organisation towards cultural competence. It is at the administrative level that the commitment to a culturally competent system of care must be embraced. The agency should have a form of self-assessment. This can only take place once the agency has determined the demographic makeup of its service area and defined the client population. It will then have some indication about directions for planning. Administrators will want to know whether their staff and governing board are representative of the population to be served. The agency can ensure that minority people are recruited and retained on the staff. The agency can include, in the interviewing process, questions about cultural differences and require work experience with minority populations before selection takes place. The agency or government department should provide training on minority issues and develop specific cultural knowledge. Training should occur in both workshop setting and on site in the community. Orientation to the minority clients's community should be mandatory. Rewards can also be built into the system for those who obtain additional training. The accessibility of services to minority communities (Owan, 1982; Flaskerud, 1986) can be improved through geographically locating services within the relevant communities in a place people frequent or recognise as a helping facility (e.g. schools, churches, temples, recreation centres, and their own homes). Clients should feel secure that they will not be rejected or punitively discharged because of their minority status. Artwork may be displayed within the facility to reflect the culture or cultures of the community. Administrative staff should have the capacity to develop new approaches or adjust existing ones so that the services fit the client rather than the client fit the service (Kumabe *et al.*, 1985). Where services are being contracted out, the government department can ensure that contractors or grantees meet certain cultural competence requirements.

Practitioner level

No cross-cultural practice can be competent unless there is a commitment from the worker to provide culturally competent services. Workers need to be aware of and to accept cultural differences. They need to be aware of their own cultural values and should have an understanding of the "dynamics of difference" in the helping process. There are at least five essential elements to becoming a culturally competent helping professional:

1. There must be an acceptance of cultural differences in the sense that each culture finds some behaviours, interactions or values more important than others.
2. There must be a purposeful self-examination of one's own cultural influences (Sherover-Marquse, 1987) on the way in which one acts and thinks (e.g. in the way that one defines family, or determines desirable life goals).
3. The "dynamics of difference" (Slaughter, 1988) must be fully understood – when one meets a client from another culture, both parties will bring culturally prescribed patterns of communication, etiquette and problem solving to that interaction and both will bring stereotypes and underlying feelings about working with someone who is "different".
4. Mainstream workers should make a conscious effort to understand the meaning of a client's behaviour within his or her cultural context, thereby adding a critical dimension to the helping process. In this way culture becomes an essential element of every evaluation.
5. The average worker cannot achieve comprehensive knowledge about every diverse cultural group so that an information base should be created containing necessary detailed information about anticipated cultural "situations".

These five elements will build a context in which cross-culturally competent practice can thrive. When professional workers understand the impact of social and cultural oppression on mental health they can begin to develop empowering interventions. For example, minority children who repeatedly receive negative messages from the media about their culture can be provided with alternative, culturally enriching experiences and these interventions can be written into treatment plans by practitioners as legitimate helping approaches.

Consumer level

It is necessary for families and associated groups that represent them to become effective advocates by preparing themselves with information about how the "dynamics of difference" operate and how a bi-cultural existence affects them. Families can play an indispensible role in protecting the mental health of their children. Groups of minority parents can also help open up lines of communication and advocate for changes to meet their needs better. Families encountering insensitive services can turn to each other for aid in interfacing with the system. As consumers become aware of services that are responsive to their cultural needs, they can encourage other minority families to use the system.

To summarise, each level of service provision can contribute to the cultural competence of the agency or system. As various attributes at different levels are implemented, the agency or system will move towards greater cultural competence. As the agency or system moves it will encounter new challenges. For example, an agency hiring minority professionals will encounter issues of cross-cultural supervision. These will then have to be addressed anew in accordance with the principles discussed above. But in this way it can be brought home to all concerned, whether psychiatrists, lawyers, legislators or other policy-makers, that policy-making or its implementation is not an exclusive or exclusionary activity, but must be undertaken in collaboration with others.

Conclusions

The ethnic minority population, which makes up 6.2 per cent of the total population, is likely to double to six million in the next 40 years. These groups of people will remain, however, very much in the minority (according to the latest census report on the subject; Ford, 1994) at less than 10 per cent of the total population. The cultural imperative in these populations is likely to become more (and not less) pressing for governments to address. Britain has to develop a consensus on policy along the lines identified in this chapter before using the law to implement or affect change. Lawyers need to lend their voice to the development of a consumer-oriented approach to the treatment of the mentally ill that correspondingly downplays the importance of professional autonomy. Otherwise, Britain's mental health system will fail to provide an effective service to its ethnic minority populations.

The revolution in the 1960s was partly effected by the changing political climate of the times, with emerging civil libertarian concerns. Lawyers, especially in the US, played their part by re-thinking who should be forcibly committed, on what grounds, for how long, and with what sort of procedural safeguards. However, that commitment to reducing the power of the government and of professional authorities in incarcerating people is only partially complete today in the absence of a matching commitment, to take a culturally based approach to these questions, that is fully cognizant of cultural motifs.

Before the 1960s, hospital personnel had exclusive control over all administrative decisions, with few incentives to terminate custody. Lawyers rarely played a role in their release. The state had the power to confine someone against his/her will by finding mental illness. Civilly committed persons were involuntarily detained in locked mental institutions for indefinite periods of time with practically no recourse to the legal process. It is essential that advocates of mentally disabled clients are cognisant of the cultural implications of what they do and one way of doing this is to make their approach more inter-disciplinarian. A practice based on cultural competence forces lawyers to adopt a multi-disciplinary approach and to evaluate the cultural effects of the lawyering process and the case's ultimate disposition. This is the level of civil rights practice that all mental health lawyers should now reach.

References

Bebbington, P., Feeney, S., Flannigan, C., Glover, G., Lewis, S. and Wing, J. (1994) Inner London collaborative audit of admissions in two health districts. II: Ethnicity and the use of the Mental Health Act. *British Journal of Psychiatry* **165**: 743–749.

Bernal, M.E., Knight, G.B., Garza, C.A., Ocampo, K.A. and Cota, M.K. (1990) The development of ethnic identity in Mexican-American children. *Hispanic Journal of Behavioral Sciences* **12**(1): 3–24.

Blom-Cooper QC, Sir Louis (1996) Foreword. In: Hoggett, B.M. *Mental Health Law*, 4th edn, p. v. London: Sweet and Maxwell.

Carter, J.H. (1982) The black aged: implications for mental health care. *Journal of the American Geriatric Society* **30**(1): 67–69.

Cope, R. (1989) The compulsory detention of Afro Caribbeans under the Mental Health Act. *New Community* **15**(3): 343–356.

Fernando, S. (1988) *Race and Culture in Psychiatry*. London: Croom Helm.

Flaskerud, J.H. (1986) The effects of culture-compatible intervention on the utilization of mental health services by minority clients. *Community and Mental Health Journal* **22**(2): 127–141.

Ford, R. (1994) UK's ethnic minorities will double in 40 years. *The Times* (London), January 20.

Grevious, C. (1985) The role of the family therapist with low income black families; *Family Therapy* **12**(2): 115–122.

Gynther, M.D. (1972) White norms and black MMPI's: a prescription for discrimination? *Psychological Bulletin* **78**(5): 386–402.

Hawkins, J.D. and Salisbury, B.R. (1983) Delinquency prevention programs for minorities of color. *Social Work Research and Abstracts* **19**(4): 5–12.

Health Committee (1993) Community Supervision Orders, House of Commons Paper, 667–1, 1992–1993 Session. London: HMSO.

Hellman, C. (1990) *Culture, Health and Illness*. Oxford: Butterworth Heinemann.

Higginbotham, H.N. (1984) *Third World Challenge to Psychiatry: Culture Accommodation and Mental Health Care*. Honolulu: University of Hawaii Press.

Hoggett, B.M. (1983) *Public Law*. Summer.

Hoggett, B.M. (1990) *Mental Health Law*, 3rd edn. London: Sweet and Maxwell.

Holdaway, S. and Allaker, J. (1990) *Race Issues in the Probation Service: A Review of Policy*. London: Association of Chief Officers of Probation.

Hune, S. (1977) US immigration policy and Asian Americans: aspects and consequences. In: *Civil Rights Issues of Asian and Pacific Americans: Myths and Realities*, pp. 283–291. Washington, DC: Government Printing Office.

Jones, B.E. and Gray, B.A. (1986) Problems in diagnosing schizophrenia and affective disorders among blacks. Hospital and Community Psychiatry **37**(1): 61–65.

Juss, S. (1997) *Discretion and Deviation in the Administration of Immigration Control*. London: Sweet and Maxwell.

Kleinman, A. and Cohen, A. (1997) Psychiatry's Global Challenge. *Scientific American*.

Kumabe, K.T., Nishida, C. and Hepworth, D.H. (eds) (1985) *Bridging Ethnocultural Diversities in Social Work and Health*. Honolulu: University of Hawaii School of Social Work.

Law, S., Rosenblatt, R. and Rosenbaum, S. (1997) *Law and the American Health Care System*. New York: Foundation Press.

Lefley, H.P. (1986) Why cross-cultural training? Applied issues in culture and mental health service delivery. In: Lefley, H.P. and Pedersen, P.B. (eds) *Cross-Cultural Training for Mental Health Professionals*, pp. 11–44. Springfield, Illinois: Charles C. Thomas.

Littlewood, R. and Lipsedge, M. (1989) *Aliens and Alienists: Ethnic Minorities and Psychiatry*. London: Unwin Hyman.

McDiarmid, G.W. (1983) Community and competence: a study of an indigenous primary prevention organization in an Alaskan village. *White Cloud Journal* **3**(1): 53–74.

McGoldrick, M., Pearce, J.K. and Giordano, J. (eds) (1982) *Ethnicity and Family Therapy*. New York: The Guilford Press.

Meinhardt, K. and Vega, W. (1987) A method for estimating under-utilization of mental health services for ethnic groups. *Hospital and Community Psychiatry* **38**(11): 1186–1190.

Mental Health Act Commission (1993) *Evidence to the Department of Health*. Nottingham: Mental Health Act Commission.

Mukherjee, S., Shukla, S., Woodle, J., Rosen, A.M. and Olarte, S. (1983) Misdiagnosis of schizophrenia in bi-polar patients: a multi ethnic comparison. *American Journal of Psychiatry* **140**(12): 1571–1574.

Neighbors, H.W. (1990) The prevention of psychopathology in African Americans: an epidemiologic perspective. *Community Mental Health Journal* **26**(2): 167–179.

Owan, T.C. (1982) Neighborhood-based mental health: an approach to overcome inequities in mental health services delivery to racial and ethnic minorities. In: Biegel, D.E. and Naparstek, A.J. (eds) *Community Support Systems and Mental Health: Practice, Policy and Research*, pp. 282–300. New York: Springer.

Pedersen, P.B. and Lefley, H.P. (1986) Introduction to cross-cultural training. In: Lefley, H.P. and Pedersen, P.B. (eds) *Cross-Cultural Training for Mental Health Professionals*, pp. 5–10. Springfield, Illinois: Charles C. Thomas.

Rogler, L.H., Malgady, R.G., Costantino, G. and Blumenthal, R. (1987) What do culturally sensitive mental health services mean?: The case of Hispanics. *American Psychologist* **42**(6): 565–570.

Rosen, H. and Frank, J.D. (1962) Negroes in psychotherapy. *American Journal of Psychiatry* 456–560.

Sherover-Marquse, R. (1987) *Liberation Theory: A Working Framework*. (Unpublished manuscript). San Francisco: Unlearning Racism Workshops.

Slaughter, D.T. (1988) Programs for racially and ethnically diverse American families: some critical issues. In: Weiss, H.B. and Jacobs, F.H. (eds) *Evaluating Family Programs*, pp. 461–476. New York: Aldien de Gruyter.

Snowden, L., Storey, C. and Clancy, T. (1989) Ethnicity and continuation in treatment at a black community mental health center. *Journal of Community Psychology* **17**: 111–118.

Szapocznik, J., Kurtines, W., Santisteban, D.A. and Rio, A.T. (1990) Interplay of advances between theory, research and application in treatment interventions aimed at behaviour problem children and adolescents. *Journal of Consulting and Clinical Psychology* **58**(6): 693–703.

Terrell, F. and Terrell, S. (1984) Race of counsellor, client sex, cultural mistrust level and premature termination from counselling among black clients. *Journal of Counselling Psychology* **31**(3): 371–375.

Vandenberg, J. and Minton, B.A. (1987) Alaska native youth: a new approach to serving emotionally disturbed children and youth. *Children Today* **16**(5): 5–18.

Williams, W.S., Ralph, J.R. and Denham, W. (1978) Black Mental Health Work Force. In: Institute for Urban Affairs and Research, *Mental Health: A Challenge to the Black Community*. Philadelphia: Dorrance.

Wong, H.Z. (1980) Treatment system considerations in the organisation of mental health services for Asian and Pacific American communities. In: *Manpower Considerations in Providing Mental Health Services to Ethnic Minority Groups*, pp. 52–59. Boulder, Colorado: Western Interstate Commission for Higher Education (WICHE).

Wu, I-Hsing and Windle, C. (1980) Ethnic specificity in the relative minority use and staffing of community mental health centers. *Community Mental Health Journal* **16**: 156–168.

Zane, N., Sue, S., Castro, F.G. and George, W. (1982) Service system models for ethnic minorities. In: Biegel, D.E. and Naparstek, A.J. (eds) *Community Support Systems and Mental Health: Practice, Policy and Research*, pp. 229–257. New York: Springer.

9

The Voluntary Sector

Joy Francis and Dora Jonathan

PROFESSIONAL VIEWPOINT

This chapter combines two different professional perspectives: that of a journalist and a mental health consultant. What concerns us both is the lack of progressive debate on the creation of viable, credible, accessible and culturally sensitive services for black people with mental health problems. Black practitioners, volunteers and service users at grassroots level are the source of rich and useful experiences, as well as practical ideas. Yet their views are not being widely sought and harnessed either by government ministers or health and local authority service commissioners.

In our respective professions, we have too readily been confronted with unsettling statements from service users and workers, saturated with fear and demoralisation over the dire state of mental health service provision in the voluntary sector. There is a great need, particularly for black organisations, to be supported in their negotiations for contracts with purchasers and applications for grants such as the National Lottery. And the long-standing divisions between white mainstream agencies and small black organisations are not inspiring confidence or useful solutions. Instead black mental health service users are stranded in the middle, often without the support and guidance they not only need but are entitled to.

While the Labour government promotes the theme of social inclusion, black mental health agencies continue to experience exclusion. They have a vital role to play, for example in the initial assessment of black clients, a role we believe needs to be extended to the NHS Trusts in care planning as part of the Care Programme Approach. Let us hope when we revisit this subject in the future that we are not forced to retread old and painfully familiar ground.

The term "black" is used in this chapter in reference to people who are oppressed by racism because of their skin colour, largely members of the African, Caribbean and Asian communities. We will not be wholly dependent on this term as we will also refer to country of origin.

With reference to our use of the terms voluntary organisations, agencies and charities, they are interchangeable. This identity confusion is at the centre of the current debate in the voluntary sector, and is fuelling a drive for charity law reform which will hopefully lead to the introduction of one unifying term (Commission on the Future of the Voluntary Sector, 1996).

Introduction

Independent, innovative, creative and pioneering are just a few of the positive terms used by the voluntary sector to describe itself. These qualities are recognised and acknowledged by the statutory sector, and are attributes voluntary organisations are keen to preserve. Heavily reliant on public goodwill, the statutory sector and, more recently, the National Lottery for funding, charities' grassroots connections with local communities places them in a pivotal position to identify key areas of need.

In theory, then, the voluntary sector should be blazing a progressive trail armed with an array of cross-cultural community-based mental health services; much-needed blueprints of good practice for others to emulate. However, the reality is less glowing. Advancements have been made with pockets of good practice dotted across the country. But these isolated role models (largely black-led) exist in isolation, deprived of adequate professional and financial support.

There is no doubt that the creation of cross-cultural mental health services is one of the most complicated and challenging areas of social policy and practice. Why? Because in today's society mental health is still a taboo and stigmatised subject, viewed with fear and misinformed suspicion (Baker and Read, 1996).

Secondly, when race enters the equation, the result is akin to a firecracker going off in a restaurant – everyone scurries towards the nearest exit. Unfortunately, some of the fleeing guests are the mental health professionals themselves. Race and mental health "is the thing that no one wants to talk about", confessed psychiatrist Elaine Murphy (Strong, 1996).

The development of culturally appropriate services in the voluntary sector is being tentatively pursued and, to some degree, hindered by a scathing national press mindful of what they see as "preventable" tragedies, such as Christopher Clunis, Stephen Laudat, Wayne Hutchinson and their victims. These black men were in the care of a range of statutory and voluntary agencies; they were once again categorised as "big, black and dangerous". Each of them asked for help but fell through defective safety nets in the community which placed themselves and others at risk.

Being bombarded with a range of highly expectant and under-funded pieces of legislation has increased the pressure already heaped on voluntary sector mental health providers. The NHS/Community Act 1990 and its much lauded principles of partnership between social services departments, voluntary sector providers and service users under the new purchaser/provider split is one example.

The implementation of care in the community has been a painful process. Its progress has been compounded by the controversy surrounding the delayed and muddled implementation of the Care Programme Approach (CPA), introduced back in 1991. Promoted as the bedrock of care in the community for people with mental health problems, its embarrassingly late implementation whipped up even more confusion. Some small black and white agencies have intermittently asked: "What is it?" and "How does it affect us?"

All of which blatantly highlights the lack of specialist training in mental health and community care for workers in the voluntary sector. Yet this very training is necessary for the successful implementation of responsibilities, resource allocation, risk assessment and reporting. Instead, staff are receiving conflicting messages about whether to send black clients into hospital or to live independently in the community. The price of a wrong decision is blame, adverse media attention and the withdrawal of a contract, possibly signalling the death knell of a voluntary agency.

"Mental health charities are being forced to fight rearguard actions instead of addressing the gaps in community care." These telling words were uttered by Chris Heginbotham, chief executive of East and North Hertfordshire Health Authority in 1996, at the annual Mental Health After Care Association conference. In short, voluntary sector mental health providers are caught between a rock and a hard place, and the cracks are beginning to show.

The Funding Culture

Short term, *ad hoc* and generally unsatisfactory funding arrangements are regularly cited as the main culprit for the scattered and under-developed cross-cultural mental health services in the voluntary sector. Apart from making it difficult to plan with the long term in mind, is it really suitable to rely on "funny money" from Urban Aid or the City Challenge for the development of mental health services?

The last Conservative government did not offer any respite on the funding front. It continually frustrated many within the voluntary sector with its blunt and persistent denial that extra resources were needed to fund community care for people with mental health problems. To solve the problem, explained the then Health Secretary Stephen Dorrell, statutory and voluntary agencies needed to apportion existing resources better (Valios and Whiteley, 1995).

The reality begs to differ. According to the Mental Health Foundation, for every £1 of the £3150 million spent on caring for mentally ill people in 1991, 91 pence went on NHS provision. Only nine pence went on local authority, private and voluntary residential and day care services. This included support at home for people in the community. And only £176 million – 3 per cent of the £5126 million community care budget covering 1992–93 – was spent on mental health services (Eaton, 1994).

In 1993, the provision of nursing and residential care for people with mental health problems by local authorities (4100 places) and the voluntary and private sector (17 500 places) absorbed an estimated £257 million. The Audit Commission has calculated that two thirds of the £1800 million spent on adult mental health services in 1992–93 was eaten up by hospital in-patient care (Chisholm *et al.*, 1997). This over-reliance on NHS provision is hardly in keeping with the basic principles of care in the community.

Many of the 300 000 people identified with severe mental health problems are being deprived of sufficient locally based mental health services (Mental Health Foundation, 1995). Despite the former Conservative government's admonishments about voluntary providers' accounting skills, it continually failed to provide the necessary information outlining its own spending on mental illness. And the lack of information on the prevalence rate of mental ill-health among black people and their take-up of services was another of its shortcomings.

Another funding pressure point is the highly competitive contract culture. A product of the new market economy ethos driving community care, it has left many voluntary providers disgruntled and shell-shocked. Complaints of being held to ransom, forced to subsidise services or compromise their charitable principles are commonplace (Francis, 1996).

A notable reaction to this trend was encapsulated in the stormy and high profile resignation of Errol Francis as director of Kensington and Chelsea Mind, London, in 1996. An advocate of culturally appropriate mental health services, he objected to the local authority's decision to cut its £300 000 service contract and grant by £64 000 (Anon., 1996a). Appalled, Francis claimed that the contract, which he refused to sign, expected volunteers to assess whether users were at risk. "Voluntary organisations are the Cinderella service. It's just expected that we will survive on a wing and a prayer" (Cooper, 1996).

Another and new source of much-needed funding is the National Lottery Charities Board (NLCB). Now in its third year, it has offered a new lease of life to many charities, but it has no reliable system in place to determine how many of its grant recipients provide mental health services for black people. Applicants have an option to tick a box indicating whether they provide services for black and other ethnic minority clients. However, there is no category to determine whether the organisation in question is black-led.

As Table 9.1 shows, this discretionary, tick-the-box system shows that, over three grant-giving rounds, a disappointing 22 organisations were identified as serving the needs of black clients. There is obviously a lot of ground to make up, an admission made by the NLCB itself.

White Voluntary Sector Mental Health Providers

One question that is often pitched at white mainstream mental health providers in the voluntary sector is, can they truly cater for the needs of black people? According to a notable number of black mental health agencies, white agencies are not doing anything for black people with mental health problems because they do not know why they should. It is out of their realm of experience, is one argument. Another is that time and

Table 9.1   National Lottery Charities Board summary by round.

Round	PR OrgName	PR Award
MA	Servol Community Trust	£476 959
	African Caribbean Community Initiative	£59 174
	Mary Seacole House	£39 529
	Vietnamese Mental Health Project	£174 130
	42nd Street Community Mental Health Resource for Young	£98 807
	Isis	£90 000
	Sheffield African Caribbean Mental Health Association	£25 000
	Creative Support	£137 880
	Nottingham Counselling Centre	£124 015
	Sahara (Asian Women's Group Mental Health)	£3 000
	Hadhari Project	£193 000
MA Total		£1 421 494
MA Count		11
MB	Asian Women's Adhikar Association	£143 068
	The Nigerian Women's Welfare Association	£44 156
MB Total		£187 224
MB Count		2
MC	RNIB (Royal National Institute for the Blind)	£296 406
	Burnley and Pendle Society of Asians Disabled	£108 132
	Shobujshathi Supplementary Education Project	£122 853
	Black Spectrum	£192 923
	Barnardo's	£391 000
	Minority Ethnic Learning Disability Initiative	£94 348
	East Park Activity Group	£26 283
	Anika Patrice Project	£143 349
	MCCR	£124 074
MC Total		£1 499 368
MC Count		9
Grand Total		£3 108 086
Grand Count		22

MA, First Round (Poverty); MB, Second Round (Youth Issues and Low Income); MC, Third Round (Health, Disability and Care).

again it is black mental health professionals who remind white providers of their responsibilities.

As large voluntary sector providers such as Mind, the National Schizo-phrenic Fellowship (NSF) and the Richmond Fellowship call themselves national organisations, they have a duty to embrace the needs of black people. Their regular appearances in the broadsheets, strong connections with politicians and royal patronage reinforces their important position in terms of policy making. But, in practice, how widely accountable are they?

A brief trawl through the historical evolution of Mind, NSF and the Richmond Fellowship yields some answers and common themes. Before 1990, their awareness of black clients ranged from non-existent to sporadic. All were jolted into action by complaints and concerns from black statutory and voluntary sector mental health professionals. The introduction of racially relevant equal opportunities policies and the employment of token black workers were commonly adopted strategies. Suspicion from the black community, users and mental health workers about the true motivations of these white agencies was another salient feature.

The experience of Mind, which has been in the forefront of mental health for 52 years, highlights some of the shortcomings inherent in mainstream service provision, particularly a penchant for missed opportunities. During the late 1980s Mind set up the Black and Ethnic Minority Development Team, funded by the now defunct Greater London Council (GLC) to look at services and resources available to black people with mental health problems. This signalled the first overt move by the charity to address race in any shape or form. But the project was short-term funded, questionably located in the south-east of England and was not integrated into the charity's mainstream work.

When the GLC funding ceased at the beginning of 1990, no attempt was made by Mind to keep the project going. This inaction was negatively received by black mental health professionals. In the same year a second chance was missed. A promotional Mind video titled *Call to Mind* only featured white people and their concerns. Three years later, after 18 months of consultation with a working group made up of black and Asian organisations and workers, Mind produced a policy – *Black and Minority Ethnic People and Mental Health*. But only last year, Mind's national director Judi Clements admitted: "In all honesty, it hasn't been fully implemented yet."

Forging relationships with black-led mental health providers is another area that has not been fully implemented by white mainstream providers. Instead tensions between the black and white mental health providers remain, particularly over the perceived ease with which white agencies attract funding to develop services for black people. Mind's own policy document hints at this trend: "Predominantly white service providers may find additional funding to do something about black people's needs." It also notes that black organisations face "considerable financial difficulties because funders feel more at ease funding better known groups like Mind".

The problem runs far deeper than this statement suggests. Black workers have cited examples of white voluntary agencies falsely securing money earmarked for black people by falsely claiming to be working with black groups and service users. But cases are difficult to prove.

Last year, a female black mental health practitioner based in a white organisation set up an independent group for black mental health survivors. By sheer chance she came across an application for government funding by a white member of staff. The application form cited her black group as a co-applicant and suggested that work would be carried out for black people assisted by the group. When she confronted the white male worker, he apologised for not asking for her permission, but the matter was not taken any further.

Later she discovered that money for advocacy work with black service users was allocated, without her knowledge, to her charity. Yet no work with this objective had materialised. Despondent, she asked not to be identified as she is still with the organisation, but she alluded to her departure in the near future as she found the situation "intolerable" and "disempowering". Widespread silence and fear is preventing this problem from attracting the attention it so desperately needs.

Most large white agencies are mindful of these experiences. "I think black organisations, understandably, continue to question the inherent racism in white organisations and suspect tokenism, or such agencies addressing black needs because there may be money or 'brownie points' in it," said Leo Sowerby, director of operations at the Richmond Fellowship.

Steps have been taken by all three providers to work more closely with black agencies. Last year Mind launched Diverse Minds, a forum made up of black and minority ethnic users, carers and workers in mental health. It will directly influence Mind's policy and campaigns as well as provide a reference point for external groups. In March 1997, the NSF's council of management adopted a statement on the needs of black people with mental health problems which it hopes all the major national charities will adopt. Only time will tell whether these seemingly good intentions lead to the manifestation of innovative and culturally sensitive mental health services.

Black Voluntary Sector Mental Health Providers

The experience of black voluntary sector mental health providers offers a sharp contrast to that of their white counterparts. They are smaller, and are generally scattered geographically. Often they are under-resourced without sturdy infrastructures and are hardly visible in the statutory and National Lottery funding queues. Black voluntary organisations have gamely shouldered the less than flattering image of being the "poor relation", as many have been forced to rely on white organisations to access funding on their behalf (Sia, 1993).

The roots to this current state of affairs stretch back to a battle-scarred history. The mid to late 1960s saw the development and seed funding of a number of small black voluntary organisations. Section 11 funding, intro-duced in the Local Government Act 1966, started the process of resourcing the black voluntary sector. The political and social climate, including the 1981 uprisings, led to a dramatic shift in the funding of the black voluntary organisations.

It signalled a move away from self-reliance to state dependency with black agencies turning to the GLC for funding. What also came to light was how short lived many black projects were, although there continues to be a dearth of information on the true state of black voluntary organisations: between 1987 and 1993 over 50 black voluntary organisations based in

London had their funding terminated. It has been widely accepted that the figure is an underestimate (Sia, 1993). Recently, more worrying examples have come to light. For example, out of 225 black voluntary organisations located in the London Borough of Lambeth 15 years ago, only 25 now remain (Jadeja, 1997).

With the charity sector in a state of flux, particularly over its identity, black mental health organisations are again losing out. Now the problem is with the traditional concept of charity. The definition is greatly at odds with the cultural and historical principles on which black voluntary organisations were founded, namely self-help and self-reliance. For example, the charitable concept of providing services for the "public good" places black mental health organisations in a quandary. They are being forced onto the sidelines as observers and are failing to reap the full benefits of charitable status because they are seen as serving only one section of the community (Sia, 1996).

Then there is the use of the term **black**. Some black agencies have found themselves challenged by statutory funders over its usage and it has been a bone of contention with the Charity Commission (Sia, 1993). Its use has also led to conflict with local authorities in the funding arena. Most social services departments and health authorities tend to stick with what they know and with people who share the same values, which euphemistically means large white mainstream voluntary agencies.

This theme also applies to charitable trusts. And although the NLCB has made some in-roads with black agencies it is still far from satisfactory. Less than 4 per cent of the £40 million allocated by the NLCB in 1995 went to black communities and has failed to implement useful ethnic monitoring and targeting systems (Fraser, 1996).

The community care principle of partnership and collaboration seems to have stalled where black mental health agencies are concerned. These are some of the reasons held up by black agencies for their failure to secure statutory contracts. But some black agencies' inexperience in costing for services has left them and their clients vulnerable. In some cases this has meant being pressured into taking on white clients with limited funding, thereby marginalising the very black people they were established to help. Or they are expected to cater for a range of black people with diverse needs such as people with Nigerian, Trinidadian, Somalian and Jamaican backgrounds – within one narrowly defined service.

A persistent claim is that when the social services funding axe falls black-led organisations are the first to feel the chop. For example, the Cassava club based in Hackney, London, has been praised by the local and health authorities, and is recognised as providing an invaluable day service for forensic clients. Yet this glowing reference did not prevent it from having its funding slashed. Attempts to raise money through alternative sources such as the NLCB have proved fruitless. It is now facing the possibility of closure leaving staff, volunteers, the community and clients in limbo.

What underpins all these developments is a crisis of credibility which afflicts black mental health agencies. Even when they provide accurate information, evidence of their work and measurable outcomes, they are still perceived as lacking in professional expertise and prone to financial mismanagement. The past four years have been peppered with unflattering stories highlighting premature closures or the sudden withdrawal of funding. Bad publicity usually ensues, bursting with allegations of infighting, financial mismanagement, a lack of resources and poor communication.

In 1994, for example, *The Guardian* reported on the closure of the Harambee organisation, a large project providing a range of diverse residential mental health services for black people in Birmingham. It was liquidated with debts fast approaching £500 000. Stories highlight a lack of user consultation, minimal delegation of responsibility and demoralisation.

More recently, in 1996, the African-Caribbean Mental Health Association in south London was on the verge of closure after 11 years because the funders – a mixture of local authorities and a local health commission – withdrew their funding and support (Anon., 1996b). Allegedly, problems stemmed from management difficulties, leading to the director's dismissal. It now exists as a mere shadow of its former self, without any funding. Many other black agencies have folded quietly, without any fanfare. The insidious implication is that black agencies are a liability, whereas white agencies are not.

Managerial ineptitude, infighting and bad practice are behind some of these failures. But there are other factors that have played a part: unrealistic demands from funders, trying to replicate a westernised Eurocentric model of management with black clients and staff; not having strong enough roots in the local community; and failing to address the insidious impact of internalised racism which, when left unchallenged, produces a self-fulfilling prophecy in line with white detractors' belief that black agencies cannot manage mental health services.

Culturally Appropriate Services: Myth or Reality?

By the time black people experiencing mental ill-health make contact with voluntary providers they are in extreme need of help and have undergone, without question, some of the most dehumanising forms of psychiatric treatment. You do not have to dig too deep to unearth the distressing statistics which have placed black people on top in the most worrying categories: brutality, racism, a tendency to be disproportionately diagnosed as schizophrenic, over-medicated and placed in seclusion.

Public acknowledgement of the need for good practice for black people with mental health problems came in June 1993 with the book *Mental Health and Britain's Black Communities* (Wilson, 1993). The first initiative of a tripartite collaboration between the King's Fund Centre, the NHS Management Executive Mental Health Task Force and the Prince of Wales Advisory Group on Disabilities, it tried to tackle mental health in relation to black communities.

It presented evidence of the difficulties that many black people face when using mainstream mental health services, and the impact of institutionalised and personalised racism. But it also documented good practice and demonstrated that much of the innovative development for black mental health emerged through black-led initiatives for those in need. These themes were built upon in an informative and optimistic publication, again from the King's Fund, entitled *Creating Solutions*. It outlined the steps that needed to be taken to develop alternatives to existing mental health service provision, primarily multi-agency partnership and the inclusion of grass-roots community groups and service users (Jennings, 1997).

There are thriving examples of good practice in action in the UK which show how delicate, time-consuming and challenging the creation of a culturally sensitive mental health service is. Although modest in number, they show what can be achieved by voluntary providers at a time when cost cutting and value for money are the driving principles behind service level agreements with health and local authorities. But they have all had to fight extremely hard to retain funding on a year to year basis.

One such project is Saheliya. Located in Edinburgh, Scotland, it caters for and is run by black women. Black is used by Saheliya in reference to non-white ethnic communities. This definition, it says, enables the organisation to respect individual cultures be they Asian, Chinese or African. The impetus for its establishment was an investigative report by the Craigen-tinny Health Project in 1991 which noted that black women were not taking up its services. Black women could not access services, it said, because of the stigma attached to mental health, race and language barriers. Among its recommendations was the need for the creation of a black women's mental health project run by black women (CHP, 1991).

In 1992, aided by a mental health specific grant, a project worker and administrative worker were employed. They carried out a survey within the community to gauge how people felt about the value of mental health services. At the time there were no black counsellors in Edinburgh so a training course was devised for volunteers with a component on racism and its role in the treatment and care of black women with mental health problems. A needs survey of black women was carried out which reported a desire for counselling and support. White mental health projects were approached and briefed on Saheliya's aims and how it would complement their existing service provision.

From initially having two staff and a group support and therapy section, Saheliya now boasts a befriending section with a project worker and 15 volunteers, a counselling section with its own project worker and two counsellors, and is on the verge of setting up a complementary therapy section. It recently appointed a Chinese sessional worker and offers practice placements for social work students. Seven crèche workers are on hand to encourage more mothers to use the project.

Initially, only a handful of black women accessed Saheliya's services. Now, 80 women use its services weekly. A guiding principle is the right for black women to determine the type of services implemented and in which direction they go. Some of the service users are full-time members of staff, befriending volunteers or are on the advisory group. Service users sit on the management committee. There is no project co-ordinator. Instead, each worker feeds into a management group.

Cultural needs are always at the forefront of Saheliya's work and it does not impose its cultural interpretations on the women. For example, women can choose whether they want to be part of a culturally mixed group or a separate group. There is an ongoing evaluation of the service to ensure that the project continues to be needs-led, a process the service users feed directly into.

Cassava is another voluntary sector project making a positive difference despite, as outlined earlier in the chapter, the possible threat of its closure. Based in the east London multi-racial borough of Hackney, it was established in the early 1990s by black mental health workers from health and social services. Distressed at the lack of creative provision for black people experiencing mental ill-health, they decided to take the matter in hand.

At first the workers, along with selected volunteers, offered their time freely to run the organisation as they only had funding for a sessional cook. Currently it provides an evening drop-in service as well as outreach support for African and Caribbean people with long-term mental health needs. The volunteers formed a management committee and, in 1994, Cassava managed to employ a part-time project co-ordinator with funding from East London and City Health Authority. But as the health authority is facing financial difficulties, their future is not secure.

As for the Future . . .

As there is no crystal ball to guide the way, the future of cross-cultural mental health services in the voluntary sector still remains uncertain. But there are some encouraging signs of activity. The finishing touches are being put to two innovative models which could shift the current debate and practice in a whole new direction, models that centre on providing a range of therapies which are culturally appropriate, accessible to the community, with staff who reflect the racial and cultural heritage of the client group, and, more importantly, show the value of partnerships in action. Initiated by the King's Fund Development Centre, the Sanctuary projects were born in 1993 as a response to the yawning gaps in mainstream mental health services for black people. The King's Fund provided funding to employ a development worker in the London boroughs of Lambeth and Hackney with three key aims: to develop a community-based crisis support service; to provide a service in which the black community would have faith and, more importantly, use; and to ensure that upon completion they would become independent black-managed agencies (Jennings, 1997).

They are now both developing along distinctly different lines in tandem with the needs identified in their respective localities. Both are on course to be open for business in 1998 and highlight the importance of truly working in partnership with statutory agencies.

Model One: Ipamo (Yoruba for "house of healing")

Ipamo is located in Lambeth, south London. With a population of 245 000, African and Caribbean people are the largest minority group in the London borough, making up 21.8 per cent or 53 432 of the total population. Poverty, substance misuse, suicide and mental ill-health are prominent in the borough (Jackson, 1997). An understanding of the social problems facing black communities in Lambeth is seen as a crucial component in the way Ipamo relates and responds to their needs.

In 1995, a director and an administrator were employed to oversee the development of Ipamo's services. Over the past two years, they have made contact with black voluntary sector mental health providers all over the country to inform them of Ipamo's objectives and to share different ways of working. Ipamo's services fall into six categories:

- Assessment Service
- Crisis Service, an alternative to in-patient care
- Family Respite
- 24 Hour Advice and Advocacy Service
- Therapy and Outreach Service drawing on the beliefs and customs of African and Caribbean communities
- Community Education and Development Programme

Plans are underway to develop an African and Caribbean Certificate of Education therapy model which will apply to this and other Ipamo services. Training has been and will be undertaken in the local community on, for example, housing estates to inform local people of mental ill-health. The plan is to raise awareness to enable black people to make the best of existing services and resources.

All Ipamo's services will be housed on one site, a large four-storey detached Victorian property in a residential area. Purchased by Lambeth Healthcare Trust from the local authority, Ipamo has renovated the property, which is graced with a tropical garden (external therapy space). Its design will reflect the local Caribbean historical influence in the locality.

A total of 31 staff including team leaders, therapists, outreach workers and advice workers will be employed to run the service. Staff will be trained in an African-centred understanding of mental illness before they start. This will avoid the pitfalls and intense pressures generated by training on the job. As the workers are expected to come from a range of disciplines, i.e. nursing and social work, attempts will be made to ensure that they are fully conversant with the Ipamo model.

As shown in Figure 9.1, there will be small team structures where each worker will be partnered with a peer support worker. Every worker will be part of a family team, guided by a senior worker. The staff team as a whole form a community under the leadership of the director.

What is striking about the Ipamo project is the level of funding it has attracted, though it has to be stressed that the money did not fall into its lap: it was a long and arduous process. From the beginning, Ipamo was determined to retain a clear identity and its independence. The funding envelope to develop Ipamo was £3.3 million through the London Implementation Zone (LIZ) from the Department of Health. The ongoing funding – £1.4 million – comes through a three-year rolling contract with the Lambeth, Southwark and Lewisham Health Association. An additional

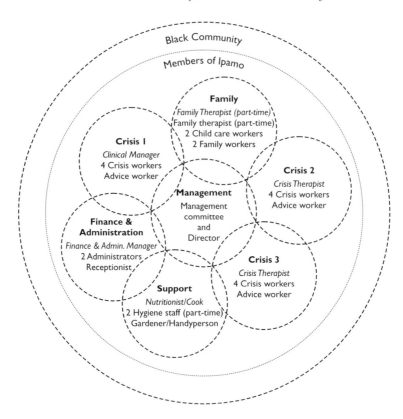

Figure 9.1   Ipamo's staff structure model (Jackson, 1997).

£70 000 in capital funds was secured from the Brixton Challenge for Ipamo's development (Jackson, 1997).

Ipamo's essential principles of mind, body, spirit and memory form a framework into which the management committee, also known as "the Elders' Council", slots. It reflects the organisation's belief that black agencies need to take responsibility for the health and well-being of black communities without being wholly dependent and constrained by Western ideas. Figure 9.2 shows how this theme enables a high level of transparency and accountability.

Ipamo is taking its message and model to a national audience. In March 1996, it held a Partnerships and Progress conference to address ways of providing effective support to black mental health workers nationally. In June 1997 it launched Safoa (Ghanaian for key), an umbrella organisation encompassing over 80 black mental health organisations in Britain.

Safoa's "birth" was celebrated during a week-long international conference, "Mental Health in the African Diaspora", from 16 to 20 June. Respected black mental health practitioners from America, the Caribbean and Africa as well as the UK aired their concerns and visions for the future of cross-cultural mental health services. Ipamo plans to hold a conference annually, and run a three-day residential course with 20 workshops for the black voluntary sector: ten for workers and ten for

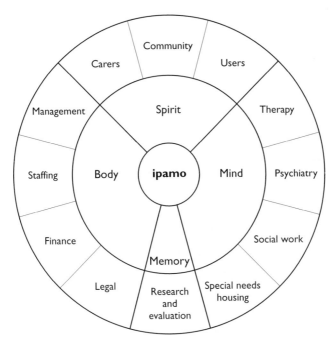

Figure 9.2 Ipamo's management committee (Elders' Council) model (Jackson, 1997).

management. Around 300 black mental health professionals are expected to attend the course each year.

Model Two: The Nile Project

The Nile Project, formerly known as the Hackney African Caribbean Crisis Service, emerged out of consultation with black users and carers as well as a range of local mental health professionals in the early 1990s. It is now based within Kush Housing Association Limited, an established, independent organisation which has been providing housing and support for black people in Hackney, east London, since 1986.

Kush recognises that, as a social landlord, it cannot ignore the needs of the wider community which go way beyond direct housing provision. The housing association is uniquely placed to use its landlord resources, management experience, and social and community rootedness to meet holistically the acute needs of the local African and Caribbean community.

Apart from being holistic, the Kush model is African-centred and intends to be appropriate in language, interventions (style and type) and diet so that care providers can meet the expressed and assessed needs of clients. It aims to work with people who, without its presence, have a high risk of being admitted to hospital, particularly those who have experienced repeated admissions or the "revolving door syndrome". There will be scope to accommodate people who have never accessed mental health services before.

The centre wants to provide an intensive service to users by working in small numbers with support from a total of 21 staff. Back-up support will be provided by trained volunteers. The idea is to work with up to six families at the centre and two families through its outreach service each week.

Key features of the service will be a rapid response to requests for its services, 24-hour provision, working with clients' cultural norms, using the local community as a therapeutic and supportive resource, carrying out direct work with the families of service users, and widely publicising the service within the African and Caribbean community.

Being responsive to crises will be another prime feature to counteract the trend for black people to be sectioned under the Mental Health Act. To tackle this there will be a crisis outreach service along with crisis intervention 24 hours a day, seven days a week. The 24-hour principle will also extend to its supported accommodation consisting of four single rooms and two family rooms backed by a staff team of nine.

Counselling and therapy, with a focus on learning patterns of relapse and the development of coping strategies, will be available. Alternative and complementary therapies will be an intrinsic part of the service. Underpinning the whole Nile Centre approach is safety within a nurturing environment. Also driving the model is a recognition of the need for adequate resources and staffing which will be bolstered by a commitment to staff training.

Ownership among staff is recognised as a crucial element. Working together to formulate a common approach to managing self-harm, violence and crises will be pursued. Plans are afoot to develop appropriate inter-agency protocols with external agencies, a clear recognition that there will be occasions when additional assistance will be needed.

Conclusion

Both black and white mental health voluntary sector providers have lessons to learn where black people and mental health services are concerned. Black agencies have to collaborate, share their experiences and successes, and devise strategies to attract funding to provide the best possible services to black people.

White voluntary agencies have to question seriously the long-term value of recruiting token black workers to address the wide-ranging needs of black people experiencing mental ill-health. The persistent presence of covert and institutional racism in mainstream voluntary agencies is barring the creation of non-medical, holistic and culturally aware services. A lack of respect for the expertise, structures and experiences of black voluntary organisations is, sadly, also apparent (Bhasin, 1997).

As more services are put out to tender by local authorities, small to medium-sized voluntary organisations will be compromised. The enduring colour-blind approach of some local and health authorities is another obstacle to be cleared and the impetus has to come from the authorities themselves. Voluntary organisations must flex their lobbying muscle to capture the attention of politicians and health and local authority commissioners. And they must drive home that they are not a cheap resource.

The Labour government has paid lip service to the disproportionate number of black people languishing within the mental health system. It has acknowledged that black people are saddled with a "double stigma". A review of mental health services by junior health minister Paul Boateng has led to a commitment to inject an estimated £500 million into mental health services, although no pointers to the creation of culturally sensitive after-care services have been provided.

Black service users are often left out of the equation, which is an incredibly irresponsible act. Their inclusion in policy formation and service creation is essential. They should be encouraged to hold user-led conferences to formulate suggestions for service delivery as well as different cultural perspectives on mental health. A central agency for the training of mental health service users could be formed. The graduates could then be despatched to work with a range of different professionals such as general practitioners and community psychiatric nurses.

As for the black voluntary sector, any new approaches must emphasise local autonomy, recognition of their cultural strength, participation, empowerment, equality, trust and flexibility to enable mental health voluntary agencies to survive into the next millennium. There has to be more accountability, sound management practices and the development of strategies which take into account past mistakes.

Many of the practices now advocated for managing the black voluntary sector, as exemplified by the Ipamo and Nile projects, need to become the norm and not the parochial exception. If these two projects are the future, then the time has come for the establishment of an over-arching national agency for black mental health. Some steps towards this end have been taken by Ipamo through the creation of Safoa.

What could a national black mental health umbrella organisation achieve? It would champion the development of new projects, support current projects to obtain funding from grant-giving trusts and the National Lottery Charities Board. It would equally be a campaigning organ as well as an advocate on black mental health concerns. This would provide agencies with the space to focus on providing much needed culturally appropriate services.

Training support would also be offered to develop skills in business planning and negotiating contracts with health authority purchasers and social services departments. It would also play a pivotal role in training committee members. An agency of this kind would undertake an evaluation of services and conduct research into what works in practice and disseminate the information nationally.

It may be that many of the practices we have advocated for the black voluntary sector are already in place in certain areas, or that agencies have developed resilient skills to cope with austere conditions. The black voluntary sector has provided some valuable lessons in the art of making such practices work and has illustrated some of the tensions and dilemmas being generated. These lessons of survival have to be shared.

References

Anon. (1996a) Charity turns down contract. *Community Care* 8–14 August, p. 5.

Anon. (1996b) Mental health association set to close. *Community Care* 25–31 January, p. 2.

Baker, S. and Read, J. (1996) *Not Just Sticks and Stones: A Survey of the Stigma, Taboos and Discrimination Experienced by People with Mental Health Problems*. London: Mind.

Bhasin, S. (1997) *My Time, My Community, Myself*. London: National Centre for Volunteering.

Chisholm, D., Knapp, M. and Lowin, A. (1997) Mental Health Services in London: Costs. In: Johnson, S. *et al.* (eds) *London's Mental Health*. London: King's Fund Publications.

CHP (1991) *Craigentinny Investigative Report*. Edinburgh: Craigentinny Health Project.

Commission on the Future of the Voluntary Sector (1996) *Meeting the Challenge of Change: Voluntary Action into the 21st Century*. London: NCVO Publications.

Cooper, C. (1996) Calm after the storm *Community Care* 22–28 August, p. 6.

Eaton, L. (1994) Why is community care failing the mentally ill? *Community Care* 30 April, p. 8.

Francis, J. (1996) Creative casualties *Community Care*. 12–18 September, p. 26.

Fraser, H. (1996) *Whose Lottery is it Anyway? – The Impact of the National Lottery on the Black Voluntary Sector*. London: Sia Publications.

Jackson, A. (1997) *Ipamo Inaugural Annual Report*. London: Ipamo.

Jadeja, K. (1997) Where is the black voluntary sector voice? *Third Sector*, 27 November, pp. 10–11.

Jennings, S. (1997) *Creating Solutions – Developing Alternatives in Black Mental Health*, 2nd edn. London: King's Fund Publications.

Mental Health Foundation (1995) *Severe Mental Illness: The Problem of Resources – Factsheet*. London: Mental Health Foundation.

Sia (1993) *Agenda 2000 – The Black Perspective, Conference Report*. London: Sia Publications.

Sia (1996) *The National Development Agency for the Black Voluntary Sector's 1994–1995 Annual Report*. London: Sia Publications.

Strong, S. (1996) On the brink of disaster. *Community Care* 22–28 February, pp. 16–17.

Valios, N. and Whiteley, P. (1995) Government rules out more mental illness cash, *Community Care* 28 September to 4 October, p. 3.

Wilson, M. (1993) *Mental Health and Britain's Black Communities*. London: King's Fund Centre.

10

An Occupational Therapist's Perspective on Developing a Culturally Sensitive Service

Georgina Foulds

Introduction

The individual who comes into contact with mental health services brings not only symptoms of illness but his/her needs, values and life-style. These dimensions of personality are developed through a person's life experience. Culture plays an integral part in this developmental experience. It shapes our understanding of illness and recovery. Culture encodes our expectations of helping service users and carers who work within these services. This chapter outlines practical approaches and developments within a community mental health team for the severely mentally ill. The challenge we face is to provide for services to meet better the needs of a diversity of cultures.

Culture, the Person and Health Services

Man is orientated to the environment principally through culture. (Jang, 1995)

Culture has an endless list of basic elements, law, customs, goals, beliefs and values. (Krefting and Krefting, 1991)

The NHS was set up in 1948 to provide a service to a fairly homogenous British population. Weller (1991) states that the NHS was geared to life-styles, family patterns, dietary habits and religious beliefs which may be neither understood by nor acceptable to many of those needing health care today. It was only in the mid-1980s that debates on community care began to focus on the importance of including ethnicity in policy. Griffiths (1988) argued that policy and action are needed to respond to the multi-racial nature of UK society. Following this, the Department of Health published a white paper in 1989, and subsequently in 1990 the NHS and Community Care Act (Department of Health, 1990) was enacted. These identified people from ethnic minorities as having particular care needs (Antony and Reed, 1990; Patients' Charter, 1991).

I write from the perspective of an occupational therapist working in a multi-disciplinary community mental health team, providing a service for people who experience severe and enduring mental health problems. The team is based in an inner-city, socially deprived area with a population of 47 000. People from ethnic minorities constitute 20–30 per cent of the population. The team is based in a "core day site" which is open from 8.00 a.m. until 6.00 p. m., Monday to Friday. Clients, once accepted by the team, can attend on a drop-in basis. Alongside this drop-in facility, structured sessions are also held. These include specialised treatment interventions, social and leisure activities. Day service activities are also held in ordinary public venues to enable people to develop their links with the community. These include sessions held at centres of adult education, women's groups, community activities and leisure pursuits.

Occupational Therapy

Occupational therapy is defined as the "science of healing by occupation" (Keilhofner, 1989). Through purposeful activities, occupational therapy helps individuals to maintain a balance of work, leisure and self-maintenance activities, to adapt to their chosen roles and to enjoy a sense of well-being (Kielhofner, 1989). The conceptual viewpoint of occupational therapy is primarily a holistic one, focusing on the individual in the context of their involvement with the physical and social world. Occupational therapy regards the human being as an open system. When the human is the system, the environment is the physical, social and cultural setting in which the system exists. It is characterised as one that cannot be reduced to the study of its parts in isolation (Kielhofner, 1989). This is an essential philosophy to perpetuate if cultural imperatives are to be truly integral to service provision. This implies that all aspects of the person need to be considered when implementing a care package, for example social, financial and educational needs. In essence this is exactly what government policy advocates, but black and ethnic minorities are not alone in their dissatisfaction with the interpretation and implementation of these policies. Occupational therapy is therefore of pivotal significance as its basic tenets are focused on this holistic system model rather than a narrower biomedical framework.

Cultural Biases in Working Practice

It is important to remember that there is as much diversity in attitudes, expectations and behaviour among minority groups in the UK as there is among the majority of indigenous white people. Rarely is culture considered in isolation from ethnicity. However, to respect cultural differences truly one must see beyond the ethnic group of an individual and know the person and the richness of their cultural heritage. We can then move towards an understanding of how illness is influenced by culture and how our interventions need to accommodate cultural sensitivities. The pitfalls of investigating culture are those of generating stereotypes rather than dissolving them. Therapists need first to analyse their own values and beliefs so as to minimise the interference with working practice (Mumford, 1994). This is part of a process of increasing empathy which must be the basis of ensuring effective social and leisure interventions. These issues are again not bounded by labels of black or white. However, cross-cultural biases do occur when any therapist neglects to consider the unique life-styles, customs and values of an individual (Chapter 2).

It is difficult for any practitioner to admit that his or her practice is discriminatory. Racism is a highly emotive issue which, when confronted, can lead to defensiveness, anger and denial. Increasing awareness and knowledge appears to be a sufficiently gentle process of challenging people's belief systems. A Community Mental Health Team increased awareness by arranging for clients to give teaching sessions on their specific religious perspectives and beliefs. They compiled fact sheets about specific religious and cultural views. These were shared with carers and the cared for (Bhui *et al.*, 1995).

A person's health beliefs may be different from those of the therapist, or symptoms may be explained in a different way. This might result in the therapist and client having different objectives, leading to non-compliance of the client and dissatisfaction on both sides (Baptiste, 1988; Krefting and Krefting, 1991). Occupational therapists aim to develop skills which enable a person to function at an optimum level, thus becoming as independent as possible. Macdonald and Rowe (1995) suggest that concepts related to personal independence/autonomy were linked to Western middle-class values. In many situations it may be better to consider the task and roles within the client's family. For example, for people with origins in the Indian subcontinent, the beliefs, family structure and respect for elders are more important than personal independence (Khamisha, 1997). Sickness and misfortune are a shared commodity; hence a solution requires a shared resolution. An individualistic intervention would lead to discord between client, family and therapists.

Within the context of a multi-disciplinary team, Bhui *et al.* (1995) found that cultural issues were not routinely included within the assessment and review system. It is important to identify, at the first point of contact with the team, a person's first language, their linguistic competence for emotional matters, dialect interference, religion and cultural identity. Attention should be paid to patterns of religious activity and cultural behaviour which interact with the presentation of and solutions to mental ill-health, or may affect the prognosis of rehabilitation (Bhui, 1994; Neeleman and Lewis, 1994). To tackle these issues within our team, a series of sensitive questions was compiled to ensure a culturally sensitive multi-disciplinary assessment. Teaching sessions and workshops were held to ensure that the team was familiar with using this tool, which aimed to obtain religious and cultural information and its implications in treatment. To ensure that a person's cultural identity continued to be included in the review of care packages, structured headings were introduced into the care programme forms: religion and culture. We adopted a variety of other strategies (Table 10.1).

Table 10.1 Action plan.

Staff training/education	User-led teaching sessions describing their specific religious perspective. Engaging in cross-cultural educational activities. Compiling fact sheets on cultural views.
Clinical practice – reducing biases	Use of culturally specific assessments and incorporating issues in review format. Use of interpreters, client-centred goal-setting, family involvement in treatment process.
Establishing links with the voluntary services	A member of staff from statutory service to be nominated as a link person to develop long-term relationship.
Developing access to complementary therapies	Carrying out a survey on users' views. Introduce a trial of therapies to service. Provide education.
Spirituality/religion	A chaplain attending the "core day site" to meet clients and provide teaching sessions for staff, including a presentation of a spirituality assessment tool. Establishing a church liaison group in local area.
Culturally sensitive day care	Displaying art and educational material; celebrating religious and cultural events; cooking multi-cultural meals; having a cultural awareness group; arranging visits to culture-specific events and places; organising cultural evenings/entertainment.

It is important that occupational therapists consider functional assessments in the context of culture so that cultural biases are avoided. These ensure accurate assessments and effective treatment planning. The Assessment of Motor and Process Skills (AMPS) is one example of such an attempt (Goldman and Fisher, 1997). It was developed for use as a cross-cultural functional assessment. Motor and process skills are fundamental to performing activities of daily living. AMPS was designed to be free from cross-cultural bias and therefore retain the same meaning when applied across cultural groups. It is a multi-layered tool which allows occupational therapists to assess global task performance and the quality of motor and process skills (Goldman and Fisher, 1997).

Links with the Voluntary Services

It is important that statutory services try to provide an all-inclusive service that accommodates the diverse cultural needs of the population it serves. The voluntary sector has largely emerged in response to this lack of such a culturally sensitive service. It is beneficial for the individuals to receive effective input from an organisation that has specialist understanding and knowledge about their ethnic background. If statutory services do not adapt, then they fail in service provision for all. It is usually presumed that this culturally sensitive intervention can be provided effectively only by people of the same ethnic origin. Ethnic matching appears to be a response to the crisis of ethnic minority service provision. However, if statutory sector workers take their responsibilities seriously, then they also should be in a position to provide effective services. How they do this seems to be the crucial question. Working with voluntary agencies is a first essential step. The voluntary sector plays an important role in this area of unmet need. Unfortunately links between the statutory and voluntary sectors are notoriously poor (Bhui *et al.*, 1995). Fears of domination and coercion that compromise principles of independent care appear to be barriers to collaboration. Staff involved in a steering group identified that better working relationships with the voluntary services would improve the access and referral process and also enable staff to obtain ideas and guidance around their working practice. It was acknowledged that this would take a long time to develop, and considered important to have one particular link person to work with each agency, to try to develop trust and effective working relationships. Even with careful planning and staff training, such plans can be disrupted by the high staff turnover that is prevalent in most inner-city mental health teams.

Developing Access to Complementary Therapies

Evidence-based practice is the current buzz word in health care. As therapists we are constantly expected to demonstrate the efficacy of the interventions we use (Culshaw, 1995). Sackett *et al.* (1996) have defined evidence-based medicine as, *"the conscientious, explicit and judicious use of current best evidence in making decisions about the care of individual patients"* (p. 470). However, the concern held about evidence-based practice is that practice will become prescriptive, lack creativity and limit a needs-led approach. It could lead to cost-cutting and "cook book practice" (Sackett *et al.*, 1996). Modern medicine has lost sight not only of the person as a human being but also of the broader environmental and socio-political context in which illness occurs. This paternalistic model of health care clashes with the voice of the user movement. People are moving away from dependence on experts and specialists, towards demanding more consumer involvement and self-reliance.

The number of people in the UK seeking complementary therapies has significantly increased in recent years. This reflects the situation in Europe, where a consumer survey showed that the popularity of complementary therapies is growing rapidly (Norton, 1995). Despite their increasing popularity, most alternative treatments are not accepted by scientific medicine. It is widely acknowledged that research investigating the effectiveness and outcomes of complementary therapies is limited, but many scientific medicines have not been rigorously evaluated either (Gutzwiller and Chrzanowski, 1986). The Mental Health Foundation report (Raleigh, 1995) recommends alternative models of care and treatment, and this is especially pertinent for some ethnic groups. I implemented a local action research project within the community mental health service to determine service users' views about the use of complementary therapies (Foulds, 1995). The demand for alternative treatments such as natural supplements, exercise and postural therapy, and physical treatments such as aromatherapy, was significantly higher among people from ethnic groups. As a result of this positive outcome, a trial of herbal treatments was introduced as part of a portfolio of alternative therapies: yoga, aromatherapy and reflexology. The queues of severely mentally ill men and women were witness to the popularity of these interventions. There was a high rate of user satisfaction:

> *It helps me to release tension.*
>
> *I feel as if my problems have been taken away.*

All of our projects were challenging as they involved a change of practice; we therefore encountered a considerable number of obstacles. The most significant hurdle was staff attitudes. It became apparent that staff required training and education around the benefits of such treatments (Foulds, 1995). Many clients self-referred, which may reflect the lack of support from staff. Randomised controlled trials are essential if we are to provide empirical evidence of the clinical efficacy, but outcome measures are not easily defined, as the healing effect of alternative therapies and the sense of well-being they introduce may not be quantifiable using currently available measures. So, do we deny our clients the one intervention which they queue up for?

The cost of providing these services might be raised as an added limitation. We introduced these therapies on the day site, not to become lifetime providers, but as an introduction for our service users; if they valued the intervention we encouraged them to proceed to find similar courses and intervention in public service settings. Hence, managers at the day site actually regard this as an effective cost-saving exercise through which our clients become motivated to seek out services which are not funded or provided by health and social services.

Spirituality/Religion

The spiritual dimension has close associations with culture. It is described and interpreted as the need for meaning, purpose and fulfilment in life (Ross, 1995). This definition refers to the totality of the person encompassing body, mind and spirit. It does not simply mean religion. It describes a belief that relates a person to the world, giving meaning to existence. It could refer to religion but could also include philosophical, psychological, sociological and political viewpoints. The role of religious or spiritual beliefs is often ignored when implementing community mental health care packages (see Chapter 5). Where religious and cultural issues do get mentioned, it is usually in connection with developing services for black and ethnic minority groups. This is confirmed by a study which found that a higher proportion of African-Caribbean people held a religious or spiritual belief than the white people. However, this same survey also suggested that those spiritual beliefs can be profoundly important for many other people (Mental Health Foundation, 1997), whether they regard themselves as religious or not.

Spiritual well-being has been defined as behavioural expressions of spiritual health, for example feeling life is a positive experience and feeling fulfilled and satisfied with life (Sims, 1994). O'Brien (1982) states that the need for spiritual integrity is a basic human need. Spiritual distress is defined as a "disruption in the life principle that pervades a person's entire being and that integrates and transcends one's biological and psychological nature" (Neal and Rodemich, 1991). This is a diagnosis that is recognised by the North American Nursing Diagnosis Association. A variety of behaviours has been associated with this condition, e.g. crying, withdrawal, preoccupation, anxiety, hostility or apathy, which could easily be mistaken for clinical depression. French psychiatrists believe in the concept of existential crisis, which is not treated with medicine. The concept of spiritual crisis does not, however, enter into DSM or ICD categories and is likely to be ignored by the more biomedical models of treatment.

Spiritual distress can occur when people experience extreme challenges in life; severe and chronic illness and its associated disabilities are indeed challenges to the integrity of the self. A diagnosis of mental illness is more than likely to induce spiritual questioning as a search for meaning. A person's illness narrative attempts to make sense of their experience of distress; people derive some satisfaction from being able to make sense of their misfortune in spiritual as well as medical and scientific terms. The stigma attached to mental illness and the exclusion from many hoped-for sources of future gratification compounds this spiritual trauma. People ask the question: "Why did this happen to me?" Is this a spiritual or a medical issue?

Much has been written about the ridicule of talking about disease as either a physical or psychological problem. Sims (1994) notes that psychiatrists are guilty of excluding spiritual considerations in their mental state assessments. The Royal College of Psychiatrists has recognised this need by stating "the need to emphasise the physical, mental and spiritual aspects in healing in the training of doctors in general and psychiatry in particular" (Kehoe *et al.*, 1992). Believing in a faith can alleviate and possibly prevent mental health problems. In a British epidemiological study, churchgoing and following a religion were found to be protective factors from vulnerability to depression (Brown and Prudo, 1981). Similarly, a 12-year review of the *American Journal of Psychiatry* and the *Archives of General Psychiatry* found that 72 per cent of religious commitments were beneficial to mental health (Larson *et al.*, 1992).

Many mental health service users value the role of the Church. A study identified that people experiencing mental health problems in the community saw the Church as the most supportive group apart from their friends. The majority of people regarded contact with religious groups as being positive. People mentioned the personal and social side of their experience, as well as their religious ones (Rose, 1996). In a local action research project we found that 74 per cent of people engaged in a community mental health service held the belief that spiritual approaches helped them cope with their mental health problems. As a result of this, the community mental health team arranged for a visiting chaplain to attend the day site. As well as establishing relationships with the clients, teaching sessions were held on spirituality, including a presentation of a spirituality assessment tool. A resource file was developed to contain information on local churches and facilities for staff and clients' use (Foulds, 1995). The team also established regular meetings with members of the local churches to discuss and feed back on any relevant issues; this was named the "Church Liaison Group". Similar measures could be taken by any mental health team where their population is predominantly of a particular religious minority. Thus although most of our African and Caribbean users were Christian, similar linkages with other religious groups should be explored.

Culturally Sensitive Day Services

Alongside the growth of the user movement, an increasing number of government initiatives emphasise the important role that service users and carers have in determining the services they receive. It is only recently that there has been a real impact on service development. Ethnic minorities are dissatisfied with existing services and seem to want little to do with statutory services. It is known that African and Caribbean groups are under-represented in user organisations and in research or collaborative initiatives with providers. Mental health service users indicate that they want: a home, enough money to live on, a meaningful day, support and friends, relief from suffering, expert specialists. Ethnic minorities fare worse on all socio-demographic indicators and hence their social and economic security is as much a part of their distress as is the specific treatment with medication. Indeed, evidence has suggested that meeting these needs has led to improved mental states (Strathdee *et al.*, 1997).

People want to engage in activities that are "useful, interesting and part of local mainstream community living" (Strathdee *et al.*, 1997). Thus, any activities provided should reflect the life of the community. When planning day services, issues such as race, culture, gender, age and religion must be considered from inception. Day care activities are poorly used by young black men (Bhui *et al.*, 1995). The specific needs of absent groups are difficult to identify, yet it remains the responsibility of our services to discover their needs by engendering trust and expressing concern about their plight if they remain isolated from appropriate care. Services tend not to acknowledge people's ethnic identity in a positive manner. It is important that ethnic identity is actively acknowledged and nurtured in policy and procedures of day care services (Table 10.1).

Conclusion

Differing ethnicity and culture creates a challenge for planning and providing culturally relevant services. This chapter describes achievements as well as barriers. Adapting to cultural needs is part of the philosophy of occupational therapy. To provide an equitable service to all those using the services, it is important that the therapist gains awareness about the beliefs, traditions, roles and life-styles of the individual. The therapist needs to gain an understanding of the impact of culture on the treatment process and client functioning. Therapists need to avoid the tendency to stereotype, perhaps first by challenging their own values and beliefs and then, secondly, by ensuring non-biased practice.

Perhaps the most fundamental challenge faced by professionals is that of understanding the service user's perspective. Surely, obstacles to providing a culturally sensitive service will be overcome if clinicians take the time to listen to the needs expressed by the person who is experiencing the mental illness.

References

Antony, P. and Reed, M. (1990) The Impact of the Griffiths Report. *International Journal of Health Care and Quality Assurance* **3**(3): 21–30.

Baptiste, S. (1988) Muriel Driver Memorial Lecture: Chronic pain, activity and culture. *Canadian Journal of Occupational Therapy* **55**(4): 179–184.

Bhui, K. (1994) *The relationship between religion and mental health.* University of London: MSc Thesis UMDS.

Bhui, K., Foulds, G., Baubin, F. and Dunn, L. (1995) Developing culturally sensitive psychiatric community services. *British Journal of Health Care Management* **1**(16): 817–822.

Brown, G.W. and Prudo, R. (1981) Psychiatric disorder in a rural and urban population 1: Aetiology of depression. *Psychological Medicine* **11**: 581–599.

Culshaw, H.M.S. (1995) Evidence-based practice for sale. *British Journal of Occupational Therapy* **58**(6): 233.

Department of Health (1990) *NHS and Community Care Act.* London: HMSO.

Foulds, G. (1995) *Developing Access to Complementary Therapies in a Continuing Care Setting.* London School of Economics: Unpublished document for Diploma Course – Innovation in Mental Health Work.

Goldman, S. and Fisher, A. (1997) Cross-cultural validation of assessment of motor and process skills. *British Journal of Occupational Therapy* **60**(2): 77–85.

Griffiths, R. (1988) *Community Care: An Agenda for Action.* London: HMSO.

Gutzwiller, F. and Chrzanowski, R. (1986) Technology assessment, impact on medical practice. *International Journal of Technical Assessment of Health Care* **2**: 99–106.

Jang, Y. (1995) Chinese culture and occupational therapy. *British Journal of Occupational Therapy* **58**(3): 103–114.

Kehoe, R., Moore, A. and Pearce, J. (1992) Developing training themes from H.R.H's delivery. *British Journal of Psychiatry* **160**: 569.

Khamisha, C. (1997) Cultural diversity in Glasgow: Part 1: Are we meeting the challenge. *British Journal of Occupational Therapy* **60**(1): 17–22.

Kielhofner, G. (1989) The model of human occupation. *British Journal of Occupational Therapy* **52**(6): 210–214.

Krefting, L.H. and Krefting, D.V. (1991) Culture influences on performance. In: Christinasen, C. and Baum, C. (eds) *Occupational Therapy, Overcoming Human Performance Deficits*, pp. 101–122. New Jersey: Slack.

Larson, D.D., Sherrill, K.A., Lyons, J.S. *et al.* (1992) Association between dimension of religious commitment and mental health reported in the *American Journal of Psychiatry* and the *Archives of General Psychiatry* 1978 through 1989. *American Journal of Psychiatry* **149**: 557–559.

Macdonald, R. and Rowe, N. (1995) Minority ethnic groups and occupational therapy, Part 2: transcultural occupational therapy, a curriculum for today's therapist. *British Journal of Occupational Therapy* **58**(7): 286–290.

Mental Health Foundation (1997) *Knowing Our Own Minds. A survey of how people in emotional distress take control of their lives.* London: Mental Health Foundation.

Mumford, D. (1994) Transcultural aspects of rehabilitation. In: Home, C. and Pullen, I. (eds) *Rehabilitation for Mental Health Problems. An Introductory Handbook.* Edinburgh: Churchill Livingstone.

Neal, P. and Rodemich, C. (1991) *Psychiatric Nursing Diagnosis Care Plans for DSM.111.R.* Boston: Jones Barlett.

Neeleman, J. and Lewis, G. (1994) Religious identity and comfort beliefs in 3 groups of psychiatric patients and a group of medical controls. *International Journal of Social Psychiatry* **40**(2): 124–134.

Norton, I. (1995) Complementary therapies in practice: the ethical issues. *Journal of Clinical Nursing* **4**: 343–348.

O'Brien, M.E. (1982) Religious faith and adjustment to long-term haemodialysis. *Journal of Religious Health* **21**: 68.

Patients' Charter (1991) *A Charter for Health; Raising the Standard.* London: HMSO.

Raleigh, V.S. (1995) *Mental Health in Black and Minority People; the Fundamental Facts.* London: The Mental Health Foundation.

Rose, D. (1996) *Living in the Community.* London: The Sainsbury Centre for Mental Health.

Ross, L. (1995) The spiritual dimension and its importance to patients' health, well-being and quality of life. Its application for nursing practice. *International Journal of Nursing Study* **32**(5): 457–468.

Sackett, D.L., Rosenburgh, W.M.C., Gray, J.A.M., Haynes, R.B. and Richardson, W.S. (1996) Evidence-based medicine: what it is and what it isn't. *British Medical Journal* **312**: 71–72.

Sims, A. (1994) Psyche. Spirit as well as Mind. *British Journal of Psychiatry* **165**: 441–46.

Strathdee, G., Thompson, K. and Carr, S. (1997) What service users want from mental health services. *Mental Health Service Development Skills Workbook.* London: The Sainsbury Centre for Mental Health.

Weller, B. (1991) Nursing in a multi-cultural world. *Nursing Standard* **5**: 30–32.

11

Mental Well-Being in a Multi-ethnic Society: Healing is as Important as Cure

Sonia Preddie and Karla Boyce-Awai

Introduction

The role of the Mental Health Nurse (MHN) is broad. These nurses work, for example, in acute and chronic psychiatric wards, secure wards and in the community in GP practices, day centres, rehabilitation centres and crisis intervention units. Nurses seek to provide a trusting relationship within which the conflicts and decisions faced by a patient are heard and resolved. Nurses help supervise medication and provide information about medication to patients and their families. Nurses also serve as a first point of contact for many patients who find doctors and other mental health professionals more distant and perhaps more threatening. Each of these roles requires specialist skills and we are by no means able to address all aspects of mental health nursing and its central role in the provision of mental health services.

In this chapter we describe contrasting experiences as black African-Caribbean nurses who provide mental health services to individuals from a diversity of cultures. We firstly explore the culture of an in-patient psychotherapy unit that reports limited referral of ethnic minority patients; we then discuss statutory community psychiatric and voluntary service provision, where most clients are of ethnic minority origin. In these two settings we discovered similarities and differences that sharply focused our thoughts on the challenges of effective service provision for ethnic minorities. Although we present our individual experiences from different therapeutic paradigms of psychotherapy and community psychiatric nursing, we feel strongly that the most powerful similarity of our work is in engagement, building trust with patients, feeling supported in our work, being given opportunities (including time) to learn more about our patients' cultures and beliefs systems. Our similar ethnic origins to African-Caribbean patients does not automatically give rise to a proficiency in the care of black and ethnic minority patients.

Psychotherapy Services and Building Alliances

The issue of evaluating generic psychotherapy services is a topical one; a recent comprehensive review found the therapeutic alliance and training of therapists of clear importance in a morass of other variables of undetermined impact (Roth and Fonagy, 1996). The need for a separate evaluation of the psychotherapeutic needs of people from ethnic minorities is controversial and has so far not been comprehensively evaluated. We examine a psychotherapeutic in-patient unit which is run along therapeutic community principles, taking a psychodynamic model. The staff are nurses with special skill in psychotherapeutic work; they determine much of the style of individual and group work. The clients are mainly white; an exploration of explanations for this generates more questions which require careful study and research.

1. Are referral sources (predominantly psychiatric consultants) not referring ethnic minority patients? How and why does this situation persist despite the considerable body of evidence that black and ethnic minority groups prefer and can utilise psychotherapies (Kareem and Littlewood, 1992; Wilson, 1993)?
2. Do people from ethnic minorities not want to enter into a process which requires a hospital admission?
3. Do we as a staff team offer an environment which is unattractive to ethnic minorities?

We intend to research the available literature, as well as draw on our personal experiences, to clarify these controversies.

An investigation of the poor referral rate of ethnic minority patients to the specialist ward was conducted by interviewing five referring consultants. We wished to explore their attitudes towards the ward, the criteria they employed to judge suitability for referrals and whether or not they had referred any ethnic minority patients. The specialist in-patient psychotherapy service comprises a unit of eleven beds, six of which are allocated to local residents. The localities for which local beds are purchased (Southwark and Lambeth) both have large ethnic minority populations (15–24 per cent). The other five beds are allocated for extra-contractual referrals (ECRs). The majority of the ECR referrals tend to come from Kent, Sussex, Salisbury and East Anglia – areas with considerably fewer ethnic minority patients. Nonetheless, survival of the unit necessitates such a policy, in view of the current climate in which economic viability supersedes the needs of local, at-risk, and mainly black populations.

In the investigation, it emerged that most consultants referred the following categories of patients to the ward:

*   people with personality disorders;
*   people who could not be helped in their present environment, and did not respond to drug treatment;
*   people who were fairly young;
*   people who exhibited self-destructive behaviour;

- people who were intelligent;
- people who were co-operative;
- people who were sociable;
- people with drug and alcohol related problems and eating disorders;
- people who had not been able to function outside hospital with the resources available.

However, hardly any ethnic minority referrals were being made. Why is this the case? An exploration of the research pertaining to ethnic minorities and psychiatry shows them to be presumed ineligible for the above nine categories (Cope, 1989; Farrington, 1993). Indeed the above criteria seem all to be based on value judgements and are readily susceptible to ethnocentric bias.

Psychotherapy services generally address people with personality difficulties. The process of diagnosis of personality disorder across cultural and linguistic boundaries is hazardous (Mezzich *et al.*, 1996). Not only is there a risk of labelling a person with a disorder, but the assessment of personality requires a detailed knowledge base of normative developmental experience, personality formation and its relationship with cultural variables. Such cultural variables include family size, culturally sanctioned ways of resolving developmental traumas, the nature and quality of attachment experiences and the real social context of maturation. The Reed report found that people from ethnic minorities, although over-represented in the medium secure units were under-represented in the category of psychopathic disorder (Reed, 1992). Mezzich *et al.* (1996) recently confirmed the impression that personality disorders are rarely diagnosed amongst African-Caribbean patients. There are few black and ethnic minority staff in special services set up to deal with people with psychopathic or personality disorders in the health and penal systems (NACRO, 1989, 1992; Reed, 1992).

One must question whether there is a universal categorisation of personality? Does personality vary between cultures? Psychoanalysts appear to think that people in society have similar formative experiences and derivative pathways, regardless of their cultural origin. The situation is much more complicated, and the reluctance of psychiatrists to diagnose personality disorder among ethnic minority patients might reflect this. That is, medical perceptions of cultural baselines in this category of diagnosis may be uncertain, and psychiatrists may be reluctant to make this diagnosis in different ethnic groups (see Chapter 3). There has been little attention paid to the role of race and culture in personality development (Chapter 2), although it is certainly linked inextricably with ethnic identity.

It is a common experience for community teams to work with black men who have been diagnosed with schizophrenia, but who are, at the same time, undergoing risk-assessment, as they are perceived as being "quietly" dangerous. In the absence of clear and valid reasoning leading to such referrals one can only assume that there is an inability to judge "character" across cultures as proficiently as one does within the same cultural group.

The World Health Organisation's findings of good-prognosis schizophrenia in developing countries supports the view that the social and cultural constructions of carefully diagnosed schizophrenia have a real impact on prognosis and on the treatment interventions to be offered. Personality factors which remain unexplored across cultural boundaries might mediate the differential vulnerability to disabling and chronic symptoms. Until these questions are more carefully studied the issue of psychotherapy service developments to suit the needs of ethnic minorities remains speculative and empirical. Such an omission precludes a critical analysis of effectiveness of psychological treatments among ethnic minorities, mirroring the same omission for psychopharmacological interventions (Chapter 6).

People from ethnic minorities hear about the oppressive treatment of patients and are suspicious of psychiatric services (Chapters 1 and 9). They are reluctant to engage with the services in the first place, and recent work shows that black severely mentally ill people become more dissatisfied with each subsequent admission (Leavey *et al.*, 1997; Parkman *et al.*, 1997). Hence ethnic minority patients, even if they come into contact with services, are likely to fall out of care. They complain less, however, in spite of suffering high levels of distressing social conditions (Lloyd and St Louis, 1996). There appears to be a long-standing "low visibility" strategy, developed to avert the prying eyes of potentially coercive social agencies. Perhaps this explains why black respondents give more information to black interviewers (Dohrenwend, 1966). The patient expectations of services and of health professionals is an essential but as yet unexplored area of concern. Our experience in this setting is that patients prefer their nurses to be from the same ethnic group. The establishment of trust is crucial.

Case Study I

A patient was referred to the ward recently. She came from Thailand but had lived in Hong Kong before coming to Britain. Her native language was Cantonese, and she had recently learned English to a very high standard. Her husband had died the year before she presented with a depressive episode for which she was admitted to hospital. She had been very close to him. While he was alive she did not learn to speak English and dealt mostly with the Chinese community. Now, a year later, she had been seeing her GP regularly with various physical problems including constipation and insomnia. The GP insisted on a referral to a psychiatrist, after which she was admitted to a busy and disturbed acute ward. She did not want to stay, attempted to kill herself on the ward and was eventually detained under the MHA. She was referred to the in-patient psychotherapy unit. Her reason for wanting to come to the unit was striking: she wanted to come because the ward was a cleaner and quieter environment. She was reluctant to talk in one-to-one sessions about how she felt emotionally, and how being on the ward would help her, but concentrated on how being in a more pleasant environment would help her. She was terrified of the groups as she felt that her English was not good enough and so she missed many groups. She negotiated discharge after three weeks, and resisted any follow up contact despite our persistence. A Malaysian Chinese nurse who worked on the unit felt that Chinese people did not wash their dirty linen in public, and that we should not expect the patient to want to discuss any psychological issues. The nurse said that, as a Cantonese speaker, she could not think of any words in Cantonese to describe psychological states in a public arena.

The in-patient psychotherapy unit environment appeared especially comforting as a haven; the interventions we offer, however, were clearly rejected by this woman. In some cultures, the idea of sharing problems may not be acceptable. In our experience, in some Nigerian sub-cultures a person who minds their own business is regarded as very desirable. People from other cultures may be unfamiliar with the concept of a therapeutic community. For them, treatment may mean going to a doctor who tells them what is wrong and what to do. They may find the idea of a place where they take responsibility for their own problems and try to help themselves a little unusual. In fact they may think the staff are being negligent, as the process does not fit their expectation of help/care. Patients from ethnic minorities may be in the minority on a ward. Given the other anxieties they have to deal with in coming to the unit, such as sharing very personal information in groups with complete strangers, this may prove to be too much. A young African woman who had been admitted to the ward stayed for about a week, after which she said, ". . . I can't stay here, there are no black people here".

This was a real issue for her, and it raised questions about how she viewed her black West Indian key nurse. As a member of a white European service, may be her key nurse's blackness had become invisible. The few black patients who do stay on the ward, it seems, often do not address issues of race. It seems that they attempt to blend in and become invisible, become white and deny their difference. Fanon (1967, p. 116) speaks of black people in white environments:

> I slip into corners, I remain silent, I strive for anonymity, for invisibility. Look, I will accept the lot, as long as no one notices me!

Recently an African-Caribbean patient proved to be an exception; in a group he expressed very powerfully his anger about his experiences as a black man in this society. The group's reception was mixed; some people considered that the issue was irrelevant, and that what was important was the psychological problems which brought him to the ward. A mixed-race patient in the group that day felt uncomfortable that the African-Caribbean man had expressed those views. The African-Caribbean patient came back the next day, saying that he believed that the ward could help him with some things but not others. Another British-born patient, of Bajan descent, expressed how embarrassed he felt when other black patients came to the ward. He himself presented himself as white middle class, in the way he spoke, the music he was interested in, not reggae and soul, but classical and jazz. He spoke about the embarrassment he felt for other blacks who were stupid, criminals, and had an appalling sense of dress. He described how he single-handedly intended to improve the image of blacks to whites, and the presence of other black patients sometimes spoiled this for him.

Psychological treatments that concentrate only on the internal world would argue that issues of race belong to the external world, and these issues do not play a central role in the therapeutic process. Intercultural therapists will argue that a therapeutic process that does not acknowledge a person's race, culture, gender and social values fragments that person. Certainly how individuals handle life's stressors is a focus of therapeutic work but it is very un-empathic to expect individuals to deal by themselves with racism, isolation and socio-economic hardship in a "more effective way". This alone is not an effective intervention, just a re-labelling of the problem as one belonging to the patient. The case study of Victoria in Kareem and Littlewood (1992) illustrates this point. Victoria speaks of her frustration with her white therapist, who made her feel that issues of racism were essentially her problem. When Victoria spoke about her feelings about being black, the therapist interpreted it as a projection of Victoria's inner chaos onto the outside world. Victoria found this approach very frustrating and terminated her treatment. Jaffar Kareem also suggests that most black people will admit the most traumatic feature of their personal lives is to be black in a white society. One of his patients, Joseph, said:

> We have been deprived of one of God's most precious gifts, the ability to "get Lost", the ability to be anonymous, the ability not to be noticed. You cannot share the depth of this feeling with anyone, especially if you are constantly reminded that you are an outsider, that you and your like are swamping this country, that always you have to pass a test. What can you do? (Kareem and Littlewood, 1992, p. 26).

Perhaps supervision registers, CPA meetings and risk-assessment monitoring are perceived to be similarly intrusive and recreate this tension.

Patients from ethnic minorities may find the power relationship in therapy unacceptable. It may remind them of other power imbalances in their lives, and they may not want it in therapy or in case management. These patients may see psychological treatments as a white middle class pursuit; they do not want to be seen as aspiring to such things. The lack of other black patients makes them feel as if they do not belong, and encourages premature termination of the therapeutic alliance. Black patients question the shortage of people from ethnic minorities and may come to the conclusion that a service which allows such a situation to occur does not have their best interests at heart. They believe that engaging with such a service involves the denial of a great part of themselves. Fanon (1967, p. 211) speaks of the negro as being ". . . constantly preoccupied with self evaluation and with the ego ideal".

Although this fear of judgement is true of any patient, regardless of race, for the patient from an ethnic minority there is the added reality of cultural stereotypes and assumptions made by the indigenous provider population. Ethnic minority patients may be anxious not to reinforce these, and present themselves in a negative light. They may be reluctant to show their vulnerabilities to whites, because of their treatment by whites in the historical past, which makes them suspicious and unsure. Jaffar Kareem, cited in Kareem and Littlewood (1992), speaks about how deep-seated feelings and rational thinking may not always go together. In his work in Israel, he asked his Jewish friends if they would consider therapy with a non-Jewish German. The reply was always the same, a German who was not Jewish must have been associated with the Nazis.

Community Services and Unmet Needs of Ethnic Minority Users

From research carried out on the setting up of the Fanon project, a black mental health voluntary sector day centre, it became apparent that the "colour blind" approach to service provision for the mentally ill in the community is not effective (Moodley, 1987). Individual clients have individual needs. It became apparent that particular cultural and socially distinct groups require tailored interventions. Their responses to why they did not use existing services were: "they were not for them"; "they were too white"; "they did not feel comfortable there".

Day hospitals were situated too near hospitals that held a lot of bad memories. We asked what facilities they did want? They wanted a place where they could feel a sense of belonging and which provided them with training in a range of work and living skills as well as recreational activities; they wanted a place where drugs would not be given, a service run by black workers only.

Case Study 2

Peter X is aged 37, with a two-year history of untreated schizophrenia. He was admitted to hospital under section 48 of the Mental Health Act, after exhibiting threatening behaviour towards the police in a south-east London car park. It appears that he had been psychotic for at least a year, with its aetiology not only in the break-up of a relationship and the death of his ex-wife, but also in poly-substance abuse. It appears that the patient had a history of persecutory and paranoid delusions stretching back some two to three years. Over the months prior to the offence, he had become increasingly suspicious, refusing to leave his house during daylight hours and eating only pre-packed food that he was able to prepare himself. He states he was carrying a knife with him the day before the offence to protect himself against a police conspiracy that he felt was partly responsible for his persecution.

This is an example of someone who lived in the community for two years untreated, and it was not until he committed an offence and was picked up by the police that the mental health services became involved. From his brief history it was obvious that Peter X and his family must have been under enormous stress from the recent bereavement they had suffered, but there was nowhere to go for help until it was too late. It is not being suggested that mental health services could certainly have prevented Peter X from committing his offence, but having somewhere for him to go, or for his relatives to seek advice about his changing behaviour, could have made a difference.

Making the Service more Culturally Sensitive

Listening to Users' Views

Clients believe that the "patch and fix" thinking is not a solution; the service must cater for their individual and cultural needs. They ask us as service providers to make changes which are healthy changes, with long-term co-operation, new and more equal working relationships, better working practices, and policies that acknowledge the voice of the user (Chapter 2).

The Service

There is a need for a definitive change in the way ethnic minorities are treated within the mental health system (Chapters 6, 9 and 16). The following service components need to be addressed:

- Seamless service – to prevent patients falling through the safety net.
- Effective partnerships between agencies – health, social services, housing, employment, etc.
- Clear risk assessments – with clearly identified outcome criteria.
- Redefinition of mental illness – taking into account individual cultural beliefs and values.
- Primary care-based service – assessments, medication use and counselling.
- Range of service – acute and special needs.
- Choice of service – rehabilitation and other specialist services.
- Clearly documented plans, policies and strategies – to achieve implementation.
- Training for mental health professionals – in race and culture awareness.
- Greater recognition of the role of the voluntary sector – in service provision.
- Black mental health teams – with a number of therapists working or trained in intercultural therapies.
- Information – advice facilities/crisis service.
- Rehabilitation – that positively values and encourages identification with the patients' own cultural or religious groups.
- Procedures – which ensure that those of different language skills and culture values can access service quickly and effectively.
- Personal choice – rather than coercion.

Psychiatry does not cater well for people from ethnic minorities. After all, many people from ethnic minorities came to this country to encounter a service that was established on principles and values which were not their own (Chapters 2 and 3). The criticisms often made by users include: "I could not make myself understood"; "There was no ethnic food." How can we constructively move forward on the basis of this knowledge?

Nurses' Influence on Access to Service

One of the basic principles of community-based service is that the service should be localised and accessible, comprehensive, and normalising in meeting the needs of the community. The role of GPs is most important and needs radically shaking up (Chapter 13). GPs are the first point of contact whenever ill-health occurs; they are not making the efforts to gain an awareness of their local community's needs and the way ethnic minorities express mental distress, in order to make appropriate referrals. GPs without cultural awareness will not be able to understand the patient and their problems. Commander *et al.* (1997) recently outlined non-detection by GPs to be greater amongst ethnic minority patients. Here is an opportunity for mental health nursing to make an impact on public mental health by close liaison with GPs. There is in progress some research on nurses working with all members of the primary care team; they give advice, do assessments, and educate the primary care team on mental health issues. More effective primary care intervention we hope averts crisis admissions that are so common amongst ethnic minorities. Moodley and Perkins (1991) suggested we improve routes into care: "Pathways into care need to become more appropriate to the needs of ethnic minorities, . . . neither too controlling nor too neglectful." They recommend that gatekeepers (i.e. GPs, social workers, nurses, police, etc.) should be trained in issues related to racism and culture. As the critical point of access to services varies by ethnic and cultural group, so the point of intervention for ethnic minorities might be different depending on their particular trust in the range of agencies that work with them.

At present there are ten nurses in the team, and three are from ethnic minorities. In the last three years, of the six doctors who have worked on the ward, one has been from an ethnic minority. Perhaps this situation conveys a message to potential service users from ethnic minorities. It must be stressed also that the token and unsupported involvement of black nurses devalues them and does not help in the long run. The danger of this in working in a multi-racial environment is that nurses from ethnic minorities may become marginalised, responsible for all ethnic minority problems, removing the onus on white nurses for taking any responsibility for multi-cultural work. The under-resourced and poorly understood task of working with ethnic minorities becomes the responsibility of the ethnic minority nurse; this arises not because of his or her skill or that he/she is the person who might engage a reluctant patient through trust, but in many instances by default because of their ethnicity. Such nurses find themselves in a position of having to take sole responsibility for failures of intervention and feel unsupported and alienated.

Conflicts of Being a Black Nurse in a White Organisation

In addition to these issues, the nurse from an ethnic minority will have to accept a certain amount of ambivalence from the ethnic minority service user. The nurse is an employee of a service that the user has historically distrusted. Service users from ethnic minorities may have greater expectations of an ethnic minority nurse; thus the nurse falls short of the perfect and idealised carer that the user expects. An ethnic minority nurse may well feel a sense of identity with ethnic minority service users, but this should not always be assumed. Generational modification of ethnic and cultural identity defies the notion that skin colour or ethnic matching is always helpful. The nurse may be perceived as having a life-style or status that is far removed from that of the user. Additionally, the internalising of negative expectations of racism means that the ethnic minority service user may feel that the nurse from an ethnic minority is not able to provide as good a service as a white nurse. What needs to be understood is that, as black professionals, we do not live all our lives in a white-dominated environment. We work within a white-dominated NHS with white colleagues, and return each day to our black lives and communities which have a different set of rules and expectations. We deal constantly with conflicts and stress, trying to remember and use appropriate behaviours at the right time and place. This cultural duality, along with a bilingual conceptualisation of our worlds, affects each person from an ethnic minority group uniquely.

Nurses who work with patients from ethnic minorities need to be aware of the issues. It is important to address cultural differences and not to deny their existence, to allow the exploration of any conflicts that arise relating to the mixed-race therapeutic relationship. It is important for all nurses to be aware of their feelings towards all cultures and ethnic groups; racist fears, wishes or assumptions may be leading to mis-perception, oppression, stereotyping or neglect of service users. White nurses need to accept that they may be mistrusted, placated, feared, ignored, incompletely confided in, or misinformed, and that these responses are rational products of people's experiences of racism. When nurses are unsure about cultural factors, it is important to use available resources to clarify the situation, that is consult members of staff from the same culture, the patient, the patient's family and other specialised agencies.

Conclusions

The current crisis in psychiatry, especially around the issue of race, will continue to grow as Britain has to face the fact that black immigrants and their descendants are making a huge demand on the profession. This demand will continue to increase as the minority population becomes more visible and numerous. Organisational politics often dominate the adoption and implementation of policies. Such an approach perpetuates neglect of ethnic minorities' health care needs.

References

Commander, M.J., Sashidharan, S.P., Odell, S.M. and Surtees, P.G. (1997) Access to mental health care in an inner city health district. 1: Pathways into and within specialist psychiatric services. *British Journal of Psychiatry* **170**: 312–316.

Cope, R. (1989) The compulsory detention of Afro-Caribbeans under the Mental Health Act. *New Community* **15**(3): 343–356.

Dohrenwend (1966), cited in Kareem and Littlewood (1992).

Fanon, F. (1967) *Black Skin, White Masks.* UK: Pluto Classic.

Farrington, A. (1993) Transcultural psychiatry, ethnic minorities and marginalization. *British Journal of Nursing* **2**(16): 805–809.

Kareem, J. and Littlewood, R. (1992) *Intercultural Therapy.* Oxford: Blackwell Science.

Leavey, D. (1997) First onset psychotic illness: patients' and relatives' satisfaction with services. *British Journal of Psychiatry* **170**: 53–57.

Lloyd, K. and St Louis, L. (1996) Common mental disorders among Africans and Caribbeans. In: *Ethnicity: An Agenda for Mental Health.* London: Gaskell.

Mezzich, J.E., Kleinman, A., Fabrega, H. and Parron, D.L. (1996) *Culture and Psychiatric Diagnosis. A DSM–IV perspective.* Washington, DC: American Psychiatric Association.

Moodley, P. (1987) The Fanon Project. *Bulletin of the Royal College of Psychiatrists* **11**: 417–418.

Moodley, P. and Perkins, R. (1991) Routes to psychiatric inpatient care in an inner London borough. *Social Psychiatry and Psychiatric Epidemiology* **26**: 47–51.

NACRO (1989) *Race and Criminal Justice. A Way Forward.* London: National Association for the Care and Resettlement of Offenders.

NACRO (1992) *Black People Working in the Criminal Justice System.* London: National Association for the Care and Resettlement of Offenders.

Parkman, S., Davies, S., Leese, M. *et al.* (1997) Ethnic differences in satisfaction with mental health services among representative people with psychosis in south London. PRISM study 4. *British Journal of Psychiatry* **171**: 260–264.

Reed, J. (1992) *Department of Health and the Home Office, Review of Health and Social Services for Mentally Disordered Offenders and Others Requiring Similar Services: Final Summary Report,* p. 3. London: DoH.

Roth, A. and Fonagy, P. (1996) *What Works and for Whom. A critical review of psychotherapy research.* New York: The Guilford Press.

Wilson, M. (1993) *Britain's Black Communities.* NHS Management Executive. Leeds: Mental Health Task Force and London: King's Fund Centre.

12

Clinical Psychology

Zenobia Nadirshaw

Introduction

This chapter discusses the views of myself and a small group of key informants who have had personal and professional experience of the nature and extent of racism and inequality issues within the study and practice of clinical psychology. It would be beyond the scope of this chapter to discuss fully the impact that inequality, injustice and disadvantage has on black and minority ethnic people; these effects are mediated through racism and the dynamics of inter-personal and organisational power. Thankfully, the more extreme, overt forms of racism as seen in the biologically based theories of the early British and American psychologists are gone, but prejudice and racism do exist within the profession. In fact, more and more people are beginning to understand that issues such as fairness, equality, equity and racism are not the result of neutral, objective and dispassionate intentions but that they are influenced by the professional's experiences and vested interest to maintain the status quo. There is unequivocal agreement that psychology has always been affected by racism of the wider society (Milner, 1990; Howitt and Owusu-Bempah, 1994). The discipline of psychology does not operate in a social, political and historical vacuum; on the contrary, it is influenced by, and in turn influences, society in a reflexive way.

Newnes (personal communication) charts the history of British clinical psychology from its foundations in medicine and religion, most notably in the psychiatry and pastoral care of the 19th century. Other commentators trace its origin to the foundation of psychology as a profession and its subsequent rise to academic prominence in the first half of this century. This route links psychology with psychiatry, the establishment of the NHS in 1948, and the significance of the psychometric school (Burton and Kagan, personal communication; Pilgrim, 1989). Clinical psychology became a separate entity within the British Psychological Society in 1958 – setting itself apart from the academic and philosophical value base of earlier days. However, the roots of clinical psychology need to be considered in conjunction with its relationship with psychiatry. Although it is a common assumption that clinical psychology and psychiatry are different and opposed, both the history and current practice suggest a mutual dependency, particularly in the context of psychiatry's varied roles within the mental health institutional setting. Clinical psychology, through its mental testing, has given psychiatry a scientific gloss, thereby acting as a supplementary profession.

Clinical psychologists, like their psychiatrist colleagues, are now funda-mental to the organisation of mental health services. They are now in a position to influence the public at large and other key decision-makers. Institutions are set up with structures and mechanisms to transfer the principle of caring into the effective provision of services. Inherent to understanding the process of setting up and co-ordinating services is the discharge of power by those who are responsible for planning and "programming" the institutions. They can determine the ethos and ideo-logical framework of the institutions, design policies and procedures and practices, delegate duties and responsibilities, determine the content and allocation of resources, define criteria for need, selection, recruitment and prioritisation.

This power, it seems, is not being used to care for black and minority ethnic communities. The under-represented are pressurised to conform to the norms, values and aspirations of the majority; individuals have to fit into major systems and institutions designed by and for white people. The effect is to continue to oppress and disadvantage the black and minority ethnic communities of Britain. Clinical psychology, like other disciplines within the mental health setting, appears to be committed to the growth of its own power and status rather than the appropriate care of the individual.

The common definition of psychology – the scientific study of behaviour and experience – appears to refer to the behaviour and experiences of a select group of people. The training values, knowledge and "technology" are still rooted in Western psychological science and minimally informed by local cultural and psychological knowledge. Inherent in this way of thinking is that one must aspire to the "normal". This presupposes that the current values held by mainstream British society are worth aspiring to, and that these values are pertinent, appropriate and relevant to all indivi-duals. In addition, concepts of normality and health in a psychologically well-adjusted person are judged against a Eurocentric perspective and background. Middle-class values dominate most of these perspectives and understanding. The teaching courses, the academic debates and dis-cussions, and the applied practice of psychology appear to be offering a single perspective on the way the world works.

Eurocentric theories, which define what is normal, implicitly, therefore, define everything else as "odd", "bizarre" or "different". It appears that value is conferred to people who look, behave and perform within an established norm. The pressures to fit people into British society's dominant cultural norms and value systems and to relinquish their "differ-entness" seem to blunt psychologists' moral sensibility to serve all sections of British society. Psychological needs of black and minority ethnic com-munities cannot be readily conceptualised in accordance with a standard service provision and delivery formula (Alladin, 1992; Nadirshaw, 1997). Psychologists have to learn to work with individuals and groups who hold unfamiliar symbolic systems, different world views, expectations and values (MacCarthy, 1988). Until such learning takes place, the psychological needs of black and minority ethnic people continue to run the risk of being ignored and devalued. Papers on ethnic minority and psychological topics are emerging gradually at the British Psychological Society's annual conferences (BPS, 1997), but the general lack of knowledge and inadequate research on the needs of minority ethnic and black communities continue to hinder the systematic provision of a comprehensive mental health service which has sound empirical foundations.

Psychology and psychologists, wittingly or unwittingly, remain part of the problem of racism, theorising about the issue of racism, "difference" at an intra-psychic level and to the exclusion of inter-group, ideological and social-structural factors. The Department of Health has funded an action research project outlining general issues for clinical psychology and minority ethnic communities (Nadirshaw, 1997), but the development of research paradigms and theories about the psychology of black people in multi-racial Britain is still urgently needed. The phenomenon of Euro-centricism, viewing mental health and ill-health with reference to norms of white cultures, the emergence of a new racism which replaces biology with culture, and inferiority with difference, continues to pathologise black people's experiences and to miss the point of the contemporary problem.

The Department of Health Supported Project

This project was undertaken to:

1. ascertain the views of black and minority ethnic users of mental health and clinical psychology services;
2. determine the extent to which practitioners and heads of psychology services were meeting the psychological needs of black and minority ethnic groups in their localities;
3. identify the future role and function of clinical psychologists;
4. guide future clinical practice and service delivery as recommended by the black and minority ethnic voluntary sector.

Sixty-five service users were interviewed, the majority from the London area. Fifty-two users of a total sample of sixty-five had had no contact or experience with clinical psychologists, and had no knowledge of the role, skill and functions of a clinical psychologist working in the mental health setting. In addition, a second group of twenty-three workers from the black voluntary sector were interviewed. Although some results are still out-standing, the overall findings offer no surprises. The general barriers preventing access to psychological services, as identified by both groups were:

*   Lack of awareness of the existence of the service.
*   Lack of information about the role of clinical psychologists within the team.
*   No information about the service (including lack of translated materials).
*   Eurocentricity of the service.

- Suspiciousness of the service and fear of being misunderstood by white psychologists.
- "Inaccessibility to psychological care".
- Length of waiting list.
- View that clinical psychology was set up for white middle-class people.

Service Development and Professional Practice

At the heart of every service is a professional ethos and ideology. This author believes that the professional's ideology by far outweighs other service-based determinants of effective psychological care for black and ethnic minority people. Certainly there are organisational challenges; these will be discussed briefly. I then intend to project a vision of how the profession of psychology can and must change if comprehensive and culturally competent mental health services are ever to be realised.

Organisational Change

The NHS has developed and refined its approach to equal opportunity by providing guidelines on issues about equal opportunity, fair recruitment, selection and overall service delivery (Chandra, 1996). Special attention has been given to needs of black and minority ethnic people. In keeping with the equal opportunity policy and practice, the British Psychological Society and its subsystems have an equal opportunity framework to address these issues (BPS, 1988, 1991). The Standing Committee for the Promotion of Equal Opportunity (SCPOE), which is directly accountable to the Council, and the Division of Clinical Psychology's "Special Interest Group in Race and Culture in Clinical Psychology" have been established. Whilst better practice has arisen from the acceptance of a wide remit of equal opportunity policy and practice, I contend that further prioritisation of black and minority ethnic people's needs is justified.

Acknowledging a multi-racial, multi-ethnic perspective alone will not suffice to challenge oppression, disadvantage and the institutional structures that put black and minority ethnic people at a disadvantage. An organisational gloss of multi-cultural initiatives obscures racist ideologies within its structures and further disguises the problem. The issue of racism must be explicitly acknowledged within the profession, as well as within the organisations that are charged with the provision of effective services for black and minority ethnic people (Alladin, 1992; Husband, 1992); just as important as this are the issues of gender and class which compound the disadvantage faced by black and ethnic minority peoples (Cline and Lunt, 1990; Williams and Watson, 1991; Shams, 1995). Culturally competent services cannot emerge from an ideology unless their operation addresses managerial change, professional clinical competence, knowledge and skills.

The British Psychological Society: An Organisational and Paradigm Shift?

The British Psychological Society needs to experience a paradigm shift – from one in which the issues of race, culture and racism are handled as if they are separate from anti-racism in the community at large, to one where they are integrated into the Society's mainstream agenda (Table 12.1). Services treat black and minority ethnic multi-racial communities as if they were homogeneous rather than acknowledging the extensive diversity that exists within and between these communities.

The author is aware that there is no single prescription for achieving these paradigm shifts. Since the production of the 1988 BPS report on *The Future of Psychological Sciences*, which recognised the multi-ethnic, multi-racial nature of Britain, the Society and the Division of Clinical Psychology have shown a willingness to tackle such issues. However, willingness has to move on from rhetoric into the world of action.

The following factors are necessary:

1. **Board level commitment and accountability.** This could take the form of a council member taking a lead on these issues, becoming a "product champion", driving these issues forward and ensuring that they do not fall off the Council's agenda. Assistance from the Society's Standing Committee for the Promotion of Equal Opportunities, and the Division of Clinical Psychology's Special Interest Group in Race and Culture in Clinical Psychology, would be of benefit to this person.
2. **Executive team leadership.** Visible leadership in the Society's sub-systems as well as in the main central office would encourage staff to

Table 12.1 A paradigm shift for the British Psychological Society.

From	To
Consultation with a representative of a notional single community.	Action with representatives of the different communities.
Providing Eurocentric models of mental health care.	Providing culturally and racially competent services.
Consideration of employment practice and service delivery.	Integration of staffing issues and provision of appropriate psychological care which is directly related to issues of equity, fairness and effectiveness to vulnerable people.
Treating black people as a problem.	Recognising their appropriate treatment as part of the overall solution to the Society's strategic plan and organisational objectives (Lunt, 1997).

integrate these issues into their work. A key senior manager could be given the responsibility of developing a coherent and effective strategy (including an implementation plan).

3. **Public participation.** Psychological policy, practice and research have to be informed by views of users and recipients of services and governed by the principles of equality, anti-discrimination and anti-racist practice. It is not good enough to rest on our role as "experts".

4. **Professionals, practitioners and teachers** have a duty to be open and accountable, to enable clients to understand the role and function of psychology and to engage in an informed manner in decision-making (Richardson, 1996).

5. **Commitment to action following consultation.** The BPS organisation has to move with the changing nature of work and service delivery. It is important to shift the firmly grounded status quo, to reveal the language of exclusion and segregation which is hiding behind the language of inclusion and elitism.

Service Developments through Teaching and Training

Training of future clinical psychologists in the subjects of cultural diversity, difference, equality and anti-racism is crucial for the role of the profession within the caring/helping world. Presently psychology students are poorly informed about such issues (Patel, personal communication). Our courses still appear to offer a single perspective, promulgating a view that there is one model in the way the world works. Textbooks of psychology continue to influence such ways of thinking (Owusu-Bempah and Howitt, 1995). Eurocentric theories define what is "normal" implicitly and define everything else as "odd", "bizarre" or indeed "non-existent". "Difference" and "diversity" become a source of confusion and destructive conflict rather than a source of learning.

Following a plea made by the author on race, culture and ethnic issues in clinical psychology training (Nadirshaw, 1993) changes have begun to creep into the existing teaching curriculum, but the new content is *ad hoc*, weak and disjointed. Psychologists must tackle racial prejudice and racism on the one hand, whilst addressing the racism of psychology on the other hand. *Ad hoc*, unco-ordinated attempts by individual psychologists, or a small group of psychologists, must make way for a more comprehensive understanding of racism at all levels within the main professional body and its different educational establishments. Lessons could be learnt from our social work colleagues in this context (CCETSW, 1991a, 1991b). Clear strategic direction needs to be provided to the accreditation and validation team and to the Committee for Training in Clinical Psychology. Clear criteria for judging courses on issues of race, culture, ethnicity and diversity must be defined and provided. Teachers, trainers, organisers of courses and curriculum and the different modules must show evidence of how they are preparing students to work within a multi-racial context, show how their students are meeting the psychological needs of black and minority ethnic communities and how their courses are organised to manage and work through the "difference" and diversity in a constructive manner.

Ideally, a long-term strategy needs to be developed to look at the short-fall in the number of clinical psychologists within the mental health setting who come from the black and minority ethnic communities of Britain. The subject matter and the content of clinical psychology must be made more attractive to students in schools and at undergraduate level. Senior black and minority ethnic psychologists could act as mentors and appropriate role models to students. Training courses could be advertised in the ethnic media. The Divisions of Clinical Psychology and Counselling Psychology could provide further details about the prerequisite requirements for specialised training with clearer expectations and definition of "relevant experience". They could validate work experience with the black and minority ethnic voluntary sector as meaningful work, as well as provide guidance on producing a well structured and typed application form for the Clearing House.

Validation and Accreditation

Systems of validation and accreditation must seek to do the following:

1. Identify the statutory/mandatory requirements for the preparation of students to work in a multi-racial context. This could include the development of a value-base unit which details the criteria, principles, elements of competence, and a clear interpretation of better and responsible practice. Supervisors must be clear about their role supervising students in such topics, and continuous professional development activities should incorporate the topics of "difference", working with diversity, equality and anti-racism principles. For too long students of psychology have been admonished for not raising these issues, although the responsibility for allowing them to remain at the margins of mainstream teaching lies with academic departments and individual colleagues.

2. Enforce the following general learning outcomes for students of clinical psychology:

    - To be aware of the bias in service provision and service delivery issues based on core assumptions about the profession.
    - To understand the history of clinical psychology and to re-visit the value base against which the work of clinical psychology can best be understood [patients rights, consent to treatment/effects of psychotropic medication, balancing the personal and political, addressing inequalities based on power and domination (Newnes and MacLachlan, 1996)].

- To have a better understanding of the barriers to psychology service as experienced by black and minority ethnic people with the mental health setting as a result of:

  (a) lack of information about available services;
  (b) suspiciousness and fear related to the use of ethnocentric psychology models which may be little meaning and impact on the black and minority ethnic people's lives;
  (c) imbalance in power relationships between the helper and the helped.

- To understand the role and responsibility of psychology services in developing appropriate and culturally-competent models of service to black and minority ethnic clients by relocating the problem from the individual to the socio-economic and socio-political nature of psychological problems.

- To understand the psychologists role as an "agent of change" in the provision and delivery of services (Webster, 1996); for example, networking with the black voluntary sector, the primary care teams, Patient's Council, use of legislation and government Acts like the Patients' Charter, Disability Discrimination Act, Race Relations Act, etc.

- To be aware of a variety of ways in which a sensitive, anti-racist perspective can be incorporated into all aspects of service delivery.

- To develop a more pluralistic approach which better reflects the psychological reality for all sections of British society, and to re-focus from the scientific to the personal framework of clinical psychology. In other words, to achieve objectivity while at the same time acknowledging and working through the powerful impact and effects of attitudes, labelling, beliefs and value systems from a white, middle class, eurocentric position.

- To understand the limitations of the current theoretical frameworks for practice and academic research which continue to follow a narrow universalist ("etic") approach, despite its limitations against the relativist ("emic") approach.

3. Ensure on-going audit of the mainstreaming of equality and anti-racist principles within the teaching curricula. Senior members of the academic teaching institutions should be charged with this responsibility. Evidence should be available of students undertaking individual or group work with clients from black and minority ethnic communities, with satisfactory supervision from trained supervisors. Steps should be taken by academic and teaching departments to increase the number of students and staff from black and ethnic minority groups (Bender and Richardson, 1990; Boyle *et al.*, 1993).

Service Provision and Service Planning

There is an urgent need within the psychology services for psycho-therapeutic and counselling for people with mental health problems who are culturally different (Nadirshaw, 1993). The colour-blind approach of "treating everyone in the same manner" overlooks the need to treat minority ethnic people with mental health problems differently and equally. Clinical psychology service providers bear the same professional responsibility for the minority ethnic community, which they are currently failing, as they do with the indigenous community. They must develop a better understanding of why factors such as race and socio-economic status unfairly disadvantage these groups. It is widely acknowledged, for example, that members of such groups are more likely to receive physical therapies and less access to talking therapies.

The 1996 Review of Strategic Policy on NHS Psychotherapy Services found that nearly half of the health authorities surveyed reported purchasing some form of psychological therapies from non-NHS agencies. The latter are often not-for-profit therapy services or charities which respond to the needs of particular groups (women, black and minority ethnic groups, gay and lesbian people). This evidence supports the author's findings (Nadirshaw, in press) that black and minority ethnic groups, like other vulnerable, disempowered groups in society, are underserved by psychological therapies. There is a common perception amongst existing psychological and counselling therapy services that members of particular South Asian communities rarely suffer from mental health problems (Nadirshaw, 1992). Stereotyped views like: "keeping it in-house", "they care for their own", "they are more psychologically robust" than the indigenous population, "move for one to somatisation" continue to reinforce the widespread belief that minority ethnic communities do not need, or do not want to use, such services. Experiences of mental health professionals (including clinical psychologists) reveal the high rate of emotional distress within these communities (Goodwin and Power, 1986; MacCarthy and Craissati, 1989; Belliapa, 1991). In fact, some psychology departments are creating part-time posts specifically to cater and provide for the psychological needs of the minority population in their local catchment area. Some projects initiated by clinical psychologists with lead responsibility already exist (Holland, personal communication; Mahtani and Marks, 1994) but they are very few and far between. Issues such as accessibility, client's choice of therapy and therapist, expectations of therapeutic goals, equity of psychological therapies across locations, efficacy of a particular therapeutic approach over another, and demonstration of a commitment to evidence-based practice in the use of psychological/counselling therapies are some of the considerations that need to be addressed within departments of psychology, counselling psychology and psychotherapy.

Despite the immense scientific growth and progress made within the field of behavioural/cognitive therapy and its application to different client populations (Kasvikis, 1995), research is needed on the best methods of delivery to black and minority ethnic client groups. Equity of service provision could be monitored by comparing the actual clients referred with the expected referral profile based on epidemiological data and socio-demography of the catchment area.

Polarisation of the debate about "mainstreaming" or "specialism" continues to be very unhelpful in psychology departments. Incorporating race and culture issues and providing for the varied and diverse needs of the local population should be part of the mainstream agenda for individual psychology departments. It is not sufficient for heads of psychology departments/mental health psychology services to opt out of responsibility for providing a meaningful and appropriate psychological service to *all* sections of their catchment population on the grounds that there are no minority ethnic communities in their localities and/or uptake of psychological services by these groups is very low. The following questions need to be posed by purchasers of psychology services within the primary and secondary mental health care settings:

1. **What steps have been taken to get to know the black and minority ethnic communities within your locality?**
2. **How user-friendly are the psychology services to these community groups, in relation to the physical setting and the information provided about the role and function of clinical psychologists? How can psychology services access black and minority ethnic communities in your locality?**
3. **How do psychology departments establish and maintain links to, and credibility in the eyes of, the community groups in relation to the inclusion of race and culture variables in their assessment methods, the tools used to gauge personality and behaviour change, the goals for therapy and in the shared values and expectations of the service?**
4. **How can a cross-cultural perspective rather than the current uniform, homogenised face of clinical psychology be offered to clients?** How can thinking in psychology reflect conceptual frameworks that recognise the complex diversity of a plural society and which provide studies about human behaviour and experience in all its socio-cultural and socio-political contexts? How can accurate assessment, meaningful understanding and appropriate interventions, within culturally contextualised constructs, be provided to students and practitioners, when working with clients who have grown up in a minority versus a majority grouping? Do you deal with differences in language and meaning? Do you find out from the family about their beliefs about their problem? Do you understand the effects of institutional inequalities? Do you know the expectations of the client? Are you aware of the implications of the use of psychometrics only? Are you aware of the impact of the assessment and therapeutic process and the implications of asking particular questions in assessment and therapy work? Do you work in a culturally respectful manner?

5. What training have the clinical psychologists received regarding working within a multi-ethnic society?

More black and minority ethnic psychologists are required to meet the multi-racial needs of Britain, and a long-term strategy needs to be developed to look at the short-falls in the number of clinical psychologists from a variety of racial and ethnic backgrounds.

However, the extent of the short-fall of psychological provision to black and minority ethnic people means that the problems will continue for some time. In the long term the solution may be a combination of (i) emphasis on contact with the black voluntary provider, (ii) more formal working and counselling concepts so that they and other interpreters have a better understanding of psychological knowledge and expertise to offer other professionals regarding the specific needs of the black and minority ethnic population, (iii) on-going training and development lectures and workshops on trans/cross-cultural issues. The subject and content of clinical psychology needs to be made more attractive to minority groups; clinical psychologists could go to meet students from schools and undergraduate courses. The working parties in training and accreditation could make more specific the pre-requirements about the work of assistant psychologist prior to training. A wide range of teaching methods could be adopted, including recommended reading of novels and autobiographies of key black people, role plays to include practice of working with interpreters and talking to children and adults about discrimination and racism in a sensitive manner; clinical presentations to consolidate theory using cultural genograms; audio or video tapes of interviews of an adult/family or child from a minority ethnic background about living and growing up in Britain or using mental health services.

Conclusion

Psychology needs to confront and be confronted with its own racism. Its tendency to react defensively to attacks on its cherished self-image needs to be questioned. The discipline and profession of clinical psychology is overwhelmingly Eurocentric as practised in Western society. The profession continues to be restricted to traditional ways of thinking and working and imposing Eurocentric psychology upon people in British society. The profession still remains concerned with its standards and status within the mental health care setting on one hand, whilst perpetuating cultural oppression, colonisation and stigmatisation to a certain section of British society on the other hand. Solutions must replace myth and old adages. Psychologists must present themselves as part of the solution and welcome opportunities to challenge racial prejudice and racism. An overall strategy for service provision, service planning and service delivery with clearly identified monitoring mechanisms must be adopted. If we do not do these things, we are "doomed to continue the boring trudge towards professional credibility and political neutrality at the expense of our humanity".

References

Alladin, W.J. (1992) Clinical psychology provision: models, policies and prospects. In: Ahmed, W.U. (ed.) *The Politics of Race and Health*. Bradford: Bradford and Ikley Community College, Race Relations Research Unit.

Belliapa, J. (1991) *Illness or Distress? Alternative Models of Mental Health*. London: Confederation of Indian Organisations.

Bender, M.P. and Richardson, A. (1990) The ethnic composition of clinical psychology in Britain. *The Psychologist* 2(6): 250–252.

Boyle, M., Baker, M., Bennet, E. and Charman, T. (1993) *Clinical Psychology Forum* June: 9–13.

BPS (1988) *The Future of Psychological Sciences: Horizons and Opportunities for British Psychology*. Leicester: British Psychological Society.

BPS (1991) *Report of the Presidential Task Force for the Promotion of Equal Opportunities*. Leicester: British Psychological Society.

BPS (1997) Proceedings of the BPS Annual Conference. *The Psychologist* 10(8).

CCETSW (1991a) *Setting the Context for Change: Anti-racist Social Work Education*. London: Central Council for Education and Training in Social Work.

CCETSW (1991b) *One Small Step Towards Racial Justice*. London: Central Council for Education and Training in Social Work.

Chandra, J. (1996) Policy and legislation In *Facing up to the Difference*. Chapter 2. London: King's Fund/Department of Health.

Cline, T. and Lunt, I. (1990) Meeting equal opportunities criteria: a review of progress in education psychology training. *Educational and Child Psychology* 7(3): 59–66.

Goodwin, A. and Power, R. (1986) Clinical psychology services for minority ethnic groups. *Clinical Psychology Forum* 5: 24–28.

Howitt, D. and Owusu-Bempah, J. (1994) *The Racism of Psychology: A Time For Change*. London: Harvester-Wheatsheaf.

Husband, C. (1992) A policy against racism. *The Psychologist* 5(9): 414–417.

Kasvikis, Y. (1995) *25 Years of Scientific Progress in Behavioural and Cognitive Therapies*, Vol. 1. Athens, Greece: Ellinika Grammatta Publisher, Akadimias 88.

Lunt, I. (1997) The Society's Colloquium and Strategic Plan. *The Psychologist* 10(8): 368–369.

MacCarthy, B. (1988) Clinical work with ethnic minorities. In: Watts, F.N. (ed.) *New Developments in Clinical Psychology*. Chichester: BPS Books, Wiley.

MacCarthy, B. and Craissati, J. (1989) Ethnic differences in response to adversity: a community sample of Bangladeshis and their indigenous neighbours. *Journal of Social Psychiatry and Psychiatric Epidemiology* 24: 196–201.

Mahtani, A. and Marks, L. (1994) Developing a primary care psychology service that is racially and culturally appropriate. *Clinical Psychology Forum* 65: 27–31.

Milner, D. (1990) *Children and Race: Ten Years On*. Sussex, UK: Ward Lock.

Nadirshaw, Z. (1992) Therapeutic practice in multi-racial Britain. *Counselling Psychology Quarterly* 5(3).

Nadirshaw, Z. (1993) The implications of equal opportunities in training in clinical psychology: a realist's view. *Clinical Psychology Forum* 54: 27–28.

Nadirshaw, Z. (1997) Different and equal: an insider's view of working with difference and diversity. Proceedings of the BPS Annual Conference. *The Psychologist* 10(8): 134.

Newnes, C. and MacLachlan, A. (1996) The anti-psychiatry placement. *Clinical Psychology Forum* 93: 24–27.

Owusu-Bempah, J. and Howitt, D. (1995) How Eurocentric psychology changes Africa. *The Psychologist* 8: 462–465.

Pilgrim, D. (1989) The rise and rise of clinical psychology. *Changes* 7(2): 44–46.

Richardson, A. (1996) Personal values: are they professional issues? *Clinical Psychology Forum* 87: 14–18.

Shams, M. (1995) Challenging inequality of opportunities: race and gender in occupational psychology. *Proceedings of BPS (Occupational Psychology) Conference*, pp. 297–301.

Webster, A. (1997) Stress and culture: working in partnership with community groups. *Clinical Psychology Forum* **105**(1): 27–30.

Williams, J.A. and Watson, G. (1991) Sexual inequality and clinical psychology training in Britain: survey report. *Feminism and Psychology* **1**(1): 78–88.

13

General Practice

Sangeeta Patel

Why do GPs need to know about Cross-cultural Mental Health Care?

The terms and conditions of service for General Medical Practitioners (GPs) require them to provide General Medical Services to all of their patients. Any person who is resident in the United Kingdom, the EEC, and from countries who have a reciprocal arrangement with Britain can received health care, free at the point of delivery, for any illness which they have developed since their arrival in the UK. People with mental health problems can use further services in primary care such as support from practice nurses, health visitors, practice counsellors and community psychiatric nurses. An increasing number of practices have direct access to practice-employed counsellors and attached community psychiatric nurses, while others would require referral through their local community mental health team. Patients usually require a referral from the GP to obtain the range of secondary care services available. However, patients who are not registered with a GP may obtain access to services through other primary care networks, such as the accident and emergency departments or genito-urinary medicine clinics. These do not give them continuity of care and patients using these services are encouraged to register with a GP.

GPs usually accept patients from within a defined local geographical area. In England, 98 per cent of people are registered with a GP; those from ethnic minority groups are not significantly under-represented on GP lists (Balarajan *et al.*, 1989; Rudat, 1994b). Patients can choose from amongst the GPs who will accept them. For both patients and GPs the choice is most commonly made according to local geography. The choice of GP may be limited for those patients for whom the GP's origin or the languages they speak is paramount: a high proportion of Asian patients are registered with Asian GPs (Balarajan *et al.*, 1989; Rudat, 1994b).

Increasingly, people are being encouraged to consult their GP with their mental health problems; this encouragement comes from a variety of sources, including health advice in the popular press and advertising, health education campaigns, such as the "Defeat Depression" Campaign (Baldwin and Priest, 1995), and personal advice from health professionals.

GPs must make an assessment of patients' problems, and decide whether to treat, refer or follow-up patients. For mental health problems, GPs manage the majority within the practice, with only a small proportion being referred to psychiatric services. Goldberg described the filters to psychiatric care: of the population at risk per year, 71 per cent consulted their GP, 31.5 per cent had a distressing episode of psychological symptoms lasting at least one week during the year, 10.5 per cent were diagnosed by their GP as having a definite mental disorder and 2.35 per cent were referred to specialist mental health services during the year (Goldberg and Huxley, 1992). Attempts to apply this model to ethnic minority groups should acknowledge that it rests on the culturally specific presupposition that individuals and their episodes of distress are equivalent, comparable and should be the focus of attention, and that this form of categorisation and diagnosis is valid. There is little consensus upon the validity of "Western" psychiatric diagnoses in other cultures (Leff, 1990; Littlewood, 1990; Krause, 1994) or of the instruments used to measure them, leaving the basis of quantitative comparisons open to question.

The proportion of South Asian and African-Caribbean patients who consult their GP for any reason has been reported to be higher than in the indigenous population (Balarajan *et al.*, 1989; Rudat, 1994b). Consultation rates with GPs for mental disorders, as described by the GP, have been reported to be lower amongst the "Southern Irish", "West Indians" and "Asians" than amongst the "Native British" (Gillam *et al.*, 1989). Furthermore, people from black and minority ethnic communities are underrepresented amongst referrals for further primary and secondary care by GPs (Pharaoh, 1995).

Cross-cultural Mental Health Service Provision by GPs

GP Knowledge

As generalists, GPs should know the important facts about common illnesses amongst their patients. Hence GPs are more likely to be aware of the central themes of psychiatric knowledge than they are aware of the limitations of psychiatric research. Much cross-cultural psychiatric research has been based upon categorisation by racial, ethnic or cultural origin, which thus creates differences between these groups. Psychiatric research, by focusing upon the more exotic and severe manifestations of psychological distress, has reified these differences (Littlewood, 1992). The emphasis in psychiatric literature upon schizophrenia and psychosis amongst African-Caribbeans, and upon somatisation, eating disorders and parasuicide amongst South Asians, reflects and reinforces the popular stereotypes of African-Caribbeans as out of control and South Asians as too controlled (with implied moral connotations; Fernando, 1991; Littlewood, 1992; Lipsedge, 1993). Negative stereotypes of ethnic minorities abound within and outside the medical profession (Gilman, 1990; Bowler, 1993). Knowledge of severe and stereotypical disorders may be uppermost in the mind of GPs under pressure to establish a working diagnosis, during consultations which may be complicated by communication difficulties and physic disorders. GPs often find working with ethnic minorities stressful. GPs and other health care workers have been reported to hold less positive views towards their Asian patients than their white patients (Ahmad *et al.*, 1991; Bowler, 1993). Prejudice and stereotypes, though powerful, are not fixed, and can be challenged by new knowledge and personal experience (Gilman, 1990). An appreciation of the meaning and context of the individuals and communities will demonstrate the superficiality of stereotypes. GPs are forced to deal with individuals and their families, often in their own context over a long period, which enables them to challenge their stereotypes.

GP Diagnostic Skills

Communication difficulties

A shared language between doctors and patients is important for the doctor to be able to make an assessment of mental health. The percentage of people who do not speak English is decreasing: in 1994, the rates amongst Indians were found to be 15 per cent (8 per cent of men), amongst Pakistanis 28 per cent and amongst the Bangladeshi community 41 per cent (Rudat, 1994a). Unfortunately, language problems are often dealt with using family members, friends or neighbours, or other workers on-site who speak the same language. These strategies are rarely appropriate or satisfactory (Pharoah, 1995). Patients and GPs need access to suitable interpreting and advocacy services, particularly in areas with a large proportion of any minority ethnic group who are not fluent in English. However, the emphasis upon language as the only inhibitor to communication has been criticised: cultural differences are often more of an impediment than language (Bowes and Domokos, 1995; Patel, 1995). While a GP of the same ethnic origin may help overcome some of the linguistic and cultural differences, these shared origins may not compensate enough for the cultural rift between doctor and patient as a result of social and biomedical training. Patients may feel that a doctor of a different ethnic origin would not understand their problems. Conversely, they may feel concerned that a doctor who does share their ethnic origins would only treat them according to their own cultural mores rathern than Western medical ones. (Indian friends have commented that they would feel more comfortable discussing mental health issues with a "white" doctor than an Indian doctor.)

The diagnosis of depression

By focusing upon issues affecting the diagnosis of depression, I hope to illustrate the complexity of cross-cultural doctor–patient negotiations. GPs have been reported to fail to make the diagnosis of depression in half of their patients (Tylee and Freeling, 1989). GPs with less knowledge or consideration of depressive illness in consultations, or those who have not elicited the cues pointing towards depression, have also been reported to be less likely to make the diagnosis (Tylee and Freeling, 1989). GPs with high proportions of patients from ethnic minorities are often those working with the least resources, for whom it is more difficult to obtain training in mental illness management (Pharoah, 1995). Doctors have more difficulty in assessing the contribution of cultural factors in patients from cultures other than their own (Helman, 1990). The presence of concurrent physical illness or initial presentation of physical symptoms, both of which are more likely in black and minority ethnic communities, have been reported to make it less likely that the GP will diagnose depression (Tylee and Freeling, 1989). People from ethnic minorities have been reported to be more likely to present their psychological symptoms somatically (Kirmayer, 1984; Mumford, 1992; Krause, 1994) and GPs may be less able to differentiate between physical and psychological components of the illness; they may perform extra physical investigations in order to reassure either themselves or the patients.

There are many connotations of mental disorder, which vary between individuals and cultures. If these connotations are negative, GPs must tread carefully to avoid offence. Doctor–patient negotiations are complex, dynamic, emotionally loaded and involve complex power dynamics, and are affected by all the preconceptions which both parties may bring. When the preconceptions are not shared or understood, then there may be a misunderstanding of intentions. For example, a GP may see a patient who is suffering from various symptoms including low mood, tiredness, poor concentration and loss of appetite amongst other symptoms that they cannot easily describe in medical terms. The GP may pick out those symptoms characteristic of depression. The patient may feel that their other symptoms have not been attended to. If they also feel that the diagnosis of depression is meaningless or has negative connotations, they may then be upset by their GP's assessment.

Early Management of Mental Illness in General Practice

There is a trend towards increasing the management of minor psychiatric morbidity in primary care. Many more GPs now have employed or attached practice counsellors (Sibbald *et al.*, 1993). Whilst support and postgraduate education for GPs is very variable, there are occasional drives to increase this, such as the national Defeat Depression Campaign, part of which was targeted at GPs (Baldwin and Priest, 1995). These are still largely based upon the majority culture, with a few exceptions. GPs have been reported to refer fewer of their patients from black and minority ethnic groups (than their white patients) to allied members of the community team. Multilingual linkworkers have been reported to see their own role as including counselling but only a small proportion of their patients are referred from GPs (Pharoah, 1995).

Patients from black and minority ethnic communities are rarely referred for psychotherapy which has been attributed to the assumption that they lack the psychological mindedness, verbal sophistication or capacity for insight (Kareem and Littlewood, 1992; Lipsedge, 1993). Racially sensitive psychotherapy has been reported to be effective (Kareem and Littlewood, 1992), but even when such facilities are available, GPs are not always aware of them (Pharoah, 1995).

Referral to Hospital by GPs

It is still often the case that GPs are involved with the care of their mentally ill patients from ethnic minorities only when they become acutely ill and require referral to hospital. African-Caribbeans and South Asians are less likely to be referred for further psychiatric or psychological treatment (Kareem and Littlewood, 1992; Lipsedge, 1993). African-Caribbeans are less likely to be referred by their GP at an early stage of illness (Owens *et al.*, 1991) and are more likely to be compulsorily admitted to hospital by the police or social services, under a section of the Mental Health Act (Moodley and Perkins, 1991). Referral to secondary psychiatric care is a complex process influenced by views of both patient and doctor. For effective and appropriate referral, various factors are important:

- the patient must present their symptoms to their GP at an early stage;
- GPs must recognise them as early symptoms of mental illness;
- both parties must appreciate the value of referral and be able to discuss concerns openly;
- both patients and GPs must have access to suitable secondary care facilities.

Unfortunately, problems can occur at every stage; when both parties do not share the same cultural assumptions, there is a wider scope for misunderstanding and resentment.

Follow-up after Discharge from Hospital

The GP is in a system of care which enables continuity and constancy, and the development of a long-term relationship with patients and their families or carers, provided that they do not move out of the GP's catchment area. The GP will often have access to the family or local support networks of those who are mentally ill and can involve them in the care and monitoring of the patients, both during the illness and afterwards to prevent recurrences. The GP, even if not involved in the initial presentation of the illness, should at least have been informed by colleagues, which will enable them to be especially aware of the early signs of relapse in individual patients. Furthermore, as the GP is the first point of call for physical problems they can monitor opportunistically for recurrences of mental illness when systematic psychiatric monitoring fails.

GPs themselves require appropriate support in the management of their ethnic minority patients who have suffered acute mental illnesses or continue to suffer with chronic mental illness. This support includes information on specific features of recurrences, treatment options available, and clear information and access to local facilities on an individual and community basis.

In my description of the current state of provision of primary care services, I have tried to illustrate some of the difficulties experienced by both patients and doctors in trying to manage cross-cultural mental health problems, and in doing so have not emphasized sufficiently the wide variations in service provision between localities or, for example, deprived and affluent areas. These differences are often greater than those differences between one cultural group of patients and another. Furthermore, space prevents me from describing the excellent service provided by many practices under these difficult conditions. In the following section, I will emphasize some of the hopes and opportunities which lie ahead for practices to improve their cross-cultural mental health care.

Future Developments

My vision is for an equitable primary health care service, accessible to all cultures, both overtly and covertly, which would enable patients to approach their GP with trust and respect, and in turn be treated with respect and understanding by someone with some knowledge of their illness and a willingness to appreciate their situation. This GP should have the ability to establish a rapport and negotiate a working diagnosis, early in the course of the illness, in order to prevent further deterioration. They should be in a position to offer effective treatment for mental illness either on or off-site, which is culturally acceptable and appropriate, ranging from advice, psychotherapy, drug treatment or formal psychiatric services and support for the patient and their carers. I have described above some of the difficulties patients and GPs face during consultations. These are surrounded by structural systems which would make it difficult for people from other cultures even when they have a perfect rapport and understanding with their GP. In this section, I will describe some strategic changes in primary care which offer opportunities to improve the mental health care of all ethnic minority groups.

Strategic Changes in Primary Care

In the early 1990s, the controversial introduction by the government of market forces into health care and decentralisation of management had marked effects upon the nature of health service provision. While they may have predisposed to the increase in the inequity of service provision, they did bring some benefits to primary care, emphasizing its role within the NHS and drawing attention to the patchy provision of secondary care services. They opened the way for those in primary care who wished to be more responsible for the secondary care services which they obtained for their patients. Unfortunately ethnic minority communities did not benefit greatly from these changes. In the main, particularly soon after these reforms were introduced, it tended to be the larger, well-organised practices that benefited the most, rather than the smaller inner-city practices serving the majority of ethnic minority populations.

Recent Changes in Primary Care

In 1996, there was a concerted governmental exercise to investigate the needs of primary care. This resulted in the release of three White Papers "Choice and Opportunity – Primary Care: the future", "A Service with Ambitions" and "Primary Care – Delivering the Future" (Department of Health, 1996a, 1996b, 1996c). Here, I shall only highlight the points which have implications for the management of cross-cultural mental health in primary care.

"Choice and Opportunity" offered more flexibility for GPs, such as the option of being salaried, rather than "self-employed", which facilitates the recruitment of GPs to work in some of the deprived inner-city areas with substantial ethnic minority populations. It also enabled the use of practice-based contracts with health authorities, which thus can be tailored to the needs of its particular population. It suggested changes to the appointment of single-handed GPs, a higher proportion of whom are involved in the care of ethnic minorities. An increased role was proposed for community pharmacies which, it suggested, may enable another avenue for the detection of early mental disorder (Department of Health, 1996a).

"A Service with Ambitions" restated the principles of the NHS as a universal, high-quality and responsive service available on the basis of clinical need. It was less specific – more a statement of government attitude rather than concrete proposals (Department of Health, 1996b).

"Primary Care – Delivering the Future" underpinned the principles of good primary care: quality, fairness, accessibility, responsiveness and efficiency. It suggested new employment options and contracts for multi-disciplinary teams which would enable cultural adaptation of services to suit the local population needs. It emphasized education and training, particularly summative assessment for general practice and changes to vocational training schemes, which present opportunities to implement cultural awareness training schemes. It suggested a review of continuing professional development led by the Chief Medical Officer and local arrangements for under-performing doctors. In research and development it promised a doubling of the spending on primary care within a new funding system, and a primary care research network to be set up within each region.

We can hope that the increased patient information, education and involvement advocated will be responsive to the needs of all cultures. There will be an extra £100 million allocated for 1997–8. It promised changes in the contracts of the workforce – the primary health care team will be included in the NHS pensions scheme: if staff are retained, it will be more worthwhile for GPs to provide them with cultural awareness training. There will be encouragement for improving GP premises, including the use of private finance initiatives. Better organised out-of-hours care and information technology using primary care development challenge funds can be used to benefit all cultures (Department of Health, 1996c).

Many of the areas covered by these White Papers are targeted at improvement of inner-city primary care, with resulting benefits to people from ethnic minorities, the majority of whom live within inner cities. In addition, they provide flexibility of employment for GPs working within inner cities, many of whom are from ethnic minorities themselves.

The Labour government, elected since these White Papers, has agreed to continue providing support for all these initiatives. Furthermore they have put a moratorium on the closure of hospitals for financial reasons and will review the situation in London. No more practices will be allowed to become fundholding and all current fundholders will have to make the transition towards locality-based commissioning. There will be further rationalisation of Health Authorities and Trusts. The White Papers have enabled the development of "Primary Care Pilots" as an alternative to locality-based commissioning bodies. At the time of writing, these pilots had not been approved, but they are anticipated to have a wide scope to act as intermediary purchasers of secondary health care; they offer practices the scope of working together in a variety of ways, as conglomerations or as federations, which can determine their own contracts for the standards of care which they feel are appropriate for their patients.

Towards the end of 1997, the Labour government published a White Paper "The New NHS: modern and dependable". The main aims of this paper were to set national standards of patient care, enforced locally, to divert funds towards patient care and to improve accessibility, quality of care of health care provision, which is more open and accountable to the public. At a local level, Primary Care Groups or Primary Care Pilot Schemes, typically serving about 10 000 patients each, will work with Health Authorities, Community Trusts and Local Authorities to commission health care and to develop and implement local "Health Improvement Programmes". Quality standards will be developed locally and nationally. From 1 April 1999, a new National Performance Framework will focus upon six areas of performance, one of which is fair access to services for patients of all social and ethnic groups. It is still unclear how effective these systems will be, but it is evident that there is currently a wide variation between the capability of different commissioning groups to make these changes effectively.

The pilots, the locality commissioning bodies and the future Primary Care Groups will have much greater flexibility and powers to negotiate services which are appropriate for their patients. This is particularly important for ethnic minority communities which have high proportions in particular localities, but smaller proportions nationally. As they are also publically accountable, there is an obligation for the bodies to represent the views of their populations. The views of ethnic minority communities that are particularly prominent in the locality will be important for the commissioning bodies. These views can be obtained by discussions with members of ethnic minority communities in, for example, focus group discussions and by inclusion of their representatives within the panels or steering groups responsible for planning or development of commissioning. As the Localities and Pilot commissioning bodies have so much more flexibility, there is no uniform structure to include ethnic minorities – the opportunities are there, but can also be lost. However, GPs themselves will often be aware of the needs of their ethnic minority populations, and through these schemes now have much more flexibility to provide appropriate services. These may include interpreting and advocacy services, or culturally appropriate counselling and psychotherapy services.

Previously, GPs were able to obtain additional services only at their own expense or through the health authority. Now GPs may be able to employ particular health workers (with an interest or expertise in the mental health care of particular ethnic minority communities) through these schemes. They also enable the provision of contracts for staff training and development, which thus can be much more clearly geared towards the needs of ethnic minority patients. I would like to see representatives of ethnic minorities working in partnership with those involved in planning, and developing specific training in primary care. If not, there is a danger of overlooking the needs of ethnic minorities yet again.

The flexibility and local nature of the provision of primary care and purchasing of secondary care would offer a potentially much more responsive service, which could be more cost-effective only if it took the needs of its ethnic minorities into account. An example is Wandsworth Community Health NHS Trust in South London, which has worked with local GPs to provide specific health promotion, dietetics and dental health promotion for people from ethnic minorities (Kendrick and Hilton, 1997).

Education for GPs

The current changes give further opportunities for the education and training of present and future GPs. Within the undergraduate curriculum, there is a change to teaching a limited core course and "special study modules" (GMC, 1991). The core course has certain central themes that run throughout the course: these can cross cultural barriers, such as the theme "Man in Society" at St George's Hospital Medical School, while the special study modules offer the opportunity for specific cross-cultural educational initiatives. More of the teaching is to take place in the community, where cultural factors are less easily suppressed than in hospital. In the future, pre-registration house officer posts will be offered in the community, where more junior doctors can learn from a more patient-centred perspective. The Royal College of General Practitioners is preparing a programme for Cultural Awareness training for GP registrars and medical students. Summative assessment for vocational trainees offers an opportunity to include cultural sensitivity in the knowledge, skills and attitudes of prospective GPs.

Postgraduate education for GPs is flexible and allows the opportunity for development of locally appropriate teaching; for example, in Croydon, we developed a study day to explore and share the issues for GPs when dealing with their patients from ethnic minority communities. In London, from 1995 to 1998, money from the London Implementation Zone Educational Initiatives has supported many GPs to receive further education; for example, one scheme employed recently trained GPs to provide locum cover for Wandsworth GPs attending weekly daytime education and audit meetings (Smith and Teague, 1996). The GPs and the academic assistant GPs who covered them were given opportunities to learn more about cross-cultural mental health care.

On a more academic level, there is a welcome trend in psychiatric literature away from describing ethnic minorities in homogeneous categories, such as "Asian", and a recognition of the limitations of standard biomedical research categories and methodology (Littlewood, 1990; Lipsedge, 1993; Krause, 1994) with a shift towards more culturally representative, meaningful research originating, for example, from focus group discussions (Bhugra *et al.*, 1997). General practice provides a good means of reaching and describing people in their own context.

Conclusions

In this short chapter, I have attempted to present a broad overview of the patchy provision of cross-cultural mental health services and problems faced by the GP, and to outline some strategic opportunities for improvement. I recognise that I have not been able to do justice to all the relevant issues: I am guilty of simplifying and reducing certain complex issues and omitting others, not least the contribution of the professions allied to medicine. While I have been optimistic about the future, I would like to add a note of caution from history which has shown that those outside the majority culture have been marginalised and discriminated against, sometimes overtly, often covertly, but mostly unconsciously, and there has been little educational or systematic support for those who would like to challenge or improve their service provision. This chapter will only prove worthwhile if it encourages those people with energy, commitment and power to use these recent opportunities to attend at last to the needs of people with mental health problems from all cultures.

References

Ahmad, W.I.U., Baker, M. and Kernohan, E.M. (1991) General practitioners' perceptions of Asian and non-Asian patients. *Family Practitioner* **8**: 52–56.
Balarajan, R., Yuen, P. and Raleigh, V.S. (1989) Ethnic differences in general practice consultations. *British Medical Journal* **299**: 958–960.

Baldwin, D.S. and Priest, R.G. (1995) The Defeat Depression Campaign. *Primary Care Psychiatry* **1**: 71–76.

Bhugra, D., Desai, M. and Baldwin, D. (1997) Asian women's perceptions of depression. *Primary Care Psychology* **3**.

Bowes, A.M. and Domokos, T.M. (1995) South Asian women and their GPs: some issues of communication. *Social Science Health* **1**: 22–33.

Bowler, I. (1993) "They're not the same as us": midwives' stereotypes of South Asian descent maternity patients. *Sociology of Health and Illness* **15**: 157–178.

Department of Health (1996a) *Choice and Opportunity – Primary Care: the future.* London: The Stationery Office Ltd.

Department of Health (1996b) *A Service with Ambitions.* London: The Stationery Office Ltd.

Department of Health (1996c) *Primary Care – Delivering the Future.* London: The Stationery Office Ltd.

Fernando, S. (1991) Racism. In: Fernando, S. (ed.) *Mental Health, Race and Cultures*, pp. 24–50. London: Macmillan.

Gilman, S. (1990) Introduction: What are stereotypes and why use texts to study them? In: Gilman, S. (ed.) *Difference and Pathology: Stereotypes of Sexuality, Race, and Madness*, pp. 15–35. London: Cornell University Press.

Gillam, S.J., Jarman, B., White, P. and Law, R. (1989) Ethnic differences in consultation rates in urban general practice. *British Medical Journal* **299**: 953–957.

GMC (1991) *Undergraduate Medical Education: The Need for Change.* London: General Medical Council.

Goldberg, D. and Huxley, P. (1992) Filters on the pathway to care. In: Goldberg, D. and Huxley, P. (eds) *Common Mental Disorders: A Bio-social Model*, pp. 30–52. London: Routledge.

Helman, C. (1990) Cross-cultural psychiatry. In: Helman, C. (ed.) *Culture, Health and Illness*, pp. 214–248. London: Wright.

Kareem, J. and Littlewood, R. (1992) *Intercultural Therapy: Themes, Interpretations and Practice.* Oxford: Blackwell.

Kendrick, T. and Hilton, S. (1997) Broader teamwork in primary care. *British Medical Journal* **314**: 672–675.

Kirmayer, L. (1984) Culture, affect and somatisation. *Transcultural Psychiatric Research Review* **21**: 159–188.

Krause, I.B. (1994) Numbers and meaning: a dialogue in cross-cultural psychiatry. *Journal of the Royal Society of Medicine* **87**: 278–282.

Leff, J. (1990) The "new cross-cultural psychiatry": a case of the baby and the bathwater. *British Journal of Psychiatry* **156**: 305–307.

Lipsedge, M. (1993) Mental health: access to care for black and ethnic minority people. In: Hopkins, A. and Bahl, V. (eds) *Access to Health Care for People from Black and Ethnic Minorities*, pp. 169–183. London: Royal College of Physicians Publications.

Littlewood, R. (1990) From categories to contexts: a decade of the "new cross-cultural psychiatry". *British Journal of Psychiatry* **156**: 308–327.

Littlewood, R. (1992) *Ideology, Camouflage or Contingency? Racism in British Psychiatry.* Presentation at "Racism and Psychiatry", conference, Montreal.

Moodley, P. and Perkins, R. (1991) Routes to psychiatric in-patient care in an inner-London borough. *Social Psychiatry and Psychiatric Epidemiology* **26**: 47–51.

Mumford, D. (1992) Detection of psychiatric disorders among Asian patients presenting with somatic symptoms. *British Journal of Hospital Medicine* **47**: 202–204.

Owens, D., Harrison, G. and Boot, D. (1991) Ethnic factors in voluntary and compulsory admissions. *Psychological Medicine* **21**: 185–196.

Patel, S. (1995) Intercultural consultations: language is not the only barrier. *British Medical Journal* **310**: 194.

Pharoah, C. (1995) *Primary Health Care for Elderly People from Black and Minority Ethnic Communities.* London: HMSO.

Rudat, K. (1994a) Demographic features. In: *Black and Minority Ethnic Groups in England, Health and Life styles*, pp. 22–40. London: Health Education Authority.

Rudat, K. (1994b) Use of health services. In: *Black and Minority Ethnic Groups in England, Health and Lifestyles*, pp. 54–78. London: Health Education Authority.

Sibbald, B., Addington-Hall, J., Brenneman, D. and Freeling, P. (1993) Counsellors in English and Welsh general practices: their nature and distribution. *British Medical Journal* **306**: 29–33.

Smith, F.R. and Teague, P.A. (1996) The Bolingbroke project. In: Entwhistle, J., Morris, J. and

Toon, P.D. (eds) *The Wider World of Education. The London Initiative Zone Educational Incentives Programme*. London: NHS Executive.

Tylee, A. and Freeling, P. (1989) The recognition, diagnosis and acknowledgement of depressive disorders by general practitioners. In: Paykel, E. and Herbst, K. (eds) *Depression: An Integrative Approach*. London: Heinemann.

14

Social Work

Shulamit Ramon

Introduction

Social work is a fairly young profession in comparison to the benchmark professions of law and medicine. It emerged simultaneously in Britain and the US at the end of the 19th century.

Non-professional social work is as old as human history, in the sense that charitable and less then charitable work with poor people, and supporting people in times of crisis and loss, have always been present in human societies in a variety of forms.

There have been many attempts to define social work, ranging from seeing it as an altruistic occupation (Timms and Timms, 1978) to supporting and ensuring the re-adjustment of people to living within acceptable social norms (Davis, 1984).

The definition that seems to me to be the most useful and comprehensive proposes that social work is a profession which offers personalised support to people suffering from problems of living, by the utilisation of psycho-social perspectives and through being an intermediary between service users and the ruling groups (Philp, 1979). This definition highlights the inherent duality and synthesis between the psychological and social dimensions of our existence which is at the core of social work. It does not overlook the social control function of social work, but puts this side by side with the caring aspect, and emphasizes the *interpreting* function of social work as the go-between rulers and users.

The distinguishing features of professional social work, in comparison with other mental health professions, are:

1. Explicit value commitments which have been translated into educational and practice policies. The central values in social work focus on people's right to respect and self-determination, in being non-judgemental about behaviour which is socially unacceptable, and in not discriminating according to age, disability, ethnicity, gender and minority sexual orientation. Thus, social work is committed to working with vulnerable, marginalised and stigmatised members of society. Empowering the client to make decisions and take greater control over his/her life is a major practical implication of the values just outlined.
2. Addressing issues and problems of living from both psychological and social perspectives. This commitment is a core theme, from

assessment, to planning interventions and re-evaluation. For example, whereas the psychiatrist assesses whether a person is suffering from mental ill-health, the social worker has to assess whether his/her state of health impacts on the psychological and social context in which he/she lives.

3. Acknowledgement of the existence of social structural frameworks. In the context of mental health social work, this would imply paying attention, for example, to people's economic circumstances as well as to their psychological state. Furthermore, within the psychological dimension a good social worker would look to understand the impact of discrimination of any type on the client's mental well-being.

The role of social work is usually perceived to be one of working within the existing structural frameworks rather than trying to be a major agent for change. This position has been criticised for being too conservative and too ready to accept the status quo (Holman, 1978; Leonard and Corrigan, 1978; Mullender and Ward, 1991).

Attention to discrimination on ethnic grounds, and to likely anti-discriminatory action, has been given within social work education and social work practice, including mental health social work, much more than in any other mental health profession (CCETSW, 1993). It has been argued, however, that the implementation of this policy has been tokenistic or misguided, especially in relation to racism awareness workshops which fostered guilt rather than positive action by white workers. The criticism may well be justified, as it is difficult for one profession to overcome successfully the ingrained discriminatory attitudes and behaviours of a society, even if these are not legally condoned.

Yet there have been some notable achievements associated with this stance, and considerable backlash.

For example, many social services departments used their Section 11 monies to employ ethnic minority workers who would not normally have the necessary qualifications to enter such posts. Local authorities keen to develop services for ethnic minorities, such as Birmingham, Bristol, Islington, Lambeth, Tower Hamlets and Newham, have done so in the field of mental health as well (see, for example, Shanti, the Fanon Centre and Cowley Road services in Lambeth). Grant monies designated for mental health were used in some places to set up services specifically for people from ethnic minorities, such as the Lambo Day Centre in Islington.

All social work courses validated by the Central Council for Education and Training in Social Work (CCETSW) have to include prominent components of the curriculum focused on discrimination and anti-discrimination, especially in relation to ethnicity. The educational portfolio of all students on the DIPSW and students on ASW (Approved Social Workers in mental health) courses has to include a section on ADP (anti-discriminatory practice).

The insistence of the CCETSW in the early 1990s that institutional discrimination does exist within social work education met with incredulity by some academics, while others accepted that this was indeed the case. The then Secretary of State for Health, Mrs Bottommly (a qualified psychiatric social worker herself), was reported to be enraged. At her insistence, the expression "equal opportunities" – a weak and faceless term – replaced those of "anti-discrimination" and "oppression".

Mental Health Social Work

Mental health social work (MHSW) has formally existed in Britain since the 1920s, with the appointment of the first social worker to the Tavistock Clinic and to Hackney Child Guidance Clinic. The role of these pioneering social workers was to take the history of the person and the family from a psychosocial perspective, to assist in the assessment as part of a multi-disciplinary team, and then to work with the adults and parents of the children on agreed aspects of psychosocial functioning.

Until 1972 MHSW developed in two parallel directions:

1. Qualified social workers worked mainly with children and their families in the community, outside hospitals. The minority of qualified social workers who worked with adults also did so from a base in the community (usually an out-patient service).
2. Unqualified social workers were based in the psychiatric hospitals, where they were first called "duly authorised officers" until, in 1959, they became "mental welfare officers".

It was only around 1972, when the large social services departments came into existence, that more qualified social workers went to work in the psychiatric hospitals.

The two groups – community and hospital – did not have a lot in common. Those working in the community with either children and their parents, or adults, focused on psychodynamic and reconnecting work. In the 1959–1983 period, the work with adults in hospitals mainly entailed contributing to the assessment leading to compulsory admission, discussing possibilities for the in-patient period and organising accommodation and benefits on discharge. Initially, qualified social workers felt that the hospitals were not therapeutic environments in which they could work on the psychosocial issues faced by in-patients. As to the statutory responsibilities, they doubted the likelihood of establishing a relationship of trust necessary for adequate work with clients while exercising coercive social control (Ramon, 1985). In addition, the numbers of qualified mental health social workers were so small up to the 1970s that they could not fill available posts; by 1961 there were only 600 such workers in the country (Jones, 1972).

Up to 1972 social workers in mental health were considered to be elite in terms of professional practice, conceptual frameworks and research within the profession (Timms, 1964; Ramon, 1985). The *Journal of Psychiatric Social Work* became the *British Journal of Social Work* in 1972.

The amalgamation of the different branches of social work into the large social services departments in 1972 was welcomed by mental health social workers, who wished to have a solid power base for social work.

By the beginning of the 1980s, however, they were disillusioned with this new base, mainly because of the preference given to child protection work over work with all other client groups, and the demand to utilise their specific expertise and skills.

Mental health social work with adults was recognised by the managers of social services departments as an important area of work requiring a well skilled workforce. This re-focus was related to the growing interest of the government in mental health issues, the proposed closure of psychiatric hospitals and the resettlement of the hospital residents in the community. Yet the subsequent course of action by the government favoured health service personnel over social workers in carrying out hospital closure and resettlement in the community (Ramon, 1992). It seemed that social workers were being used to perform more overtly controlling functions, as reflected in the increase of statutory roles for social workers in child protection, and in having a government keener than ever before on strong social control mechanisms for populations perceived as "deviant", "unproductive" and hence "undeserving".

The wish to include a psychosocial perspective came particularly from those interested in the human rights dimension of the legislation, such as Leo Gostin, the then legal adviser of Mind (Gostin, 1976), and the British Association of Social Workers. The psychosocial approach was perceived as a necessary antidote to the dominant psychiatric model, which despite professed eclecticism (Clare, 1976) did not include this approach in either understanding and interpreting mental illness, or in central intervention strategies.

Most of the issues faced by social workers in working with people from ethnic minorities do not differ in essence from those faced by other mental health professionals. These have been adequately covered by Bhui and Christie (1996).

From the social work perspective, all of these issues are founded in the marginal position of ethnic minorities in our society. This understanding does not imply that there are no additional factors which are important to know and act upon. However, adopting a psychosocial approach means that both reparative and preventive work have to take account of the psychological and social dimensions that are specific to the place of ethnic minorities (Farrar and Sircar, 1986). Pertaining to everyday practice, this has meant being trained to be sensitive to the possibilities of (Farrar and Sircar, 1986; Fenton and Sadiq-Sangster, 1996):

- misdiagnosis of risk due to misreading of cultural difference;
- identifying factors within ordinary living which heighten stress and may lead to mental illness, where preventive action may be required (e.g. domestic violence, high level of unemployment among young African-Caribbean men, arranged marriages for young women who may not wish to follow this custom, racial harassment);

- culture-specific factors which are associated with the significance given to certain events and relationships by the person, her/his family and their community, and which may tilt a person from experiencing stress to experiencing mental illness; for example, if a woman feels prevented from seeking lay support when depressed because of the way she is treated by her husband, within the norms of her community, she may also feel that she cannot seek professional help, because of real or assumed cultural barriers between her and mental health professionals;
- the impact of being in a minority/marginalised position, to the development and maintenance of mental distress and illness (e.g. people who are unsure or unhappy with their ethnic identity, people with more than one ethnic identity, the interaction of ethnicity and sexual identity, the place of religion).

Recent Developments

A considerable, and growing, part of the work of social workers in mental health is ensuring that people are getting the benefits they are entitled to and guiding them in the search for accommodation and meaningful day activities.

In working with ethnic minorities, this has entailed:

1. After the Nationality Act in the 1980s, ensuring that people with the right to British nationality had it legally recognised.
2. Working on resettlement of people from ethnic minorities has led in some places to establishing group homes for black people and Jewish people.
3. The development of advocacy within mental health has also led to some projects which focused on people from ethnic minorities, such as the Mary Seacole House project in Liverpool (BASW, 1997). In this project service users and volunteers who were not users were trained to become peer advocates in Mental Health Review Tribunals, case conferences and police stations.

Some of the best known and the more successful projects of involving users in planning and running services have been initiated by social workers, and are located within social services departments (Hennelly, 1990).

The issue of physical and sexual abuse is one which has taxed social workers not only in relation to child protection, but also in the context of mental health (Mullender and Ward, 1991; Perlberg and Miller, 1992).

The issue of abuse is particularly emotive within ethnic minority groups which pride themselves as being morally superior to the majority, and where revelations of such abuse are perceived as giving further ammunition to those who have negative attitudes towards the minority group. Thus when the Black Sisters of Southall spoke publicly about the existence of domestic violence and sexual abuse within their Asian community, they were reprimanded by the community's traditional leadership (Sahgal and Yuval-Davis, 1992). For white social workers (or any other white worker), working with these victims within their community becomes particularly demanding.

Legislation-based Mental Health Social Work

The 1982–1983 Amendments to the Mental Health Act 1959

The 1982 Amendments of the 1959 Mental Health Act in England and Wales and the 1983 similar Scottish Act cemented a new role for social workers in mental health (Barnes *et al.*, 1990).

This change of heart was not reflected at all in the 1982 Barclay report on the roles and tasks of social workers, which came out in favour of generic, locality based, social work teams.

The Act has formally established the existence of Approved Social Workers (ASWs) who receive specialised training of sixty days after two years of post-qualifying work in order to carry out the following tasks:

1. Assess people at the point of request for compulsory admission in terms of risk to themselves and others, and in terms of whether hospitalisation can be prevented by the use of the least restrictive alternative locations and forms of interventions.
2. Recommend a course of action, which has the same legal status as the recommendation provided by the psychiatrist.
    This power signifies a major departure from past tradition. In everyday reality it has meant that social workers and psychiatrists have either to find common ground or to rely on second opinions, such as that of two psychiatrists over-ruling the recommendation of the social worker, or asking relatives to apply for the admission.
3. Provide reports for Mental Health Review Tribunals when patients either appeal before the tribunal or their status is reviewed by the tribunal. The report by social workers has to focus on the realistic possibilities for safe living for the patient and relevant others in the community where the person would be discharged.
4. Provide a follow-up during the post-discharge in the community period to people who have been admitted on a compulsory basis.
5. Social workers are members of the Mental Health Act Commission, also established within the 1982 amendments (as are other professions).

Acting as ASWs has meant the following:

1. MHSWs are doing a lot more assessment and much less of other aspects of their work.
2. They are thus also more engaged at the controlling edge of social work and mental health work.
3. They are therefore also more in contact with members of ethnic

minorities who fall into the over-represented categories outlined by Bhui and Christie (1996).

4. They are largely prevented from fulfilling the task of indicating and weighing the least restrictive alternatives as too few such facilities exist in the country.

5. The task of providing an effective follow-up is seriously curtailed by too few ASWs and the time taken up by assessments.

6. Being an ASW is now perceived as a respected and desirable status within the profession. This was not the case in the first few years after the law came into effect, as the increase in statutory work was perceived as a threat to the more caring and counselling work carried out by social workers. The change in status reflects, therefore, a shift in attitude within social work: the additional power is welcomed and its use justified on the grounds that other professions make worse use of similar powers.

The evidence on the role of ASWs in relation to clients from ethnic minorities builds up a picture very similar to the experience of mainstream psychiatry (Barnes *et al.*, 1990).

Within the framework of the latest Criminal Justice law, ASWs also act as "appropriate adults" for people in police custody who are judged to be vulnerable. Some of these people suffer from mental illness, or learning difficulties, or could be vulnerable when under the influence of drugs or alcohol. In any case, the legislators have opted not to call in lawyers, doctors or nurses, but for social workers to act as a buffer between the police and these people. This reflects well the intermediary role mentioned in the definition of social work outlined above.

The Community Care Act 1990

This Act, applied since 1993 within social services departments, has had considerable impact on mental health social work. Most MHSWs have become designated care managers, some of whom may also be ASWs. Rationing considerations have meant that only people with serious mental illness are considered for care management, and that preventive work has been greatly reduced.

Furthermore, although care management has been interpreted differently by different authorities, the majority have opted to use it as a tool of assessment and planning, rather than of intervention based on the strengths model. The focus on assessment and planning is directly related to perceived lack of resources to do anything else, as well as to the preferred governmental line.

The Act states that care management should be focused on identifying and meeting people's needs, rather than fitting people into existing services. This intention is to be welcomed, even if the reality of rationing has so far enabled at best only limited choice for some users, and no choice for others.

It further states that users and carers have to be consulted. People from ethnic minorities and their needs are mentioned in one sentence in the paper that led to the Act – the Griffith report of 1988 (Community Care: Agenda for Action) (Watters, 1996). However, the Act does not provide guidelines about the nature and process of consultation. A minority of social services authorities have gone for innovative ways of encouraging genuine participation by users and carers, including users of mental health services, at both the individual and group levels (e.g. Derbyshire, Newcastle). Usually such initiatives have been jointly undertaken with the local health authorities. The majority of authorities have done little beyond paying lip service towards consultation at either level. For example, although users have to see their care plan, most authorities do so without previous formal consultation and without the necessary preparation which would enable users to state with confidence their preferences; consequently most users do not even remember being shown their care plan, let alone have a copy of it, or feel ownership of the plan. The same applies to relatives who act as informal carers.

The Community Care Act has also introduced a split between purchasing and providing. Although social services departments have delayed such a split, most care managers have been designated as purchasers whereas ASWs and other mental health social workers (e.g. those few still working in children and family consultation centres) have become providers. Most social workers doubt the usefulness of this split.

Social workers are also expected to record unmet needs, which could in theory feed into the purchasing plans. In principle this is a positive idea, which in reality depends on the readiness of the purchasers to take notice of these records.

Social workers have bitterly complained about the increase in paperwork and the decrease in time given to direct work with clients, especially counselling, as a result of the implementation of the Community Care Act. There is nothing in the spirit of the Act which dictates these two outcomes; they are the by-product of a climate of rationing and of a strong belief in the usefulness of managerial models in social services and social work. Both of these elements are anathema to the value given in social work to investing time and energy in developing professional relationships with clients and to the social mandate of supporting vulnerable people. The implementation of the Act has also fostered the rapid development of the private for-profit sector (especially in housing and forensic services) and of the not-for-profit sector (housing and day care), while social services facilities have been forced to close down. Social workers are concerned about the accountability of the non-public sector services.

Some clients have benefited substantially from the implementation of the Community Care Act, where individualised needs and choice have been taken seriously. So far, we lack evidence as to the specific impact of the Act on clients from ethnic minorities who use mental health services (Watters, 1996).

Issues for Social Workers in Multi-disciplinary Work

Recently attention has been given to multi-disciplinary collaboration in statutory work. A disproportionate number of public inquiries related to homicide in the last five years have focused on black men. Findings have been used by journalists and pressure groups such as Schizophrenia A National Emergency (SANE) to demonise young black men suffering from mental illness (Ramon, 1996). Interestingly, SANE regards social workers as symbolic of professionals who are no good, as they do not wish to use hospitals as a first resort, and do not adhere to the biological model of mental illness.

Although disagreements between psychiatrists and social workers on recommendations for compulsory admission are known to exist, curiously there is no research on the degree of disagreement, and how disagreements are handled. Anecdotal evidence varies according to who is telling the tale.

Social workers use their seniors in cases of disagreement, and are furious when the GP goes behind their back and invites two psychiatrists to over-rule their recommendations. They locate the disagreements in having a different perspective on mental illness and problems of living; namely as they do not adhere necessarily to the disease model they can see a wider variety of options than psychiatrists which explain strange behaviour. GPs and psychiatrists have little patience with social workers who disagree with their views, arguing that anyway social workers do not understand much about mental illness.

Yet the law does not expect social workers to ascertain in their assessment whether the person suffers from mental illness or not, but to concern themselves with the issues of risk and location of intervention at the point of crisis. Therefore, whether social workers' knowledge of mental illness is sufficient or not is immaterial, as long as they are able to recognise the risk entailed in mental illness.

Most of the recent scandals and subsequent inquiries have highlighted how difficult it is to assess the risk accurately, and prevent it from becoming a danger for all of the mental health professionals.

The lack of good multiprofessional collaboration has been identified as one major issue in allowing users of mental health services to fall through the safety net and to get to the point of murder or suicide.

From the perspective of social work, such collaboration is made difficult and at times impossible, not only because of the underlying differences in perspective just outlined, but also by the lack of hospital beds at crucial times, and the lack of non-hospital crisis facilities, staffed by both medical and non-medical personnel. The latter point is also picked up by service users. The introduction of the Care Programme Approach (CPA) for people with serious mental illness, in which the co-ordinator can be only from the NHS, is seen by social workers as a further regression into the biological and medical models of mental illness.

Working with Carers

Traditionally, social workers focused on family work in mental health. As the statutory load increased, less family work has been undertaken. Social workers in the 1960s and 1970s followed, more than any other mental health professionals, the view that family dynamics can cause mental illness. This has been interpreted by carers – and psychiatrists – as a belief that the parents have caused the mental illness of their offspring. This interpretation is far wide of the mark – the dynamics of a relationship may lead to mental illness without any intentional action on the part of any of the participants in such a relationship.

For ethnic minority relatives, social workers have become the symbol of the professionals who take away their chilren. Relatives do not register that social workers are:

- very reluctant to do so and see the removal of children as their failure (Thoburn, 1988);
- are often found guilty of not taking children away before serious abuse has taken place in a number of inquiries;
- are also those who return children to their parents after arduous work.

Future Developments

To contemplate the future, we need to begin by having a good grasp of what the major stakeholders want.

We do have clear indications of what users want, even if the degree of representativeness of the expressed views remains uncertain. The feedback from ethnic minority users (albeit insufficient) gives the same pointers as that from other users (Wilson, 1993).

Users want:

1. to be treated with respect, and for their version to be seen as valid as that of any other stakeholder;
2. services that are easily accessed by them, mostly non-medical, and not in a hospital setting (Rogers *et al.*, 1993); this pertains especially to crisis and respite services;
3. much more attention to be given to their employment and education prospects than is the case presently;
4. access to counselling and complementary therapies, reduction in the use of medication, attention to side-effects of medication;
5. fuller information about the range of available interventions;
6. to have a clear say in decisions concerning their lives.

Ethnic minority users point out the continuation of the discrimination they suffer in other spheres of life within psychiatry too (e.g. higher rates of use of section 136 by the police to detain people from black ethnic minorities; Wilson, 1994). Some of them would like to have services only for members of a specific ethnic minority, where workers too would be from ethnic minorities.

Carers want:

1. to be valued by professionals, including social workers. They wish to be acknowledged as the crucial co-workers which they are, which implies being listened to, having their accounts taken seriously, being consulted, and being party to shared information;
2. easy access to hospital beds and for psychiatric wards to continue to exist;
3. for quicker admission than is currently possible;
4. tangible support;
5. an end to the discrimination (against ethnic minorities) and lack of respect by professionals (including social workers) which they have experienced.

Carers (mainly mothers) were the activists who led to the establishment of the Afro-Caribbean Mental Health Association in Brixton. The general public, egged on by the media and some representatives of relatives' organisations, seem to want a quiet life in which those who suffer from mental illness, and are a potential risk to others, are committed to closed hospital wards indefinitely.

The current intolerance of non-biological approaches to mental illness provides a paradoxical answer to the proposed merger of health and social care and its ability to provide a unified, "integrated" mental health service in England, Wales and Scotland (Northern Ireland has had such a service since 1993). In such a climate a unification will only mean that psychosocial approaches to mental illness will be even more marginalised by those who adhere to biological approaches than is currently the case, when the latter have to respect the autonomy of social workers. This pessimistic reading of the situation is partly based on the views of social workers in Northern Ireland, who feel discouraged by being part of the unified service (Campbell, 1996).

The dominance of the biological approach also bodes badly for the development of a fresh approach to ethnic minority mental health issues, because from this perspective ethnicity, social or psychological factors are of little significance to the understanding of and intervention in mental health problems. There is an urgent need, therefore, to inform the public better and work systematically to undo the harm caused by SANE, mentioned above, especially to the public image of young black men suffering from mental illness.

All mental health professionals, but particularly psychiatrists and GPs, need to be prepared for changes in attitudes, information and skills in their work with sufferers from serious mental illness, especially those from ethnic minorities. Unless there is a shift from a biological to a truly bio-psycho-social model of psychiatry, people from ethnic minorities will continue to be treated as second-class citizens.

Such changes take a long time to achieve, and are best targeted at the basic training level of all mental health professionals.

Much of the mental ill-health experienced by ethnic minorities relates to being discriminated against socially and to being marginalised. It is not realistic to expect mental health professionals, including social workers, to be able to change the belief system of society and the structural factors which lie behind it. However, each professional group can expect its members to address these issues within its own remit, to work on changing the belief system and mitigate the effect of the structural issues. Professions have often shaped public opinion, not merely reflected it, as demonstrated by the attitudinal change in relation to child abuse, or to the resettlement of long-term residents from psychiatric hospitals. Social workers have done so more than any other professional group, but still need to do better in the future.

Within social work there is an urgent need for the following:

- More sensitive training about the roots of discrimination, the obstacles it creates for ethnic minorities in everyday life (particularly in the context of mental distress), and how to create new, realistic, opportunities for such service users.
- Many more opportunities and resources for group work and community work within social work, as a way of enabling users and carers mutually to support each other, raising awareness of shared issues, and allowing social workers to use their skills as initial leaders of such projects, while encouraging users and carers to take on the leadership in subsequent phases (Mullender and Ward, 1991).
- Advocacy systems in which people from ethnic minorities can be represented by advocates of their choice. This would be a very positive step, but one which would need to be part of a new Mental Health Act, and apply to admission assessments as well as to other components of the system.

All mental health professionals can (and should) lobby their professional organisations for structural, legislative and policy changes. However, a shared vision based on the belief in equality of opportunities combined with respect for cultural differences would be a pre-requisite for such lobbying.

We also have to find more effective ways for the voice of users and carers from ethnic minorities to be heard by the public and the professionals. Existing accountability systems within health and social care leave a lot to be desired in terms of eliciting this voice, listening to it, and implementing the desired changes. Although social services are currently more accountable to the local population than the health service is, such listening has happened in too few places (Brandon, 1997). Suitable legislation could promote local forums for users and carers and the means to ensure that they are truly representative of the local population.

One burning issue is whether mental health services for ethnic minority people should be separated from those offered to the majority, or whether the thrust of the effort should go to ensuring greater sensitivity to the specific issues which these people have within ordinary services, which mostly have white workers and white users. Separatist services are usually created on the assumption of their temporary nature, i.e. until the attitude of the majority changes. Therefore, the issues at stake are what works best in terms of changing this attitude and how to minimise the suffering of ethnic minority people in the time it takes for this change to come about. One solution for the reduction in suffering is to have separatist services. Indeed, some of the best services for ethnic minorities within the mental health system are offered only by separatist services (e.g. Shalvata in London for the Jewish community or the Afro-Caribbean Association in Manchester). It is regrettable that there is little collaboration among such services, despite the obvious shared interest and the mutual benefits to which such a collaboration could lead. The lack of such a broad coalition reflects the narrowness of separatist services, as well as the gap between white and black, and richer and poorer ethnic minorities. Having such services also delays the urgency of change by the majority, and marginalises services for ethnic minorities (Watters, 1996).

Of the different propositions for the future outlined above, the creation of a strong voice for users and carers from ethnic minorities seems to be the most urgent step to take, not only from the perspective of social work but of the mental health system as a whole. Social workers could play a positive role in supporting such a voice, given their experience in setting up user-empowerment initiatives in Britain. However, for mental health social workers to act in a more empowering way there would be a drastic reduction in bureaucracy, and social workers need less statutory work or more workers, so that time and energy can be freed for them to engage at greater depth with members of ethnic minorities and with mental health issues in general.

References

Barnes, M., Bowl, R. and Fisher, M. (1990) *Sectioned: Social Services and the 1983 Mental Health Act*. London: Routledge.

BASW (British Association of Social Workers) (1997) *Pulling Together – Social and Health Care*. Health Related Social Work Centenary Conference, 13 May 1996, Birmingham.

Bhui, K. and Christie, Y. (1996) Purchasing mental health services for black people. In: Thornicroft, G. and Strathdee, G. (eds) *Commissioning Mental Health Services*. London: HMSO.

Brandon, D. (1997) Confusion and hypocrisy rule as common values melt. *Professional Social Work* **4**: 11–13.

Campbell, J. (1996) Northern Ireland: one model of integrated services. In: Ramon, S. (ed.) *International Perspectives on Health Social Work in the 1990s*, pp. 77–84. Sheffield: ATSWE Publications.

CCETSW (1993) *Ethnicity and Mental Health Social Work*. London: Central Council for Education and Training in Social Work.

Clare, A. (1976) *Psychiatry in Dissent*. London: Tavistock.

Davis, M. (1984) *The Essential Social Worker: A Guide to Positive Practice*. Aldershot: Wildwood House.

Farrar, N. and Sircar, I. (1986) Social work with Asian families in a psychiatric setting. In: Coombe, and V. Little, A. (eds) *Race and Social Work: A Guide to Training*. London: Routledge.

Fenton, S. and Sadiq-Sangster, A. (1996) Culture, relativism and the expression of mental distress: South Asian women in Britain. *Sociology of Health and Illness* **18**(1): 66–85.

Gostin, L. (1976) *A Human Condition*. Leeds: Mind Publications.

Hennelley, R. (1990) Mental health resource centres. In: Ramon, S. (ed.) *Psychiatry in Transition: British and Italian Experiences*, pp. 208–218. London: Pluto Press.

Holman, R. (1978) *Poverty: Explanation of Social Deprivation*. Brighton: Martin Robertson.

Jones, K. (1972) *The History of the British Mental Health Services*. London: Routledge.

Leonard, P. and Corrigan, P. (1978) *Social Work under Capitalism*. London: Macmillan.

Mullender, A. and Ward, D. (1991) *Self-directed Groupwork*. London: Whiting and Birch.

Perlberg, R. and Miller, A. (eds) (1992) *Power and Gender in Families*. London: Routledge.

Philp, M. (1979) Notes on knowledge in social work. *Sociological Review* 27(1): 83–111.

Ramon, S. (1985) *Psychiatry in Britain: Meaning and Policy*. Croom Helm.

Ramon, S. (1992) The workers' perspective: living with ambivalence and ambiguity. In: Ramon, S. (ed.) *Psychiatric Hospital Closure: Myths and Realities*, pp. 83–121. London: Chapman Hall.

Ramon, S. (1996) A scandalous category: media representations of people suffering from mental illness. In: Ramon, S. (ed.) *Mental Health in Europe*, pp. 186–210. London: Mind/Macmillan.

Rogers, A., Pilgrim, D. and Lacey, R. (1993) *Experiencing Psychiatry: Users' Views of Services*. London: Mind/Macmillan.

Sahgal, G. and Yuval-Davis, N. (eds) (1992) *Refusing Holy Orders: Women and Fundamentalism in Britain*. London: Virago.

Thoburn, J. (1988) *Captive Clients*. Aldershot: Wildwood House.

Timms, N. (1964) *Psychiatric Social Work*. London: Routledge.

Timms, N. and Timms, R. (1978) *Perspectives in Social Work*. London: Routledge.

Watters, C. (1996) Representations and realities: black people, community care and mental illness. In: Ahmed, W. and Atkin, W. (eds) *Race and Community Care*. Milton Keynes: Open University Press.

Wilson, M. (1993) *Mental Health and Britain's Black Communities*. London: NHS Management Executive, Mental Health Task Force and King's Fund Centre.

Wilson, M. (1994) *Black Mental Health: A Dialogue for Change*. London: NHS Management Executive, Mental Health Task Force.

Part IV

Planning, Policy and Managing Change

15

Government Policy and Ethnic Minority Mental Health

Dele Olajide

Introduction

It is apposite to review government policies with respect to ethnic minority groups on the 50th anniversary of the birth of the National Health Service (NHS).

At the inception of the NHS, British society was relatively homogeneous with a negligible ethnic minority population. There was a political consensus following the Second World War to provide universal health care for all at the point of contact, with no financial barriers. There was great expectation that a healthy population would provide the required workforce to regenerate the damaged infrastructure which followed the devastation of the war. It was also assumed that, with improvement in the health of the workforce, less demand would be placed on the NHS in the long term. The NHS was therefore formed when there was a strong sense of social conscience and a reasonably cohesive society.

Fifty years on, society has become fragmented and less cohesive. People now live longer as a result of improved socio-economic conditions and significant advances in medical science. The increasing cost of health care has become a vigorous subject of debate and rationing is no longer a taboo subject. In most developed countries, not only does health care now represent between 5 and 12 per cent of the Gross National Product (GNP), but the rate of increase of health care significantly exceeds economic growth.

The NHS, as the largest employer in Europe, has a duty to lead by example in terms of provision of equitable care for all citizens, equality of opportunity for its workforce and anti-discriminatory practices worthy of emulation by other employers.

This chapter will focus on government policies as they affect people from ethnic minority communities. In the context of this chapter, ethnic minorities are defined as those of Asian, Caribbean and African descent because they stand out as "different" from other ethnic groups. We recognise that other minority groups may have negotiated successfully or are at various stages of negotiating some of the issues that are raised in this chapter. Ultimately, the aim of the NHS must be to provide services which all members of the multi-cultural society will feel comfortable in using, while retaining the choice of access to whichever services they feel best fulfil their needs. NHS policies and practices have traditionally adopted the view that the needs of the minority ethnic groups can be met by using a universal model of service provision which is "colour blind". Only now are policy-makers beginning to realize that a universal model of service provision can not work in a multi-cultural society, without creating inequalities in terms of access and unmet needs due to demonstrable health variations across various groups in society.

Socio-demography

There is a view of the ethnic minority society as a monolithic "out group" because of apparent similarities in skin pigmentation, migration from similar geographical regions and religious beliefs. There are significant inter-ethnic and intra-ethnic group differences which make such assumptions fallacious. The unique cultural attributes between groups risk being lost when they are lobbed together as a group with similar needs, assumptions generally based on historical cultural stereotypes. This diversity is also demonstrated in the pattern of the geographical distribution of the various ethnic minorities in England (Table 15.1) and suggest that policies aimed at ethnic minorities ought to take into account such distributions if they are to be successful. The 1991 Census indicated that the ethnic minorities under consideration now constitute approximately 6.2 per cent of the population of England and Wales (OPCS, 1991). It further showed that 59 per cent of those who defined themselves as black Caribbean live in the Greater London area. Black Africans on the other hand are to be found predominantly in Greater London (79 per cent). In contrast, only 9 per cent of those who described themselves as Indian live in inner London while 33 per cent live in outer London. Now, compare this with the Bangladeshi population of whom 45 per cent live in inner London and 9 per cent live in outer London. The Chinese are by far the most widely dispersed ethnic group with 40 per cent residing in Greater London and 43 per cent spread out in different parts of England.

Such geographical distribution suggests that London and the Metropolitan cities with significant ethnic minority communities need radically to re-think strategies of mental health care delivery to cater effectively for these populations. This is a major challenge which service planners ignore at peril to their organizations and society at large. The traditional model of mental health care delivery is inappropriate to these communities and their needs can not be made to fit the majority norm of appropriate service. At the moment, regardless of the level of funding in these areas, there is inadequate uptake from, and non-cost-effective service provision to, these minority communities.

Table 15.2 shows that ethnic minorities constitute more than 5 per cent of the population in the following areas: inner and outer London, West

Table 15.1 Percentage distribution of ethnic groups (Source: 1991 Census).

Population	All Ethnic	Black Caribbean	Black African	Black Other	Indian	Pakistani	Bangladeshi	Chinese	Asian Other
Inner London	22	36	53	29	9	7	45	20	24
Outer London	24	23	26	18	33	13	9	20	36
West Midlands	13	15	2	9	17	20	11	4	5
West Yorkshire	6	3	1	4	4	18	4	3	2
Greater Manchester	5	3	3	5	4	11	7	6	3
Leicestershire	3	1	1	1	9	1	1	1	2
Bedfordshire	2	2	1	2	2	3	4	1	1
Berkshire	2	2	1	2	2	3	0	2	2
Rest of England	23	15	12	30	20	24	19	43	25

Table 15.2 Ethnic groups as a percentage of the local population.

Population	Total Ethnic	Black Caribbean	Black African	Black Other	Indian	Pakistani	Bangladeshi	Chinese	Asian Other
Inner London	25.6	7.1	4.4	2	3	1.2	2.8	1.1	1.8
Outer London	16.9	2.7	1.3	0.8	6.5	1.4	0.4	0.7	1.6
West Midlands	14.6	2.8	0.2	0.6	5.5	3.5	0.7	0.2	0.4
Leicestershire	11.1	0.6	0.1	0.3	8.4	0.4	0.2	0.2	0.4
Bedfordshire	9.9	1.8	0.2	0.5	2.7	2.3	1.1	0.3	0.3
West Yorkshire	8.1	0.7	0.1	0.3	1.7	4	0.3	0.2	0.2
Berkshire	7.6	1	0.3	0.4	2.6	1.9	0.1	0.3	0.5
Greater Manchester	5.9	0.7	0.2	0.4	1.2	2	0.5	0.3	0.2
England	6.2	1.1	0.4	0.4	1.8	1	0.5	0.3	0.4

Midlands, Leicestershire, Bedfordshire, West Yorkshire, Berkshire and Greater Manchester.

We have highlighted these variations at the outset as they have significant implications for strategic planning of services for these groups if policies are to be translated to cost-effective actions. We would advocate that government policies and initiatives are *targeted* at these areas where their impact is likely to yield maximum returns, as a result of the greater unmet need, high motivation for change and the potential for such initiatives to provide value for money. We are advocating a policy shift from "the big bang" national initiatives which achieve maximum political publicity with no enduring shift in professional and public attitudes, to a "focused targeting" which may be low key but sustainable because the community, as a result of vested self-interest, can become a partner in effecting change. Any lessons learnt from such initiatives can be adapted and transplanted to other ethnic groups. This way, changes are incremental and sustainable.

Age Distribution of Ethnic Minorities

Figure 15.1 shows that the growth rate of ethnic minorities is higher than that of the indigenous population in all age groups except those of 45 years and above. The fastest growth rate is in the 5–15 year-olds, who are vulnerable to exclusion from school and brushes with the law for minor criminal offences. Those in the 16–44 age group are over-represented in both the psychiatric and criminal justice systems (McGovern and Cope, 1987; DoH and HO, 1992; Koffman *et al.*, 1997). What can we learn from this population structure with reference to mental health strategies?

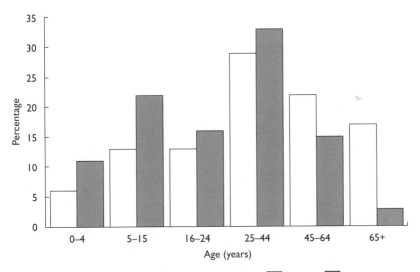

Figure 15.1   Age of ethnic groups in the UK 1991. ☐ White, ■ Black.

1. That a policy of mental health promotion targeted at the 5–15 age group is likely to lead to an increased awareness of mental health issues and a willingness to access help at an earlier stage of mental distress. Such policy will need to involve other agencies such as education, employment and the criminal justice services.
2. That the current population of psychiatric patients, who are predominantly in the population band of 25–44 years, if not adequately managed will become chronic long-term patients revolving between mental health services and the criminal justice system (Richie *et al.*, 1994). The problems will be compounded in the Metropolitan areas unless effective alliances are forged between housing (to reduce homelessness), employment (effective employment rehabilitation), education (adult education initiatives) and a re-configuration of services which relies less on acute beds but on a range of provision that developed to meet the local needs of the population.
3. The problem of ethnic minority populations over 65, while not a major issue now, will need to be addressed in the next century. Hitherto, there has been a reverse migration back to the country of origin by first-generation migrants, but as the socio-economic conditions of their country of origin become more parlous, there will be little incentive for reverse migration in the future. If the population trend continues, the age of second-generation migrants will increase at a higher rate than that of their indigenous counterparts. This age group will not have the option of reverse migration as they are citizens of this country without the option of a second country. Again, the geographical distribution as shown in Table 15.2 will mean that certain regions of England and Wales will need to develop strategies to deal with the special needs of these populations.

Relevant Mental Health Policies, 1959–1998

While significant and sometimes radical changes have occurred in mental health service delivery in the last four decades (Table 15.3), most of these changes have not focused on the needs of ethnic minorities as their needs are subsumed under the general "culture free" universalist model of care provision. The universalist model presupposes that a good-enough service for the majority population will also be appropriate for minority groups. Implicit in such an assumption is the conclusion that policy-makers are either ignorant of the heterogeneity of this group or are guilty of arrogance borne out of a belief (a relic from the colonial past) that they know what is best for ethnic minority groups. Another possible explanation may be discerned from the observation that policies are often driven by political imperatives. Too high a profile given to ethnic minority issues might be construed by the majority population as a sign of affirmative action, when there are inequalities for everyone in health care, especially in socio-

Table 15.3 Landmark NHS policies of relevance to mental health 1959–1998.

1959	Mental Health Act.
1975	*Better Services for the Mentally Ill*. Ministry of Health White Paper based on the Audit Commission.
1976	*Joint Care Planning: Health and Local Authorities*. DHSS Circular.
1981	*Care in Action. A Handbook of Policies and Priorities for Health and Personal Social Services in England*. DHSS.
1982	*Korner Report* – Collection and use of information on hospital and clinical activity.
1983	Mental Health Act.
	Care in the Community. DHSS Consultative Document.
1986	*Making a Reality of Community Care*. Audit Commission Report.
1988	*Community Care: Agenda for Action*. Sir Roy Griffiths.
	The Report of the Committee of Inquiry into the Care and After-care of Sharon Campbell.
1990	NHS and Community Care Act.
	House of Commons Social Services Committee Report on Community Care.
	Community Care in the Next Decade and Beyond.
	White Paper: DH Guidance on Care Programme Approach.
1992	Mental Illness Key Area in DoH Health of the Nation.
	DH White Paper, Joint Department of Health and Home Office Review of Services for Mentally Disordered Offenders.
1993	*Mental Illness Key Area Handbook*.
	Secretary of State's 10 point plan.
	*Mental Health and Britain's Black Communities: Tripartite collaboration between NHS-ME, King's Fund and The Prince of Wales Advisory Group on Disability.
1994	*Richie Report on the care of Christopher Clunis.
	Guidance on establishing supervision registers [HSG(94)5].
	Guidance on discharge of mentally disordered people and their continuing care in the community [HSG(94)27].
	*Mental Health Task Force – London Project and Regional Race Programmes.
	*Black Mental Health – A Dialogue for Change.
	*NHS Executive Letter EL(94)77: Collection of Ethnic Group Data for Admitted Patients.
	*Establishment of NHS Ethnic Health Unit.
1995	Mental Health (Patients in the Community) Act
	Mental Health – Towards a Better Understanding. Health of the Nation Public Information booklet for ethnic minorities users and their carers.
1997	The new NHS: Modern. Dependable.

* Policies directed at ethnic minorities.

economically deprived areas. In such a climate of competing needs, it is easy to see how policies can be skewed in favour of the majority population.

The advent of the Community Care Act 1990 led to a public awakening of their need to co-exist in the same neighbourhood with patients released into the community, who had hitherto been hidden away from public gaze in the well meaning, but outdated, Victorian asylums. Mental illness, as one of the five key areas in *The Health of the Nation* (DoH, 1992), also highlighted this hitherto neglected area of health. The publication of the Richie Report (1994) on the badly managed care of Christopher Clunis (who killed

Jonathan Zito, a total stranger) highlighted the pitfalls of care in the community and mobilised critical attitude – both lay and professional – towards this desirable but untested social experiment. This tragic event and other headline incidents triggered a flurry of policy response with the introduction of the supervision register [HSG(94)5], a renewed emphasis on the moribund 1989 Care Programme Approach (CPA) and the enactment of the Mental Health (Patients in the Community) Act 1995 [HSG(96)11].

It may be a pure coincidence, but 1994 saw the mental health of ethnic minorities catapulted to the top of the national political agenda.

Health of the Nation

The NHS has set an evidence-based health strategy which encompasses where and how people are cared for and with what aims and goals in view. This strategy should ensure that policy is grounded in the known epidemiology of mental disorders whether the sufferers are located in specialist services, in primary care, in schools, in the workplace or in prisons. Such a strategy requires close inter-agency working and also requires an effective and co-ordinated framework of prevention and mental health promotion (Annual Report of CMO, 1995).

These objectives are articulated in the *Health of the Nation: Mental Illness Key Area Handbook* (DoH, 1993) as follows:

- to reduce the incidence and prevalence of mental disorder;
- to reduce the mortality (both from suicide and from deaths from physical illness) associated with mental disorder;
- to reduce the extent and severity of other problems associated with mental disorders such as poor physical health, impaired psychological and social functioning, poor social circumstances and family burden;
- to ensure the delivery of appropriate services and interventions; and
- to reverse the public's negative perceptions of mental illness by countering fear, ignorance and creating a more positive social climate in which people are encouraged to seek help.

The picture painted above is far rosier than the experience of the average mental health user from ethnic minorities. The prevalence of psychosis in African-Caribbeans is 3–6 times higher than that of the indigenous population, and probably closer to that of Irish immigrants (Dean *et al.*, 1981; Cochrane and Bal, 1989; King *et al.*, 1994; Bracken *et al.*, 1998). Despite the higher prevalence of psychosis in African-Caribbeans, there is increasing evidence of a better prognosis (Mckenzie *et al.*, 1995), although several studies indicate greater use of the Mental Health Act (Owens *et al.*, 1991; King *et al.*, 1994; Koffman *et al.*, 1997; Takei *et al.*, 1998) and greater admission into secure units (Browne, 1990). The most worrying statistic is the tendency for African-Caribbean patients to end up in prison or secure units once they have entered the mental health care system (King *et al.*, 1994;

Takei *et al.*, 1998). Although we lack good data at present, the body of available evidence appears to point to a systematic failure of the mental health and social after-care system to deal with these individuals once they are received into these systems. The causes of this alarming situation are multifarious and need unpacking if we are to rectify the damaging effect of mental health care on patients from ethnic minorities.

While researchers have been busy studying psychoses among African-Caribbeans to the exclusion of other forms of mental disorder, a parallel activity has been preoccupying them with the Asian population. There have been suggestions that the suicide rate is higher among this population, based principally on population projections (Raleigh, S., *et al.*, 1990; Raleigh, V., 1992). A more recent study (Neelman, *et al.*, 1997) also found a higher rate of suicide in younger women from the Indian subcontinent compared to all other ethnic groups. The debate with respect to a higher incidence of suicide in Asians is often muddied by using deliberate self-harm (DSH) as a proxy for suicide.

The prospective study by King *et al.* (1994) and the point prevalence study carried out in the former North and South Thames Regions on all in-patients on a census day (Koffman, *et al.*, 1997) indicate a higher prevalence of schizophrenia among **all ethnic groups** when compared with the indigenous population. The notion of an epidemic of schizophrenia in black Caribbeans is beginning to creep into scientific discourse without any critical appraisal of the evidence. The evidence offered for this so-called epidemic arose from hospital statistics mainly from the geographical areas with a large black Caribbean population, and was not derived from population studies (e.g. Wing and Hailey, 1972; Rwegellera, 1977; Bebbington *et al.*, 1981). The paucity of in-patient statistics on depression or anxiety disorders in the same geographical area has not been used to explain the absence of these conditions in the African-Caribbean (Nazroo, 1997). A large-scale, multi-centre study using similar methodology to that employed in the US Epidemiological Catchment Area studies is more likely to provide reliable answers to the question of higher rates of psychoses in ethnic minority communities (Adebimpe, 1994).

We shall now examine specific government initiatives directed at the ethnic minority communities and the impact, if any, on the issues that such policies set out to address.

Mental Health Task Force

The Mental Health Task Force, set up in 1992, focused its attention from January 1993 to December 1994 on the twelve inner London DHAs and their associated social services departments. It also undertook a consultation exercise with black mental health groups and organisations, and published a booklet, *Mental Health – A dialogue for a change*, as well as a video, *Different Cultures – Different Needs*. Sadly, the outpourings of recommendations and initiatives generated by the Mental Health Task Force were quietly shelved with its demise.

NHS Ethnic Health Unit

The NHS Ethnic Health Unit (NHS-EHU), a quango, was established in 1994, based in Leeds and given a 3-year lifespan. It was given the mammoth task of advising the NHS Executive Board, the Regional Offices (ROs), NHS Trusts, primary health care teams and voluntary organisations on the very broad and nebulous subject of "ethnic minority health". It was expected to achieve these disparate goals through: (i) developing quality standard tools for Performance Management Directorates; (ii) commissioning projects to assist purchasers to "increase the effectiveness of consultation and communication with their local black and minority ethnic groups"; (iii) producing a checklist for health authorities and GPs to "develop and provide comprehensive primary care for local minority ethnic groups"; and (iv) "developing a strategy that will enhance communication between the NHS and black and minority ethnic organisations".

Of particular relevance to mental health was the task of monitoring the collection of Ethnic Group Data for Admitted Patients introduced in 1994 and made mandatory from 1 April 1995 (see below). With such wide-ranging objectives, it is hardly surprising that the EHU made little impact in its short lifespan. There are cynics within the ethnic minority community who believe that organisations such as the EHU were set up to fail, by virtue of the scale of the task and the time that was given to achieve it.

Collection of Ethnic Group Data for Admitted Patients

In an attempt to understand the pathways within mental health care, the NHS Executive letter of November 1994 [EL(94)77] provided guidance for the collection of ethnicity data for all in-patients with effect from 1 April 1995. The Hospital Episode Statistics (HES) record information on all episodes of patient treatment in England purchased by the NHS. An episode is defined as a period of treatment in a specific hospital provider while under the care of a particular consultant.

Information on each episode is collected by individual hospitals and passed via the Health Authority to the Office of National Statistics (ONS) on a regular basis. As HES provide detailed information on hospital service utilisation, patient characteristics, diagnoses and any procedures carried out, they are an invaluable source of information at both Health Authority and Trust levels in determining the level of morbidity, service uptake and hence relevance to the local population. At the time of writing (January 1998), ethnic group data collection was patchy even in those areas with high ethnic minority populations. Clearly, this is where the Regional Offices through the Performance Directorates need to insist that Health Authorities include ethnic data collection in the minimum data set (mds) and that this is audited with penalty for poor performance. Perhaps it is time for the NHS Executive to revisit this subject again to find out why, two years after data collection was made mandatory, little action has taken place.

The overuse of sections of the MHA also requires monitoring and the Mental Health Act Commission has made this one of its twelve medium-term goals.

Staff Recruitment and Retention in the NHS

"I want to stress that taking action to promote equality in employment is not just a matter of moral justice or of fairness to people from minority ethnic groups. It is good, sound common sense, and it makes business sense too." Thus spoke Virginia Bottomley as Secretary of State for Health when launching "Ethnic Minority Staff in the NHS: A Programme of Action" (NHSME, 1993). Most professionals from ethnic minority communities working in the NHS would agree that little has changed since the programme was launched. The glass ceiling is still firmly in place to prevent career advancement for all black professionals working in the NHS. Like ethnic minority patients who suffer from the double jeopardy of mental illness and racism, so their professional careers suffer from the universal low morale in the NHS, and the problem of poor opportunity for career advancement.

There are still too few ethnic minority senior nurse managers despite their significant representation at lower levels. Health Authority and Trust Executives from ethnic minorities are still a rarity even in areas with large ethnic minority populations. Approximately 5 per cent of non-Executive Directors in the NHS are from ethnic minority backgrounds. This is an under-representation of the group as a percentage of the population, and yet there are areas where the ethnic minority population is as high as 40 per cent of the local population. There is no justifiable explanation for such anomalies. It can not be that there are not enough qualified professionals out there to do the job; one has to assume a lack of political will to make it happen. If the government is serious about providing services that are relevant to the local community with improved uptake, and which provide value for money, it must make both moral and economic sense to mobilise the ethnic minority manpower resources available within its workforce in order to achieve the desired goals. It is also the case that a demoralised workforce makes poor spokespersons for the NHS in their communities. This raises the question of recruitment from these communities. Why join an organization where you are not valued?

When faced with a dearth of females in the workforce, the government launched Opportunity 2000 with remarkable success. Perhaps it is time that a similar programme was undertaken with respect to ethnic minority professionals to ensure that we are not still struggling with this problem in the next millennium.

There has been a mechanism in place for monitoring the ethnicity of the NHS workforce since 1993. Perhaps the newly formed NHS Equal Opportunities Unit (combining gender, race and disability) will take a more critical look at its remit to ensure that the eight goals of the programme of action (recruitment and selection; staff development; racial harassment;

appointments to NHS Boards; service delivery; doctors; nurses; and management training) are rigorously monitored. The NHS Excutive could boost the equal opportunity programme by establishing schemes such as "Investors In People (IIP)" for employers who practise an active equal opportunity programme among their workforce. Currently, most employ-ers proclaim themselves "working towards equal opportunity" which is meaningless jargon and a smokescreen for inaction.

The Way Forward

This chapter does not seek to give the impression that nothing has changed in the past two decades or that change will not happen. On the contrary, changes have taken place, sometimes by default or in response to headline incidents. *Ad hoc* change cannot be managed and gives the impression of damage-limitation. Change is inevitable but it must be championed from the centre in order to let those in the field know that it is in their interest, and that of the population which they serve. The status quo is no longer tenable in a multi-cultural society in which we all have a stake.

Government can act as an agent for change in the following domains.

Primary Prevention

Meltzer *et al.* (1995) have demonstrated a correlation between mental health and poor housing, poor education, unemployment, living in council accom-modation, single parenthood and being alone in the general population. It would be surprising if these same factors were not correlated with mental ill-health in ethnic minorities.

The present government has shown some understanding of this by appointing a minister with responsibility for public health. Health promo-tion should be targeted at those at greatest risk, such as under-achieving teenagers at school, the young single parent, the unemployed and margin-alised youth in inner cities, and the homeless. The improvement of environ-mental factors such as poor housing, poor education and unemployment can lead to an increased quality of life, as well as breaking the cycle of prison and psychiatric services which is frequently the fate of the most vulnerable in these groups. More research both in primary prevention and the alleviation of these social factors is required if we are to gain better understanding of the causal relationships between mental ill-health and socio-economic deprivation.

Secondary Prevention

Secondary prevention may be realised by means of early identification of mental health problems in high-risk groups, followed by appropriate inter-vention in the form of:

- accessible information;
- psycho-social support;
- identification of problems related to acculturation;
- socialising of the children of migrant families at an early stage;
- promoting better communication between users and care-givers, through better training of all professionals in cultural issues and the use of interpreters where necessary;
- improved opportunities for education of people from ethnic minorities in the mental health professions (a case needs to be made to address the dearth of black Caribbean graduates in the health professions);
- increased attention to cross-cultural approaches to psychiatry, psychology, nursing and social work.

Wider Social Obligations

- Ensure equal access to employment and educational opportunities as well as to mental health services. Failure to provide equal access leads to alienation and marginalisation of ethnic minorities and a feeling among individuals that they are subjected to institutional racism. This can lead to anger, resentment and a sense of insecurity, which in turn lead to social dissension with adverse effects on the mental health of all sections of society.
- It is important for the wider community to accept ethnic minority groups as integral parts of the total society and also for ethnic minorities to accept the need to live in harmony with the host community. It is essential for ethnic minority communities to maintain a sense of identity and pride in their individual cultures. This will allow each ethnic minority group to achieve a balance between maintaining its own cultural identity and becoming fully integrated into a wider multi-cultural society. This will enhance the self-esteem of ethnic minority groups.

The Criminal Justice System

Government policies and how they are implemented can exert undue pressure on ethnic minority families in a way that the indigenous society does not appreciate (e.g. immigration policy, policing style and the penal system). The resulting sense of insecurity in many ethnic minority communities can inadvertently promote mental ill-health. The above recommendations require effective partnership between government and its various agencies on the one hand and the society as a whole on the other hand. The initiative for transforming Britain into a multi-cultural society at ease with itself is the responsibility of all citizens, but politicians must have the vision to manage the change process so that those who feel most threatened by change are not marginalised or allowed to arrest the pace of change.

References

Adebimpe, V.R. (1994) Race, racism and epidemiological surveys. *Hospital and Community Psychiatry* **45**(1): 27–31.

Bebbington, P.E., Hurry, J. and Tennant, C. (1981) Psychiatric disorders in selected immigrant groups in Camberwell. *Social Psychiatry* **16**: 43–51.

Bracken, P.J., Greenslade, L., Griffin, B. and Smyth, M. (1998) Mental health and ethnicity: an Irish dimension. *British Journal of Psychiatry* **172**: 103–105.

Browne, D. (1990) *Black People, Mental Health and the Courts*. Report by Commission for Racial Equality and Afro-Caribbean Mental Health Commission.

Chief Medical Officer (1995) *On the State of the Public Health*: Annual Report. London: HMSO.

Cochrane, R. and Bal, S.S. (1989) Mental hospital admission rates of immigrants to England: a comparison of 1971 and 1981. *Social Psychiatry and Psychiatric Epidemiology* **24**: 2–11.

Dean, G., Walsh, D., Downing, H. and Shelly, E. (1981) First admissions of native-born and immigrants to psychiatric hospitals in south-east England 1976. *British Journal of Psychiatry* **139**: 506–512.

Department of Health (1989) *Caring for People with a Mental Illness*: The Care Programme Approach. (Abstract)

Department of Health (1992) *The Health of the Nation: A Strategy for Health in England*. London: HMSO.

Department of Health (1993) *The Health of the Nation: Key Area Handbook – Mental Illness*. London: HMSO.

Department of Health (1994) *Black Mental Health – A Dialogue for Change*. NHSE: Mental Health Task Force.

Glover, G. and Malcolm, G. (1988) The prevalence of depot neuroleptic treatment among West-Indians and Asians in the London borough of Newham. *Social Psychiatry and Psychiatric Epidemiology* **23**: 281–284.

King, M., Coker, E., Leavy, G., Hoare, A. and Johnson-Sabine, E. (1994) Incidence of psychotic illness in London: a comparison of ethnic groups. *British Medical Journal* **309**: 1115–1119.

Koffman, J., Fulop, N.J., Pashley, D. and Coleman, K. (1997) Ethnicity and use of acute psychiatric beds: one day survey in North and South Thames Regions. *British Journal of Psychiatry* **171**: 238–241.

Lloyd, K. and Moodley, P. (1992) Psychotropic medication and ethnicity: an inpatient survey. *Social Psychiatry and Psychiatric Epidemiology* **27**: 95–101.

McGovern, D. and Cope, R. (1987) The compulsory detention of males of different ethnic groups, with special reference to offender patients. *British Journal of Psychiatry* **150**: 505–512.

Mckenzie, K., van Os, J., Fahy, T., Jones, P., Harvey, I., Toone, B. and Murray, R. (1995) Psychosis with good prognosis in African-Caribbean people now living in the UK. *British Medical Journal* **311**: 1325–1328.

Meltzer, H., Gill, B., Petticrew, M. and Hinds, K. (1995) The prevalence of psychiatric morbidity among adults living in private households. OPCS Surveys of Psychiatric Morbidity in Great Britain: report 1. London: HMSO.

Nazroo, J.Y. (1997) *Ethnicity and Mental Health: findings from a national community survey.*

NHSME (1993) *Ethnic Minority Staff in the NHS: A Programme of Action.*

Office of Population Censuses and Surveys (1991) London: HMSO.

Owens, D., Harrison, G. and Boot, D. (1991) Ethnic factors in voluntary and compulsory admissions. *Psychological Medicine* **21**: 185–196.

Raleigh, V.S. and Balarajan, R. (1992) Suicide levels and trends among immigrants in England and Wales. *Health Trends* **24**: 91–94.

Raleigh, S.V., Bulusu, L. and Balarajan, R. (1990) Suicides among immigrants from the Indian sub continent. *British Journal of Psychiatry* **156**: 46–50.

Richie, J., Dick, D. and Lingham, R. (1994) *The Report of the Inquiry into the Care and Treatment of Christopher Clunis*. London: HMSO.

Rwegellera, G.G.C. (1977) Psychiatric morbidity among West Africans and West Indians living in London. *Psychological Medicine* **7**: 317–329.

Takei, N., Persand, R., Woodruff, P., Brockington, I. and Murray, R.M. (1998) First episodes of psychosis in Afro-Caribbean and white people: an 18-year follow-up population based study. *British Journal of Psychiatry* **172**: xxx–xxx.

Wing, J.K. and Hailey, A.M. (1972) *Evaluating a Community Psychiatric Service: The Camberwell Register 1964–1971*. London: Oxford University Press.

16

Social Analysis: Policy and Managerial Issues

Frank Ledwith and Charles Husband

Introduction

This chapter will advance a series of propositions, outline relevant results from a recent research project on organisational factors in the provision of community mental health services for minority ethnic groups, and make some recommendations for the future development of such services, with added comments on broader social and economic policy issues. We adopt a systems approach which sees organisational change in collective terms, not based on individual change. Similarly we take as read a view, which is developed in a full report of our research (Husband *et al.*, 1997) that racism is primarily a collective, organisational problem, not just an expression of psychological and social pathology in a few individuals.

As is outlined elsewhere in this volume there is ample evidence that, nationally in Britain, mental health services are culturally inappropriate, oppressive and unacceptable to minority ethnic groups. Sadly there is little indication of a clear government policy direction to remedy the situation: the Mental Health volume within the Health of the Nation targets suggests, as the only specific proposals for change, more culturally appropriate food and the employment of more minority ethnic staff. Given the scale of the problems of discrimination, this seems a seriously inadequate response.

Since 1979 there have been massive changes in public services in Britain, with the privatisation of most utilities, and the introduction of market mechanisms in health and social services and (to some extent) in education. Within the NHS, the largest employer in Europe, there has been the introduction of general management, increased involvement of doctors in management, the purchaser–provider split and the introduction of GP fundholding. In spite of all these changes there is little sign of the diminution of the power of (mainly hospital) doctor providers to determine what services are to be offered (Harrison *et al.*, 1992) or of greater responsiveness to the needs for inter-agency working in community servicesm (Audit Commission, 1986). In fact, as Smith *et al.* (1993) point out, government directives towards joint working are contradicted by the introduction of market mechanisms which promote competition between providers.

Our research examined community mental health services as these affect the majority of clients/patients. We found relatively little research and theory available to help us understand how community health services work even within the NHS, on which most research has concentrated. Most commentators on NHS management (for example, Ham, 1992; Allsop, 1995; Klein, 1995) concentrate on hospital management. Ackroyd (1995) outlined a very useful framework for understanding the management of the NHS in terms of a tripartite structure: professional, bureaucratic and political (at local and national level). He suggested that the NHS is organisationally incoherent and therefore in theory unmanageable but has been made to work by habits of mutual adjustment between the three arms of governance. There has been even less research into the links between community and primary care services which, including pharmaceuticals, consume around one third of the NHS budget. As the Audit Commission (1986) pointed out, clients have complex needs which may vary over time yet the services offered essentially consist of discrete "boxes" into which clients are fitted. As a consequence of various agencies working to separate budgets, the total cost of care may be much higher than it need be. The NHS and Community Care Act 1990 removed social security funding from the equation but health and social services purchasing is still very incoherent in regard to mental health purchasing (Audit Commission, 1994). Flynn *et al.* (1996) have carried out ground-breaking research on what they call "the ethnography of purchasing and providing" community health services. They point out that the type and time scales of intervention are quite different from those of hospital services and require much more of a "relational market" approach, relying on mutual trust which is threatened by the idealised, self-interested market behaviour of "economic man". Soothill *et al.* (1995), in a ground-breaking book, outline some valuable guidance in noting:

- there are many possible models of inter-agency management (Hugman, 1995);
- particular legislation has had a considerable impact on services such as child protection and community care of the elderly (Hugman, 1995);
- the tribe-like behaviour of professional groups who show an affinity for collaborative working mainly with "their own kind" (Beattie, 1995);
- the resistance to innovation of professionally dominated organisations which can best be countered by a user-led approach (Cole and Perides, 1995).

It is remarkable that *all* the authors so far cited give little or no mention of the role of the voluntary sector and lay care in discussion of community care in spite of the fact that there are nearly 7 million lay carers in Britain who, if paid at an hourly rate at the European Union minimum decency level, would cost ten times as much as the professional care at present provided (Nolan *et al.*, 1996).

Research Findings

Thus it can be seen that the research we carried out in Camchester (a pseudonym) on "inter-agency collaboration in the provision of mental health services for ethnic minorities" had to be planned without much in the way of adequate formal theory. We accepted that the term "mental health services" is a misnomer or euphemism for "mental ill-health services" and that mental health is influenced by a vast range of determinants ranging from intracellular processes in the brain to "the state of civilisation". We accepted too that there are and have been furious debates as to the meaning of mental illnesses, with explanations ranging from the biological/medical views of disordered brain chemistry and/or hormonal balance to those that present psychiatry as an instrument of ethnic, gender and class oppression. The concepts of "race" and ethnicity are the subject of much analysis and debate, and we live in a society which consists of many cultures and many substantial minority ethnic groups. We therefore adopted a simple approach of investigating the *perceptions* of the services provided amongst those managing or providing services. In essence we were asking simple questions which could be roughly summarised as "What are you trying to do and how well are things going?", in relation to services generally and then specifically for members of minority ethnic groups.

Due to previous contacts and the prestige of a university research project, we were able to begin our work by interviewing the very senior staff in health and social services. Thereafter we were able to progress down the organisation to what we called the "foot-soldiers" who actually provide services in the statutory and voluntary sectors. We also surveyed published literature and gathered information on good practice across Britain and interviewed a number of religious leaders in the mosques and some "alternative" healers. We were given time by a lot of very busy people who were often astonishingly frank with us about their problems and their difficulties in collaborative working. We held a number of sessions where we fed our conclusions back to our respondents which were in some cases critical. In all cases we had open and fruitful discussions without any serious or irreparable disagreements, which gave us confidence in the validity of our conclusions.

We found that services for members of minority ethnic communities were frankly inadequate: minority ethnic clients were much under-represented as users of services yet there was ample evidence of high levels of need. Within general practice there were well documented reports of high levels of postnatal depression, of general anxiety and depression, and of psychosexual problems. In addition community initiatives such as breast cancer screening had suggested high levels of social isolation and depression. There was a large and growing incidence of deliberate self-harm in young minority ethnic women. There had been a number of special initiatives over the years to develop better services for minority ethnic groups but it was widely accepted that these had not resulted in clear and lasting benefits. In discussing the extent of inter-agency collaboration, it was clear that there were some very well developed links, for example between GPs and psychiatrists or between health service counsellors and voluntary sector agencies. Overall the range and extent of such collaboration was limited.

Taking a wider perspective and thinking of the tripartite division of organisational power referred to above (political, managerial and professional), the political aspect was predominant. National policies were the most potent force in shifting the service, with two contradictory policies being pursued with vigour: the demand for greater priority to be given to the needs of those with severe mental illness and yet pressing for ever more fundholding amongst GPs who have little engagement with the needs of this (small) group in comparison with the large caseload of the "worried well". Fundholding GPs had the financial power to demand particular services from health and social services staff and can thus impose their own priorities. These contradictory forces of central government priorities and local purchasing power generated very real pressures within the mental health system. It had already been fractured into health and social service providers, in what the authors describe as the "two way stretch" (Ledwith, 1996). It is therefore not surprising that senior and "foot-soldier" staff felt relatively powerless to influence policy and were consequently demoralised by the fragmentation of well established, multi-disciplinary teams. As a consequence of the "two way stretch" the teams were increasingly unable to set their own agenda in relation to service delivery. Indeed high levels of stress and fragile, or collapsed, morale were very evident within the "foot-soldier" interview data. Nonetheless there were a number of examples of clear and decisive local leadership to plan and implement new forms of service, originating primarily in the NHS provider Trust and in social services. We found that the formal planning processes between the health provider, social services and the health authority purchaser had little impact on the pattern of service development.

With regard to the needs of minority ethnic clients, locally there was little sustained political pressure for improvement of mental health services and thus relatively little managerial attention was given to it, particularly by the health authority purchaser. Professionally there had been leadership within a long-standing specialist cross-cultural psychiatry unit, but the unit had an ambiguous status within the larger service. It had few staff and there was confusion amongst GPs as to the criteria for referral to the specialist unit instead of to the local, generic services. Nationally it is clear that the areas with best practice have strong minority ethnic voluntary services which provide accessible and acceptable broad-spectrum services and, in addition, allow for the skills and career development of minority ethnic staff. It was therefore disappointing to see how undeveloped the services were locally with some history, sadly, of patriarchal opposition to services directed at women.

It was our conclusion that, unless there are some substantial changes in national policy, prospects for the minority ethnic volunary sector do not look bright for a number of reasons:

- In an expert seminar, reviewing national trends in voluntary sector mental health services for minority ethnic clients, it was suggested that there was a good deal of professional and managerial prejudice against minority ethnic voluntary organisations who were expected to provide services "on the cheap" without proper funding for infrastructure development, yet were regarded as having poor financial management.

- The new "contract culture" of health and social services meant that voluntary organisations were being restricted in the range of services to be offered and the range of clients to whom they could be offered: their strength lies in the ability to deal with all areas of need, yet this was being undermined by contracts for particular services (for example, counselling) to particular clients (those diagnosed as having a mental illness).

- The Health Authority had little experience of funding voluntary sector organisations and was legally prevented from giving grants. Social services had much more experience and understanding of voluntary sector funding yet their budgets were being severely cut, with annual budget decreases of 6–8 per cent.

- Alongside tightening or reductions in general budgets, there had been the growth of Mental Illness Specific Grants, with social services receiving 70 per cent of funding from central government for particular, innovative projects, which could include the voluntary sector. Such grants, however, should be seen against overall reductions in budgets: typically they were for a limited duration of 2–3 years, just enough time to become established and then have to be disbanded unless taken on under mainstream funding, which was unlikely whilst many statutorily required services were in jeopardy.

However, from the field of public housing, there is evidence that much can be achieved with sustained and earmarked funding for minority ethnic issues. The Housing Corporation had pursued a 10-year strategy (sadly discontinued in 1996) of funding black housing associations which led to the growth of a number of strong and developing, well managed black organisations providing housing to members of minority ethnic groups. It is clear that sustained effort involving serious amounts of money can do much to alleviate the effects of institutional racism and promote the interests of minority ethnic groups.

Effective Mental Ill-health Services

It is clear that those who are in a state of "dis-ease", mentally and emotionally, might benefit from skilled "talking cure" help, from medication, and maybe from hospital care away from family and work commitments. There are, however, possible iatrogenic effects of such care: professional–lay relationships are characterised by imbalances of power. Where such imbalances impair the capacity for autonomous functioning and even disrupt existing social networks (Pattmore, 1987), then the effects might be to leave the client/patient even more prone to "dis-ease". There is ample research evidence that mental ill-health is exacerbated by poverty, poor housing, by lack of adequate social support and by disruption of social circumstances occasioned, for example, by unemployment or forced migration (Goldberg and Huxley, 1980; Blaxter, 1990; Benzeval *et al.*, 1995). However, it is clear that such mental ill-health can be not just the effect but also the cause of social difficulties in terms of impaired skills to negotiate with bureaucracies, in increased inter-personal conflict, loss of secure housing and of jobs, reduced income and may involve conflicts with the law. It is therefore clear that mental ill-health services should provide advocacy support for individuals to enable their social and civil rights to be protected, a role that does not sit easily with professional, medical roles. It follows therefore that mental ill-health services should seek to provide a range of services for any individual client over an extended time without requiring them to find their own way through the maze of community support services.

These are general statements of need which are true for everyone. In addition there are special needs for members of minority ethnic groups where the belief systems may be very different from those of the majority white population: for example a perceived greater unity of mind, body and social being, plus experience of being discriminated against in daily life, in employment, in housing and in interactions with statutory agencies. In addition there may be considerable disjunctions between different generations as the younger people acculturate much more to the values and mores of the majority society in regard to such issues as rights to individual autonomy. Different generations of minority ethnic people and the two genders may thus have different needs for generic versus specialist minority ethnic services, for gender-specific care, for medical versus "talking cure" care, for more or less help with negotiating the bureaucratic jumble of statutory services. Statutory services such as health and social services are large organisations with powerful built-in self-sustaining mechanisms which result in a strong resistance to change and with boundaries guarded by professionals. Within such organisations, change will typically occur only slowly, over decades rather than over years. In addition increased collaboration with relevant agencies such as housing, education (both school and community based), the police and criminal justice system will be slow to develop.

Resolving the Policy Contradictions

It is patently obvious that organisations cannot go in two opposite directions at once unless extra staff are provided. It is therefore vital that the government resolves the policy contradictions between placing greater emphasis on the severely mentally ill and promoting GP autonomy, which fragments any coherence in purchasing. There can be no doubt that there is a need for clear direction to maintain the severely ill as a high priority yet to be aware of the value of early action to avoid the worst effects of any downward spiral. By definition such people are demanding of time and typically show, at best, gradual improvement. They are thus often avoided (probably without any conscious plan) by busy, over-worked professional staff. Without clear direction, community staff are likely to "drift away" towards the worried well, particularly to young, attractive and articulate clients. GP fundholding is bound to lead to a two-tier service if it is effective in providing and obtaining better services for patients than obtained prior to fundholding. Since fundholding is restricted to larger group practices with adequate infrastructure, it is less likely to be implemented in inner city practices, where most members of minority ethnic minorities reside and where single-handed and two-doctor practices are the norm. It follows, therefore, that fundholding in general practice, unless it becomes universal, will be against the interests of minority ethnic groups. There is little evidence that there have been substantial benefits in patient care attributable to fundholding (Audit Commission, 1995) though it can be suggested that it may have allowed substantial innovation by a minority of practitioners.

It is our conclusion that, to remove the policy contradictions and better serve the interests of minority ethnic groups, it would be better to abolish GP fundholding or, at the very least, to remove mental health funding from its remit.

The Development of Inter-cultural Communicative Competence

In spite of widespread acceptance of ethnic diversity evidenced by the huge (8 per cent annually) growth in foreign leisure travel, professional practice finds it hard to adapt. "If they want treatment in 'our' service they had better be like us" are statements majority ethnic professionals find it easier to say than "I have great difficulties in working with this client". As Kim (1992) has pointed out, "stress is part and parcel of inter-cultural encounters . . . To be inter-culturally competent means to be able to manage such stress, regain the internal balance, and carry out the communication . . . to successful interaction outcomes." There is considerable ethnic diversity throughout Britain. Those who equate ethnicity with skin colour may deny this but there are "hidden minorities" such as Jewish, East European and Irish communities, the latter with the worst health profile in terms of hospitalisation for depression (in women) and rates of alcoholism (in men). Kim (1992) distinguishes between **communicative competence** (in relation to a specific cultural group) and **inter-cultural communicative competence** which would enable people to be flexible and creative in meeting the challenges of any cross-cultural interaction. We would suggest that when such general competencies are meshed with a knowledge base in relation to a particular ethnic group then there is the development of **transcultural communicative competence**.

The essential characteristic of such generic competence is **adaptability**, which can be expressed in cognitive, affective and behavioural dimensions. In cognition it is expressed as a refusal to be dogmatic or insist on reducing new experiences to familiar and safe categories, a willingness to learn, to change ways of thinking. In the affective dimension such adaptability requires the ability to express a positive and open emotional engagement and control of anxiety. In the behavioural dimension such adaptability may be expressed in action, though it is acknowledged how difficult this can be. "Do as I say" is an easier prescription to utter than "Do as I do". Initial training is an obvious place to introduce a proper foundation for professional practice but a great investment in initial training can be undermined by the "professional" scorn of the old guard in the practice setting. Given the inter-professional, inter-agency nature of mental ill-health care, there is a need for intra- and inter-organisational development based on the purposive development and implementation of shared values and purpose (Senge, 1991). As suggested above, institutional structures and political imperatives are critical in the determination of health needs and the shape of service provision. On the one hand it can be confidently asserted that no single profession or agency has shown a consistent and adequate response to minority ethnic mental ill-health needs, yet, on the other hand, all agencies have some levels of commitment, skills, and individual and organisational competencies to provide for such needs. It follows therefore that the skills are widely dispersed but need to be harnessed.

As noted above, in health and social work there is ample evidence of racism in the professions (defined as a generalised discriminatory practice, not as the egregious and clearly expressed verbal abuse and mistreatment); there is also evidence of inadequate training to enable all, or even the majority of staff, to claim competence in working with minority ethnic clients (CCETSW, 1991; Gerrish *et al.*, 1996). Additionally it is clear that promoting the mental health needs of minority ethnic clients is still heavily dependent on the initiative and commitment of a few individuals (typically from minority ethnic backgrounds themselves). Training transculturally competent individual practitioners would not necessarily address the failure of statutory and non-statutory mental health agencies to develop an adequate institutional response to minority ethnic needs. Declaring individuals, or even small under-resourced specialist units, to be responsible for addressing such needs is doomed to failure – passing the buck in place of proper institutional policy.

Promoting Organisational Change

To be effective in promoting organisational change, it is vital to understand the basic "physiology" of what makes institutions "tick". As Senge (1991) and many other theorists and practitioners have suggested (for example, Griffiths, 1983), organisations change only when the inputs to them change.

There are changes which can be made in the *process* of organisations. In the case of the shift towards the seriously mentally ill, the government has monitored performance criteria of the severity grading of patients/clients treated. The development of indicators of "patient centred" aspects of quality has proved elusive and requires more thought and research. In the meantime the input which would make the most difference in the short term would be more effective feedback from users and carers on the acceptability and effectiveness of mental ill-health care organisations. In this way the successes and failures in transcultural communicative competence can be documented and acted upon. To do this there needs to be properly stratified and representative surveys of minority ethnic groups' views which are then actioned *at the most senior levels in the organisations, avoiding the dangers of tokenism.* In addition, there are examples of good practice where voluntary sector staff are involved as expert consultants to help statutory sector staff understand the social context of individual clients' dis-ease and to develop a more rounded approach to assessment and treatment. Implicit in such an approach would be the requirement for a more coherent structure for the purchasing of services, a requirement that has been acknowledged by central government (DoH, 1997).

In regard to **structures** of organisations clearly there need to be efforts to promote the employment of more workers from minority ethnic backgrounds. This, however, would be a longer-term project. Clearly the implementation of equal opportunities policies will be vital but they need to be backed up by measures to ensure appropriate training and career development paths within organisations which provide better support for the heavy load of responsibility carried by such staff. In regard to blurring the boundaries between professional and lay care the role of the voluntary sector is crucial since it would not be so bound by the professionally policied boundaries of practice found in the statutory sector. "Low-level" support services within community support teams, which have been developed by a number of social services departments, point the way to more effectively overcoming the boundaries between "professional" and "care assistants" and between statutory and voluntary sectors. Such blurring could help the move towards a more "bottom heavy" skill mix as suggested by the Audit Commission (1994).

The Way Forward

The usual response to a clear demonstration of inadequacy in services provided is to suggest that more money is needed. We are suggesting no such thing and indeed would suggest that more of the same would be of little benefit to members of minority ethnic groups, for whom present services are mostly seriously inappropriate and unacceptable. Indeed our suggestions of an increased role for the voluntary sector and empowering of lay people would require a redirection rather than any necessary increase in funding. Going beyond the shape of mental ill-health services as they are now, we suggest that there could be several strands of a new approach, both at the conceptual level and at the level of national policy.

At the conceptual level we would challenge the euphemistic elision of "mental health" with "mental illness" which we have had to accept whilst talking about services and discussing these with our respondents. We would agree with Tudor (1996) on the importance of separating the continuum of "mental illness/disorder" from the continuum of degrees of "mental health". At a basic level such a separation would enable the acceptance of the idea of promoting the mental health of those diagnosed as "mentally ill". As Tudor (1996) points out, services for such people mostly seek to *manage* patients, both in hospital and community settings, "to keep them occupied", often with a subsidiary aim of promoting low levels of expressed emotion. If a more mental health approach were adopted, then service quality could be less focused on process and more on outcomes, for example the number of "mentally ill" people living in their own homes as tenants and holding "real" jobs.

At a wider level, the separation of mental health and mental illness would enable the removal of mental health from a narrow medical model and an examination of the wider context of mental health and how to protect and promote it. It would then be possible to start from basic questions about what mental health is, which have been answered in a number of ways, as outlined by Tudor (1996). A simple version was provided by Freud who suggested that the essence of mental health is "to love well and to work well". We would wish to extend the term "work" beyond the comfortable assumptions of middle-class theorising which take the availability of adequately paid work for granted. In this way we would seek to make links between concepts of mental health and those macro-economic policies that dominate the world order.

Fryer (1995) summarises a mass of evidence amassed since the 1930s in countries such as Austria, Britain and the United States which indicate that unemployment leads to mental distress, apathy, helplessness, and social isolation and disintegration. As important is his comment that re-employment does not solve the problem since there are important issues of "quasi-employment" where people feel forced to take jobs in which their skills and talents are seriously under-employed and under-valued. Hartley *et al.* (1991) have summarised the studies in Israel, the Netherlands and the UK which show that job insecurity is associated with impaired mental health (shown by increased psychosomatic symptoms and depression). The particular relevance to the present theme is that high levels of un-employment increase the exclusion of minorities from the labour market with subsequent marginalisation, impoverishment and consequent damage to mental health (Sinfield, 1992). The increasing impoverishment of women in current high unemployment policies has been well documented (Ledwith, 1997) and there is ample evidence that minority ethnic groups are more likely to be unemployed at any and all levels of educational qualifications (Thomas, 1995). Therefore the mental health of minority ethnic groups is particularly likely to be damaged by current economic policies which regard full employment as inimical to the interests of "more important" aims of low inflation, and low government spending enshrined in the stability criteria of European Monetary Union.

The essence of mental health promotion at local level lies in consideration of people within communities. There would thus be a need to reorient the focus and roles of community mental health centres (or teams) (CMHCs). Firstly it is known that these are heavily dominated by health staff, headed in nearly 50 per cent of cases by "physicians" with no examples of management by a social services employee or voluntary sector worker (Tudor, 1996, p. 119). In fact the term "community" as the title of such teams is misleading unless seen within usual "NHS speak" in which everything not in hospital is seen as community services. As noted by Tudor (1996, p. 120), "CMHCs rarely engage in substantial community development activity, such as developing self-help groups or engaging with community action groups and are rarely accountable to local people through management groups or other structures." Certainly such teams could be reoriented towards a social network model as has been developed extensively in the USA and Canada with local examples in the Wirral on Merseyside (Ledwith, 1993). Within such a model the team members would seek to identify and mobilise local resources of buildings and people, in particular harnessing the energy of volunteers and local voluntary sector organisations. Whilst such an approach would be considered novel for CMHC staff, it would be regarded as standard by those involved in community education, particularly in those inspired by the transformative vision of Paulo Freire who sought to enable community groups to understand the nature of the oppression they suffered and to act collectively to challenge it (Lovett, 1975; Ritchie *et al.*, 1994; Ledwith, 1997). There are thus alliances that can and should be made locally between CMHCs and Community Education, who in turn would need to make better links with Citizens Advice Bureaux (Paris and Player, 1993) in order to ensure that clients obtain the welfare benefits to which they are entitled. The Green Paper (DoH, 1997) expressed concern over "a restricted model of care" arising from NHS leadership. We can be more blunt in suggesting that the medical model of individual treatment must be made a small (though vital in extremis) part of the spectrum of services which should be dominated by a social integrative model within which social services staff (if adequately funded) are much better trained and qualified to take the lead. The recent proposal by the Secretary of State for Health for "health action zones", bringing together NHS bodies and local authorities, community and voluntary groups and others in an inter-professional, inter-agency collaboration, is similar to the framework for mental health services envisioned here.

It has no doubt been noticeable that the analysis so far presented in this section of "The Way Forward" has dealt mostly with mental health in general without particular emphasis on minority ethnic groups. The reason for this is that advocacy of a mental health approach with a wider social perspective inherently suggests the need for marginalisation and oppression to be taken into consideration. Where such advocacy would have particular focus would be in insisting on positive action to develop long-term partnerships with minority ethnic voluntary groups who have shown so many examples of user-focused good practice and have been an active and effective challenge to the individual pathology models of so much health service practice.

However, radical reshaping of mental health services cannot operate in isolation from the wider context of social policy and the management of ethnic diversity in Britain (Husband, 1996). With the politics of devolution within the United Kingdom nurturing etho-nationalisms and the previous Conservative government's erosion of commitment to meaningful multi-culturalism still to be corrected, it would be naive to assume that British social policy is formulated within a political culture that positively embraces ethnic diversity. If health policies are to anticipate and plan for ethnic diversity, rather than engage in *ad hoc*, retrospective gestures, then the fabric of British political consciousness must incorporate an acceptance of "differentiated citizenship" (Kymlycka, 1995) wherein the state recognises the logic of treating people differently in order to treat them equally. Universalist provision that does not plan for ethnic diversity is in essence assimilationist and discriminatory. The ideas relating to an equitable and acceptable mental health service outlined in this chapter cannot thrive in a context of ethnocentric and paternalist concepts of citizenship.

There is thus a need, at the highest policy level, to comprehend the real significance of ethnic diversity, for the re-formulation of concepts of mental health and mental illness and the development of more appropriate services. There is now no lack of knowledge on the issue. Rather there is an institutional, professional and political resistance to incorporate the reality of ethnic diversity into determining service delivery. If there is to be a political push from the top, our research suggests that there is a need for a coherent articulation of minority ethnic community concerns to rise from the base of the mental ill-health care pyramid. Minority ethnic users, professionals and activists have all generated distinctive critiques of the current system of care. The present minimal policy response argues loudly that these critical voices have not achieved meaningful political leverage. The process of constructing a potent, minority ethnic force within national health care policy formulation remains relevant and urgent. Unless such pressure is exerted, the demands of the mainstream and majority population will continue to dominate. If this were to happen, then Britain would be a much poorer country culturally and socially in failing to accept the challenges to conventional, majority culture thinking posed by the rich diversity of multi-ethnic culture. Within professions there are severe challenges to be faced, particularly to the hegemony of psychiatrists who, as is typical of doctors, have considerable, negative power to block change (Harrison *et al.*, 1992). If minority ethnic clients are given the opportunity to "vote with their feet" and select the services they find most appropriate, then it would necessarily follow that the racism evident in much psychiatric practice would be challenged. The availability of alternative models of care are thus vital to enabling the services to change to more appropriate forms.

References

Ackroyd, S. (1995) Nurses, management and morale: a diagnosis of decline in the NHS hospital services. In: Soothill, K., Mackay, L. and Webb, C. (eds) *Interprofessional Relations in Health Care*, pp. 222–238. London: Edward Arnold.

Allsop, J. (1995) *Health Policy and the NHS*. London: Longman.

Audit Commission (1986) *Making a Reality of Community Care*. London: HMSO.

Audit Commission (1994) *Finding a Place: A Review of Mental Health Services for Adults*. London: HMSO.

Audit Commission (1995) *Practice Makes Perfect*. London: HMSO.

Beattie, A. (1995) War and peace among the health tribes. In: Soothill, K. Mackay, L., and Webb, C. (eds) *Interprofessional Relations in Health Care*, pp. 11–30. London: Edward Arnold.

Benzeval, M., Judge, K. and Whitehead, M. (1995) *Tackling Inequalities in Health: An Agenda for Action*. London: King's Fund.

Blaxter, M. (1990) *Health and Lifestyle*. London: Tavistock/Routledge.

CCETSW (1991) *Setting the Context for Change: Anti-racist Social Work Education*. London: Central Council for Education and Training in Social Work.

Cole, M. and Perides, M. (1995) Managing values and organisational climate in a multi-professional setting. In: Soothill, K., Mackay, L. and Webb, C. (eds) *Interprofessional Relations in Health Care*, pp. 61–80. London: Edward Arnold.

DoH (1997) *Developing Partnerships in Mental Health*. London: Department of Health.

Flynn, R., Williams, G. and Pickard, S. (1996) *Markets and Networks: Contracting in Community Health Services*. Buckingham: Open University Press.

Fryer, D. (1995) Benefit Agency? *The Psychologist* **June**: 265–272.

Gerrish, K., Husband, C. and Mackenzie, J. (1996) *Nursing for a Multi-ethnic Society*. Buckingham: Open University Press.

Goldberg, D. and Huxley, P. (1980) *Mental Illness in the Community*. London: Tavistock.

Griffiths, R. (1983) *The NHS Management Inquiry Report*. London: HMSO.

Ham, C. (1992) *Health Policy in Britain*, 3rd edn. Basingstoke: Macmillan.

Harrison, S., Hunter, D.J., Marnoch, G. and Pollitt, C. (1992) *Just Managing: Power and Culture in the NHS*. Basingstoke: Macmillan.

Hartley, J.F. *et al.* (1991) *Job Insecurity: Coping with Jobs at Risk*. London: Sage.

Hugman, R. (1995) Contested territory and community services. In: Soothill, K., Mackay, L. and Webb, C. (eds) *Interprofessional Relations in Health Care*, pp. 31–45. London: Edward Arnold.

Husband, C. (1996) Defining and containing diversity: the right to be understood. In: Ahmad, W.I.U. and Atkin, K. (eds) *Race and Community Care*. Buckingham: Open University Press.

Kim, Y.Y. (1992) Intercultural communication competence: a systems theoretic view. In: Gundykunst, W.B. and Kim, Y.Y. (eds) *Readings in Communication with Strangers*. New York: McGraw-Hill.

Klein, R. (1995) *The New Politics of the NHS*, 3rd edn. London: Longman.

Kymlycka, W. (1995) *Multicultural Citizenship*. Oxford: Clarendon Press.

Ledwith, F. (1993) Social support and social therapy. *Lancaster and Westmoreland Medical Journal* **1**(12): 323–325.

Ledwith, F. (1996) *Health Matters* **Autumn**: 10.

Ledwith, F., Husband, C. and Karmani, A. (1997) *Promoting Inter-agency Mental Health Provision for Ethnic Minorities*. Ethnicity and Social Policy Unit, University of Bradford. Final Report to NHS Executive, Northern and Yorkshire Region.

Ledwith, M. (1997) *Participation in Transformation: Towards a Working Model of Community Empowerment*. Birmingham: Venture Press.

Lovett, T. (1975) *Adult Education, Community Development and the Working Class*. Nottingham University: Department of Education.

Nolan, M., Grant, G. and Keady, J. (1996) *Understanding Family Care*. Buckingham: Open University Press.

Paris, J. and Player, D. (1993) "Citizens" advice in general practice. *British Medical Journal* **306**: 1518–1520.

Pattmore, C. (1987) *Living After Mental Illness: Innovatory Services*. London: Croom Helm.

Ritchie, C., Taket, A. and Bryant, J. (1994) *Community Works*. Sheffield Hallam University: Pavic Publications.

Senge, P. (1991) *The Art and Practice of the Learning Organisation*. New York: Century Business.

Sinfield, A. (1992) The impact of unemployment on welfare. In: Kolberg, J.E. and Ferge, Z. (eds) *Social Policy in a Changing World*. Frankfurt: Campus.

Smith, R., Easter, L., Harrison, L. *et al*. (1993) *Working Together for Better Community Care*. Bristol University: SAUS.

Soothill, K., Mackay, L. and Webb, C. (1995) *Interprofessional Relations in Health Care*. London: Edward Arnold.

Thomas, J. (1995) New Britains: Briton and its people in facts and figures. *Observer*, **January 28**, p. 16.

Tudor, K. (1996) *Mental Health Promotion: Paradigms and Practice*. London: Routledge.

17

Managing for Cultural Competence

Jeff Chandra

Introduction

People from minority ethnic communities have lived in Europe for over a millennium. Since the end of the Second World War, a significant proportion of black and minority ethnic people have migrated to Europe from ex-colonial countries, settling primarily in cities where goods and services were most readily available. In the UK, for example, people from black and minority ethnic communities account for 6.2 per cent of the total population but are concentrated in urban centres such as London, Leicester, Birmingham and Bradford. In the London Borough of Brent minority ethnic people make up nearly 45 per cent of all residents. Nationally, there are seventeen other cities and boroughs with minority ethnic populations greater than 20 per cent.

As they became an increasingly significant part of the UK population, differences in their patterns of illness and disease, compared with those seen in the indigenous white population, were observed by health care workers, although this information was not formally collected or systematically studied. More recently, there have been attempts to identify these differences. The result has been an increasing body of evidence which suggests that distinct patterns of illness are found amongst people from different racial, ethnic, cultural and religious backgrounds and that health care provision must be adapted to take account of the needs of minority ethnic groups.

There is clear evidence that the effects of racism, both institutional and individual, taken together with racial and cultural differences, has meant that minority ethnic people have poorer overall health outcomes in terms of morbidity and mortality than the general population and experience significantly greater difficulties in accessing appropriate health services. Based on this evidence, the government has attempted to address the specific health needs of minority ethnic communities, through its policies and its guidelines for the National Health Service (NHS). However, the implementation of such policies and practices by some Trusts, health authorities and social services departments has not been consistent and has not necessarily led to more appropriate and accessible services. There now exists a substantial amount of research about the ways in which the mental health needs of black and minority ethnic communities, in particular, are not met by many professionals working in the health and care systems.

For example, the incidence of diagnosed schizophrenia and other mental health problems attributed to black and minority ethnic communities is an area of significant diagnostic ambiguity. Indeed some observers see it as indicative of the more general way in which the system treats people from minority communities.

Research evidence shows that people from black and minority ethnic communities may manifest different patterns of illness and may have greater difficulty accessing some services. Notwithstanding the publication of guides such as Balarajan and Raleigh's *Ethnicity and Health* (July 1993), *Black Mental Health – A Dialogue for Change* (1994) published by the Department of Health's Mental Health Task Force and Chandra's *Facing Up to Difference* (1996), there remains a continuing concern that many white health care professionals are often ill prepared to treat patients from cultures other than their own. The gap in cultural understanding is particularly acute in the treatment of mental illness.

There is much evidence, some of it controversial, based on research studies about the mental health experiences of black and minority ethnic communities. In particular, Sashidharan (1989), Dutt (1991) and Mumford (1992) have highlighted key issues related to the diagnosis and treatment of mental illness in black and minority ethnic people. Unfortunately, this work has not been disseminated widely enough to make a significant impact.

The lack of proper understanding of culturally specific issues has had direct consequences. Where mental health assessment and treatment is required, there is evidence that patients from ethnic minority groups, especially African-Caribbean people, enter psychiatric services via the criminal justice system rather than through GP referrals, although they are no more likely to be detained under the Mental Health Act 1983 (Rwegellera, 1977; Harrison *et al.*, 1988).

Although the greater number of court compulsory admissions for African-Caribbean people may be accounted for by higher rates of psychotic illness and/or by late intervention leading to the involvement of emergency services, these are not the only factors. Racial stereotyping, by which young African-Caribbean men, for example, are perceived as disturbed and threatening, could be a factor, as could the reticence of this group to use GP services routinely.

Notwithstanding the development work which has already taken place, the over-representation of patients from black and minority ethnic groups compulsorily admitted under the Mental Health Act 1983, their difficulty in accessing primary care services, problems of communication (including inappropriate interpretation services), commonly held perceptions of black and minority ethnic people suffering distress as difficult or "strange", and institutional and individual racism, all point to a clear need for a systematic and determined approach to making services culturally competent.

The Management Task

Effective management of health care systems requires a thorough understanding of the needs and wants of patients and carers, as well as the ability to organise appropriate and effective service responses to those needs and wants. There is little doubt that mental health services in the UK are at a very early stage of understanding the needs and wants of what is now a very diverse multi-cultural community.

Any serious attempt at making mental health services culturally competent requires a root and branch examination of the mental health care system as a whole. Whilst all the staff groups and professions working in mental health have an important role to play, it is a unique role of managers to ensure that all parts of the system work together as a coherent whole. It is necessary, first of all, that managers understand the evidence linking ethnicity and mental health so that they have a grasp of the issues that require to be addressed in order to provide "equitable" services. The existence of individual and institutional racism needs to be recognised and confronted. The second key task is to appreciate that what is likely to be needed is not a "quick fix" (none exists) but rather a change in the culture of their organisation which can be achieved only with sustained effort over a period of time, because what is required is not just a change of policies and procedures but changes to the response of staff to black and minority ethnic patients. If this change follows from changes in staff attitudes, so much the better.

In brief, management needs to take a strategic approach which encompasses the entire gamut of organisational variables such as:

- revisions to service strategies, policies and procedures;
- development of service specifications which go with the grain of the religious and cultural beliefs of minority groups;
- the pro-active involvement of users, carers and the minority community itself in shaping and monitoring services;
- development of specific quality standards;
- ensuring that the organisation's staffing reflects the diversity of the community being served.

This chapter sets out some of the ways in which management can contribute to the provision of culturally competent mental health services.

Strategic Focus

The research for *Facing up to Difference* (Chandra, 1996) showed that, nationally, most activity to address minority ethnic health issues is through short-term, time-limited projects, often funded by short-term grants. Such work has an important role but there is a conspicuous lack of a strategic approach by commissioners and providers of mental health services. The challenge for the health service is to integrate the ethnic dimension within the mainstream commissioning and business planning processes of health authorities, Trusts and primary care groups. For those working in the field of ethnicity and health this, of course, has been a long-standing aspiration, but the evidence shows that there is much that remains to be done. A successful strategy is likely to be one where the key players have been involved in its creation and are clear about the shared objectives that are to be achieved. Here again, the evidence shows that there is often poor co-ordination of approaches between commissioners and providers of health services and in particular between primary, community and secondary care providers of services.

The voluntary sector, particularly black voluntary groups, has a crucial role to play in mental health services. Where these groups exist they have the potential to add realism and specificity to the strategic planning process because they are likely to be in close contact with users and carers of mental health services. They may well actually provide services and, if this is so, commissioning organisations may well have a provider organisation which has a head start in delivering a culturally competent service to a section of its population. Indeed, a strategic objective of significant benefit would be supporting such organisations to become organisationally and financially robust enough to play a significant long-term role in service provision and development. Even where the organisation is primarily focused on advocacy for their community, their involvement in service development is conducive to adding relevance and credibility to the service planning process.

A strategic focus for mental health services would require that all the key stakeholders identified above jointly address the key mental health issues which stand out for black and minority communities. These include issues of access to services, appropriateness of existing services and of course acceptability, and this cannot be done without a sound understanding of the cultural and health belief systems amongst those communities. This is where the involvement of users and the community itself in the process of service planning and provision becomes vital.

Involving Users and Carers

One of the most frequent criticisms of the NHS by black and minority ethnic groups is not lack of consultation but that consultation is not followed by action. Undertaking another round of consultations without acknowledging previously expressed views is likely to be perceived as yet another manifestation of NHS "deafness" to local voices. Therefore, the key task for managers in mental health services is not just to establish effective mechanisms for involving users and carers but to ensure that there is regular feedback in response to the views and comments being expressed by users, carers and community representatives. There are a number of key points at which users and carers need to be involved.

- At the **planning** stage, involvement will ensure that services meet real needs rather than needs based on stereotypes and "common knowledge".
- In **service delivery** black and minority ethnic service users must have confidence that service providers communicate with them effectively, treat them with respect, build on individual strengths and meet individual needs. On-going liaison with groups of service users can help achieve this sensitivity at the individual level. For some services it may be appropriate to encourage and facilitate service users to deliver services such as advocacy.
- Involving users in **monitoring** and **evaluating** services is an effective way of obtaining feedback on whether services are genuinely culturally competent.

The approach to involving users and carers also requires careful thought. Any such approach must recognise that:

- racism and its resultant indirect and direct discrimination is a real experience for users and carers;
- many black and minority ethnic people do not use services so "non-users" or "potential users" should be consulted;
- there is a great cultural, religious and linguistic diversity within black and minority ethnic groups with some different needs and some common needs; any strategy should be targeted to the particular minority ethnic group being consulted;
- the priorities of black and minority ethnic service users may contrast with local epidemiological information about the illness/disease which should be their primary concern.

Effective involvement with users and carers takes time, particularly where community groups do not have well developed "representatives". Some key steps in planning a user involvement process include:

1. Determining the aims and purposes of the consultation so that all parties are clear about the process as well as likely outcomes.
2. Examining what consultation and participation mechanisms already exist and evaluating how effective these are in involving black and minority ethnic communities in a meaningful way.
3. Developing a strategy which is an integral part of the organisation's processes and which is regularly evaluated.

Improving Communications

There is extensive evidence that communication problems affect accessibility to health care and can mean less appropriate services (including potentially serious misdiagnosis), and frustration and delay for all concerned. Excessive reliance is still placed on relatives – often young children – to bridge the communications gap.

The survey relating to black and minority ethnic groups, *Health and Lifestyles* (HEA, 1994), included a section on languages spoken. The key findings of that survey were as follows:

- Although most South Asians can speak some English, only about three out of ten (32 per cent) of Indians and one out of ten (10 per cent) of Bangladeshis considered English to be their main spoken language.
- Women were less likely than men to speak English and only a small proportion of those aged 50 or over considered English to be their main spoken language.
- About one quarter (24 per cent) of Indians and almost half (48 per cent) of Bangladeshis were unable to read English; smaller proportions were unable to read any language.

This research confirms that language is a significant barrier to the provision of appropriate and culturally competent health services. It goes without saying that the social, cultural and medical complexities around mental health issues make the importance of good clear communications between patients and professional staff even more important. In particular, the use of relatives to assist in communications between patients and professional staff introduces a potentially damaging conflict between the patient's wishes and those interpreting for them. A fundamental task therefore in the creation of a culturally competent service is the provision of skilled help which bridges the communication gap between patients and mental health services. Indeed, perhaps more than in many other services, there is the need for advocacy on behalf of patients as opposed to purely technical interpreting or indeed link working, although both these latter services also have a role to play. The main aspects of advocacy are:

- it facilitates linguistic and cultural communication between the service user and the health professional;
- it advises other health professionals on, and ensures delivery of, appropriate health care acceptable to the particular needs of the service user including adherence to differing religious, cultural or dietary norms and requirements;
- it provides information, advice and support to the service user to enable them to be fully informed about their medical condition, to be able to voice their rights and expectations, to know their rights, and to be able to make informed choices;
- it acts on behalf of, and in the interests of, the service user;
- it advises the service user about and ensures access to other professional agencies regarding their health-related needs.

It is the job of managers to ensure that such help is provided within a clear policy context. A policy for communication needs to identify the quality standards to which the services will operate, the professional development needs of those providing the advocacy support, in what circumstances relatives are to be used or not used for interpreting support and what role other staff in the service have in providing interpreting services.

The other aspects of communications is information on mental health and mental health services for users and carers, provided in a culturally and linguistically acceptable way. So far as patient information is concerned there is still extensive and undue reliance placed on written materials. Some of this material is counter-productive because the translations do not take account of the relevant cultural and linguistic subtleties. On the other hand, there is good evidence that information provided in audio and video tape formats in community languages, developed in full consultation with relevant communities, reaches many more people than written information. Several health services also use community language radio stations, television and newspapers to reach local black and minority ethnic communities. There is no doubt that much more open and public discussion of mental health within the minority ethnic communities needs to be fostered to cut through the stigma, fear and secrecy that sometimes exists around mental health issues within the different communities.

Staffing the Service for Cultural Competence

Although some improvements have been achieved over recent years, discrimination on the grounds of ethnicity, race and colour remains an unattractive feature of NHS employment practice in many places. This is despite the public policy stance which recognises that the case for equal opportunities is not simply a moral one. One of the most effective ways of achieving culturally competent services is to recruit, train and retain staff from the ethnic minority communities themselves. During 1992 and 1993 the then Secretary of State for Health chaired a task force to develop a national framework for attracting, retaining and developing black and minority ethnic staff in the NHS. This initiative recognised that the NHS had not achieved much progress, despite many years of exhortation and reports, for example the King's Fund Task Force on Equal Opportunities, together with some highly publicised cases of proven racial discrimination. The report of the Secretary of State's Task Force on Staffing was published as *Ethnic Minority Staff in the NHS: A Programme of Action* [EL(94)12]. At the launch of the document the Secretary of State said:

> I want to stress that taking action to promote equality in employment is not just a matter of moral justice or a fairness to people from minority groups. It is good sound common sense and it makes business sense too.

This document remains national policy and a system of recording ethnicity of staff with national returns was put in place to monitor developments.

However, a survey of NHS staff undertaken in 1997 by the Manufacturing, Science and Finance Trade Union found a dismal picture. Some NHS Trusts in areas with large ethnic minority populations admitted that their workforces were entirely white. Almost 170 Trusts failed to complete the monitoring returns and *NHS Trusts in Leicester and Bradford admitted that they did not have any black or Asian staff at all.* It is also the case that where ethnic minority staff are employed they are generally at the lower echelons of the professional or staff group and conversely very few black and minority staff are in senior decision-making positions at Chief Executive or Executive Director level on NHS Trust and Health Authority Boards.

A key management task therefore is to ensure that mental health purchasers and providers have within their number skilled staff from the communities for which services are being provided. Primarily, the achievement of this objective is not a matter of new policy because there is extensive policy advice and guidance available on equal opportunities from the NHS Executive, the Commission for Racial Equality and similar bodies. The task is one of putting this high on the management agenda and ensuring that the anti-discriminatory values which most NHS organisations appear to espouse are evident through the actions of managers and staff within the organisation, particularly those involved in the recruitment, selection, training and development of staff. It is a legitimate and necessary matter for the NHS Trust or Health Authority Board to identify the current ethnic makeup of its staff and to receive regular progress reports on the achievement of its equal opportunity targets, one of which must be to reflect in its staffing the ethnic makeup of the population served. This is indeed one of the goals set out in *Programme of Action* as one of the eight goals contained in that document.

There has often been debate about whether purchasers have any right to influence providers on matters of staffing. In the face of a massive failure to move towards equitable staffing of the NHS, such discussion merely lends weight to those who argue that the NHS is irredeemably racist. Given that staffing and service delivery are inextricably linked, purchasers have every reason to demand that their providers address staff imbalances which prevent them from providing culturally competent mental health services which are appropriate, accessible and acceptable to *all* the communities served.

The point about staffing, of course, does not just apply to recruitment and selection of staff from black and minority ethnic groups. It is incumbent on managers to ensure that all staff who are providing services to a culturally diverse community are equipped with the tools to do so in a sensitive manner. Training that can equip health professionals with more knowledge, information and sensitivity in providing services to black and minority ethnic communities can be broadly divided into three approaches:

- Cultural awareness training.
- Race awareness training.
- Anti-discriminatory training.

Before provider and purchaser agencies commission or undertake training for staff it is important that they fully understand the differences, advantages and disadvantages of each of these approaches. In general terms **cultural awareness training** aims to provide information on the customs, habits and life-style of black and minority ethnic people living in Britain for the purpose of understanding their culture. Such training has severe limitations because it can reinforce simple stereotypes such as the notion that all the ethnic groups behave in similar ways, the different culture of groups explains why they find many services inappropriate and it makes the assumption that if you have professionals trained in cultural knowledge then you can provide a culturally competent service.

Race awareness training aims to raise awareness of racism and its implications with the hope of changing individual racist attitudes and behaviour. Such training can focus on individual and personal racism and ignore institutionalised racism. Institutional racism can be tackled by central government and its agents, e.g. NHS Executive (NHSE), its Regional Offices, Health Authorities and NHS Trusts. The way in which such training is carried out can sometimes create guilt and resentment in white trainees which is not the most positive emotional motive for attitudinal and behavioural change. Nevertheless, personal change can be fostered by Trusts by making issues of equality a part of managers' individual performance review and also by service specification by purchasers.

Anti-discriminatory training has at its core the notion that people can only judge actions not attitudes. Appropriate behaviour is precisely what organisations need to encourage through their values, policies and procedures. On balance it is the anti-discriminatory model which has the potential for significantly altering the behaviour of staff provided it is carried right through the organisation in a systematic way and the feedback from staff, users and carers used to evaluate whether the training has had the desired effect.

Setting Standards

Quality standards are the means to an end. The end is to ensure that health services are accessible, appropriate and culturally competent to meet the needs of black and minority ethnic communities. Reference has already been made earlier to the need for a strategic approach to the planning of services and an integral part of this is the need to establish clear standards which can be monitored. *Facing Up to Difference* (Chandra, 1996) includes a range of quality standards in relation to ethnicity and health covering ethnic monitoring, communications and information, religious and spiritual needs, bereavement, gender, diet, personal care, anti-discriminatory training, employment and complaints. Of course, not all these are automatically relevant to mental health services but a number of the standards set out could be adapted with benefit in most mental health provision. Conceptually, it is possible to consider quality standards on the basis of Figure 17.1. This shows four concentric circles and each circle is explained below.

Statutory standards – the inner circle

The relevant sections of the Race Relations Act 1976, such as Section 20, make it unlawful to discriminate in the provision of services on racial

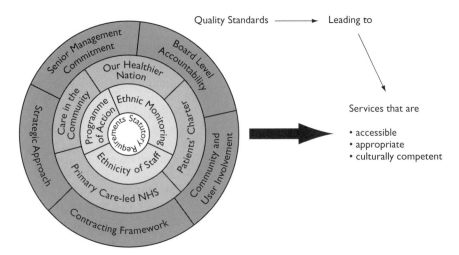

Figure 17.1   A framework for quality standards for mental health. Inner circle: statutory standards; second circle: mandatory standards; third circle: contractual standards; fourth circle: organisational standards.

grounds. The requirement to adhere to this should be explicit in service specifications for mental health services.

Mandatory standards – the second circle

Contracts should also specify the need to meet the mandatory requirement of the health service in relation to ethnicity and health. Two of these requirements relate to the collection of data to help in the planning and provision of culturally competent services.

- Ethnic monitoring of staff.
- Collection of ethnic group data for admitted patients, EL(94)77.

Contractual standards – the third circle

It is at this point that the standards referred to earlier, for example in relation to respecting the privacy and dignity, cultural and religious beliefs of patients, need to be specified within contracts and specifications for service provision.

Organisational standards – the outer circle

The organisational arrangements which improve the prospect of achieving culturally competent services are included within the circle. Examples of such arrangements include board level accountability for ensuring that the needs of ethnic minorities are being addressed, senior management commitment to ensuring an effective dialogue with users and carers of mental health services and the development of a strategic approach to

Table 17.1 An example of quality standards.

Point of delivery	Quality standard
Primary care	Provide and disseminate literature about nature of mental illness and the roles of services at all key contact points for service users and potential users (in appropriate languages).
	Undertake targeted outreach work to raise awareness of issues, services and roles of professionals in conjunction with CMHTs, interpreters, linkworkers and black voluntary sector providers.
In-patient admission	A clear admissions policy and procedures to be in place which specifies the assessment procedure. Ethnicity recorded as per EL(94)77. The language, age, sex and religion of all clients to be noted.
	Patients and/or relatives/carers will be given verbal information (to be reinforced in a written format/audio tapes) on admission about:
	<ul><li>hospital facilities;</li><li>complaints procedures;</li><li>legal status on admission and rights;</li><li>professional roles;</li><li>rights to advocacy and interpreting.</li></ul>
Assessment	Explanations to be supported by relevant written/audio material in relevant languages.
	An advocacy/interpreter to be offered.
	Each patient (and carer if appropriate) will be involved in the development of her/his care plan. Each care plan must have therapeutic, recreational, social and rehabilitation components.
	Care plans will be reviewed at planned regular intervals. A timetable of review dates will be drawn up and adhered to. Patients will be given advance notice of the date and given the opportunity to attend and/or be represented by a relative/friend or advocate.
Treatment	A planned programme of activities on and off the ward to be in place. This must involve "therapeutic" interaction of patients with nursing, paramedical and appropriate black provider's staff.
	Programme to be regularly reviewed and reviews recorded.
Discharge	Unit to have a written discharge policy which specifies:
	<ul><li>all discharged patients to be notified/referred to GP;</li><li>all relevant agencies, including key black providers, to be notified;</li><li>discharge follow-up procedures to be undertaken by relevant staff with the appropriate language, cultural skills/or staff to be accompanied by an advocate/interpreter;</li><li>agreed CPA procedure prior to discharge;</li><li>named key worker and contact point.</li></ul>

achieving the change that is required. At the time of writing the NHSE is considering a quality award for organisations that can display excellence in the field of equality, both in terms of service provision and also staffing. Statutory and voluntary sector mental health services for black and minority ethnic communities need quality standards and monitoring mechanisms as the majority of changes required to improve access and sensitivity are changes to practices. Table 17.1 sets out a framework for some of the specific standards that might be included within contracts for mental health services.

Concluding Comments

Mental health services are in transition from models based around in-patient care towards treatment and care within the community. Managers already face a challenging task in ensuring that risk is minimised to patients and carers as this historically significant shift is made. However, for black and minority ethnic communities this transition will have been a failure if the known difficulties of access, inappropriate service provision and acceptability are not addressed, to say nothing of the known epidemiological variations in mental health care.

There is, of course, a need for considerable further research in order to learn more about the reasons for those variations as well as to evaluate effective service provision for different minority groups. Nevertheless, there is enough sound information available to demonstrate that effective action can be taken to overcome the barriers that currently exist. The task for managers is to ensure that the whole organisation is aware of the information about the needs of black and minority community services, such as the cultural and religious factors which are particularly relevant in making services appropriate and acceptable; and to organise the resources available in a way which ensures that these are considered an integral part of the management and service provision task rather than as an after-thought.

References

Balarajan, R. and Raleigh, S.V. (1993) *Ethnicity and Health – A Guide for the NHS*. London: Department of Health.

Chandra, J. (1996) *Facing Up to Difference*. London: Department of Health and King's Fund.

Dutt, G.C. (1991) How cultural beliefs hamper psychiatric treatment. *Overseas Doctors Association News*, August/September.

Harrison, G. *et al.* (1988) A prospective study of severe mental disorder in Afro-Caribbean patients. *Psychological Medicine* 18(3).

HEA (1994) *Health and Lifestyles Survey; Black and Minority Ethnic Groups in England*. London: Health Education Authority.

Mumford, D.B. (1992) Detection of psychiatric disorders among Asian patients presenting with somatic symptoms. *British Journal of Hospital Medicine* 47: 202–204.

Rwegellera, G.G.C. (1977) Psychiatric morbidity among West Africans and West Indians living in London. *Psychological Medicine* 7: 317–329.

Sashidharan, S. (1989) Race and Mental Health 2: Schizophrenic – or just black? *Community Care* **783**.

NHS Executive [EL(94)12] *Ethnic Minority Staff in the NHS: A Programme of Action*.

NHS Executive [EL(94)77] *Collection of Ethnic Group Data for Admitted Patients*.

NHS Mental Health Task Force (1994) *Black Mental Health – A Dialogue for Change*. London: Department of Health.

18

The Purchasing Commissioner

Peter Gluckman

A Short Guide to Commissioning (Purchasing)

The commissioning of services, whether in health care (by health authorities, GPs or (in future) primary care groups) or in local authorities (by social services departments), consists essentially of making an assessment of need for the population for which that commissioner is responsible. For example, the commissioner for mental health ensures that services are provided to meet the assessed need for people with mental ill-health. For black and ethnic minority populations, services need to be culturally sensitive and relevant. It is the commissioner's job to ensure that culturally sensitive services provided by culturally competent professionals are in place.

An Unexpected Pattern of Patient Care for Ethnic and Cultural Minorities

The impact of ethnicity and culture on those commissioning mental health services is striking. The local health and social care system, whether simply inherited or carefully constructed, treats thousands of people a year, but seems at times out of tune with the needs of parts of the population and is criticised by them. Service users, carers, families and communities identify deficiencies in attitudes and responsiveness, and at times outright discrimination.

For these groups, the techniques of public health epidemiology, the expertise of providers and even access to primary care are problematic. Like a dye released into a complex river system flowing over rocks and through channels, the progress of patients from ethnic minorities and different cultural groups through mental health services shows some unexpected currents: under-representation in primary care for depression and more minor disorders; involvement of GPs sometimes only at the time of sectioning under the Mental Health Act 1983; the almost complete lack of black people in psychotherapy and other talking therapies; the over-representation of young black males compulsorily admitted to adult psychiatric wards; use of heavy medication; high levels of suicide in young Asian women; and the disproportionate presence of ethnic minorities in the three Special Hospitals. Even discounting possible misdiagnosis due to racial stereotyping and lack of cultural awareness, the over-representation of different ethnic minorities in acute mental health services indicates a very high level of mental distress in those groups.

Financial allocations are determined by a weighted capitation formula assuming only relatively minor variations in need from the average across the country. The commissioner of mental health services has to balance the conflicting needs of ethnic and cultural minorities and the majority population with the wider priorities of the health authority for services other than mental health.

At conferences on the needs of ethnic and cultural minorities, the commissioner is at first surprised then encouraged by the extensive research available about how to meet these needs. Yet it seems difficult to create shifts across mental health services as a whole to respond to the literature other than in pilot and demonstration areas. Similarly, the commissioner in reviewing her or his own progress towards culturally sensitive commissioning notes that any change or development is largely at the margin, with mainstream services difficult to affect.

At What Stages Does a System Consider the Needs of Minorities?

Ethnic and minority cultural groups tend to have lower incomes, reduced employment and educational opportunities, inadequate housing and poorer nutrition. As a result their health status, wherever as individuals they enter the NHS, will be compromised. To the extent that those inequalities can be addressed and reversed so health status will be improved.

The increasing emphasis on collaboration, public health in a broad sense and reducing inequalities could have a major impact over time on the mental well-being of ethnic and cultural minorities (NHS Executive, 1997).

Returning to the shorter term, it is only recently that the maturity of the commissioner/provider system has allowed the serious consideration of ethnic and cultural minority health issues. The period 1986–1995 saw few systematic and mainstream approaches to the needs of these minorities, although there were a number of interesting and innovative projects established during this time. The mental health strategies that began to emerge from the new purchasing health authorities between 1994 and 1996 addressed the issues and concerns around ethnic and cultural mental health issues but mainly identified action yet to come as subject to additional funding. Great structural change in the NHS (and possibly in other parts of the public sector too) particularly disadvantages and impacts upon ethnic and cultural minorities. Only a sustained focus on the complex, subtle and sensitive issues of ethnicity, cultural diversity and mental health will enable any change in the wider system.

Identifying the strengths of the fading NHS "internal market" system and building on them, while acknowledging its real weaknesses and trying to exclude or at least to minimise them, will help commissioners to make progress even as the new national framework evolves. That framework, as set out in the White Paper "The New NHS" (Department of Health, 1997, pp. 24–31), will benefit mental health service users as it is based on integrated care and partnership.

Strengths and Weaknesses of the Commissioning System (Purchaser/Provider)

The principal **strengths** of the purchaser/provider split are as follows:

1. It moves the focus of attention from the interests of the institution to the needs of the population. Within the overall population it is possible to identify its various components and communities, and to determine how and to what extent mainstream services can be culturally attuned to become responsive to a wider range of need and the extent to which, if any, specific targeted services need to be established.
2. It is potentially public health led. With the focus on the population a much stronger element of health status as opposed to health service can occur. While this approach inevitably links to longer-term plans and action it gives the opportunity for partnerships with ethnic and cultural minorities to develop. It allows engagement in the planning and delivery of services to occur and provides a realistic chance for links with other agencies and sectors that impact on health status, not necessarily led by the NHS but supported by its knowledge and expertise.
3. It enables understanding of the role and contributions of other sectors and agencies in the wider system, e.g. local authorities, voluntary agencies and the private sector, and gives those contributions full recognition.
4. It creates the opportunity away from day-to-day operational management to investigate the needs of different and smaller populations and for individuals and organisations to articulate those needs.

The main **weaknesses** of the purchaser/provider split are as follows:

1. The distance it can create between purchasers and people delivering services.
2. Legitimisation of behaviour which is not in the interest of patients by emphasising competition between institutions rather than collaboration around patients' needs.
3. Perverse incentives to maximise income rather than drive down costs.
4. The purchasing health authority can seem remote and bureaucratic, particularly to ethnic and cultural minority communities experiencing disadvantage in their everyday lives in general, and in access to health services in particular.

A continuing shortcoming of the NHS at both national level and locally has been the inability of the service to implement the Department of Health's requirement (NHS Executive, 1994) for ethnic monitoring, which has been successfully carried out by many local authorities for 20 years. As a result, our knowledge across the service of differential access to services by ethnic and cultural minorities is incomplete and a key aspect of the epidemiology of local populations is not available. A clear national framework to which health authorities, trusts and GPs are held accountable is a particular need. Irrefutable evidence about differential access by black and ethnic minorities to mental health services would create a knowledgeable environment for people to change their approach and services.

Maturity and Plurality in Commissioning for Minority Needs

There has been, in the maturing purchaser/provider system, an increasing number of purchasers. These include health authorities, GPs and local authorities (in some instances). Even with the reduction of commissioning bodies envisaged in the White Paper "The New NHS" (Department of Health, 1997, p. 16) there will still be many commissioners operating in each health authority area.

Within any system, the history of responses to minority ethnic and cultural needs is that they are understood (eventually); the organisation becomes sufficiently developed to address those needs; then that work comes to an abrupt stop when those public institutions are abolished, merged and recreated. It is essential therefore that the primary care groups, however they evolve, recognise the needs of ethnic and minority cultural groups and continue the work already begun. Those needs must not be put on hold once again while a new organisational process unfolds, this time involving GPs, community nurses and social services departments with legitimately divergent views about what is commissioning and what is their part in it.

For a mental health provider serving a multi-cultural catchment area, attuning its services to cultural differences will have to be done as purchasing continues to be devolved to primary care groups. They will have to take those cultural needs into their commissioning plans. In turn these plans have to be part of each health authority's health improvement programme.

As primary care groups' commissioning extends to the wider primary health care team, they have a great potential to link with local community and voluntary groups, while establishing effective links with local social services and housing offices. Primary care group commissioning could enhance the sensitivity of primary care and specialist mental health services to ethnic and cultural diversity. An alternative view is that the effort (by GPs, community nurses, mental health trusts, health authorities and others) to make a success of primary care group commissioning for existing acute and community mental health services will once again divert attention from the needs of ethnic and cultural minority groups. It is essential to avoid this unwanted outcome.

For the mental health commissioner who increasingly will be carrying out her/his work in conjunction with GPs and other primary care staff, there is a particular and specific responsibility to ensure that the frustrating history of recognition, submergence and then final re-acknowledgement of ethnic and cultural mental health issues does not happen again. This caution reflects the experience of seeing the theory behind two previous White Papers in 1989 unfold in practice (Department of Health, 1989a, 1989b). The theory ran that if health authorities focused on the needs of the population, then the needs of black and ethnic minorities would be included. To some extent this is true, but there has been disappointment and little evidence of material improvement so far in the health of black and ethnic minorities as a result of previous NHS changes.

Each health authority will need to ensure that, as part of the development of its health improvement programme for its population, primary care groups take on as a core task a public health and needs-based assessment (including that for their minority patients and their mental health needs) which informs their commissioning plans.

In some localities, ethnic and cultural minority groups will be the majority of the population; in others the proportion may be very small. Even in localities with a large minority population there may be many communities represented within it. One interesting feature of demographic change in some areas in recent years has been the move away from preponderance by African-Caribbeans of West Indian descent or people of Asian origin from India and Pakistan to a far greater diversity: West Africans, North Africans, Africans from Somalia, Eritrea, Rwanda and the Congo, populations from newer members of the European Union (Spain and Portugal), people from Eastern Europe and former countries of Yugoslavia and the USSR, and refugees and asylum seekers. These include traumatised people who have come from areas of war and torture. Communication in a multiplicity of languages becomes necessary.

National Policy, Population Need and Local Response

While these changes in the demographic structure impact on the health and the social care system as a whole, they is particularly poignant when trying to commission mental health services for this new, disparate and needy range of populations. From the perspective of a general practice or mental health Trust it seems that just as they are beginning to understand the needs of, and orientate their services towards, ethnic and cultural minorities, newer populations arrive with different requirements for targeting and delivering services.

In this context, health authorities have to fulfil two equally pressing national requirements. These are:

1. to support and develop the central place of primary care in the delivery of mental health services to the population;
2. to concentrate resources on those in greatest need, often through specialist mental health NHS Trusts.

Both of these are excellent policies, but the tension and contradiction between them is not yet fully integrated at national level and consequently locally commissioners struggle to make it work. At the same time there has been an increasingly strong torrent of national guidance and requirements to health authorities, Trusts, local authorities and GPs around managing the mental health system. Success in implementing this range of policy initiatives has been patchy.

The sustained recent emphasis on mental health at national level has benefited ethnic and cultural minorities. There is now much more understanding and use of research evidence at local level and there are many individual pilots and projects around ethnic and cultural mental health issues. This knowledge is not being pushed forward on a sustained or co-ordinated basis. Although it will take time for the government's overall policy framework for the NHS to evolve, it is essential to maintain mental health and the needs of ethnic and cultural minorities as top priority through the coming changes.

With the current emphasis on collaboration and primary care group commissioning, it is important that each health authority, working in partnership with other agencies, defines its individual role. One essential role is that of "ringholding"; understanding the whole system and how it works; facilitating links and alliances to remove blocks; and improving every agency's capacity to contribute. In the current pluralistic, fragmented and evolving system only the health authority has the responsibility for an overview of what is happening across the whole population. Its role is to lead and facilitate strategic change rather than the change that can be created better by primary care groups or the Trusts. In mental health these changes are driven by the following:

1. Increasing empowerment and knowledge of individual service users, their carers, families and minority communities about services, drugs and interventions.
2. Impact of mental health on primary care resources which have yet fully to respond to the needs of black and ethnic minorities.
3. Increasing level of severe mental ill-health among some children and young people, particularly those from minority groups.
4. Growing scale and severity in the level of serious mental illness among adults, among whom black and minority patients are over-represented.
5. Large proportion of severely mentally ill adults with a dual diagnosis, i.e. also linked to alcohol and drug misuse.
6. Large numbers of elderly people with either severe depression or dementia.
7. Public anxiety and concern about spectacular failures of the system.

8. Skill shortage in key clinical and professional groups where black and minority ethnic staff are under-represented.
9. Lead role for local authorities and community care legislation for the mentally ill living in the community.
10. Shortage of appropriately supported housing tenures and schemes for people who do not need to be in NHS accommodation but who are not able to sustain totally independent living. Black and minority ethnic groups find it difficult to access such accommodation as it exists.
11. Developing role of the voluntary sector both as a "commissioner without budget" (as advocate, campaigner and educator for mental health in general and for ethnic and cultural minorities in particular) and as provider of innovative and niche services for certain aspects of service for those populations.
12. Impact of new drugs and therapies.
13. Impact of caring for mentally disordered offenders within the NHS and the consequent skewing of development funds away from community-based services for the wider mentally ill population. Patients from black and minority communities are over-represented in this high need group, many of whom could be cared for in other settings.
14. Proposed move of patients from the three Special Hospitals (Ashworth, Broadmoor and Rampton) into less secure community settings and the need to ensure financial sustainability for receiving health authorities so that other general community and acute services, whether in mental health or general hospital settings, are not cut.
15. The change in the employment structure particularly in inner cities where increasingly information technology, flexible learning and good communication skills are pre-requisites of finding and keeping a job. This development is allied with the virtual disappearance of large parts of manufacturing industry and other manual occupations which provided a range of useful jobs where individuals could work for a period, depart and take up equivalent employment elsewhere. Responsibility for meaningful daytime activity is not clear, very expensive and largely absent. To the extent that black and minority communities suffer from inequalities in educational opportunities it will be more difficult for them to secure new jobs created by economic changes.

Long-term Needs, Short-term Funding

The current mental health service configuration across health and social care, however excellent or deficient, cannot be sustained. It is largely supported by:

- the temporary funding of double running costs where long-stay institutions have been closed and replaced by mental health community facilities;

- the mental illness specific grant which is vital funding but not permanent;
- the Mental Health Challenge Fund;
- central government grants to help pay for the care of mentally disordered offenders;
- in London, the use of London Implementation Zone funding for developments in primary care-based mental health services;
- the use of three-year joint finance funds allocated by joint consultative committees which sustain much of the black voluntary sector;
- welcome but short-lived national initiatives, e.g. NHS National Ethnic Health Advisory Group.

If this short-term targeted funding were reduced or ended, large sections of the community mental health services, developments in mental health services in primary care, joint projects with local authorities and support for innovation in the voluntary sector would cease. Much of this new funding has particularly benefited ethnic and cultural minorities. It is from Mental Health Challenge Funding, mental illness specific grant, primary health care pump priming and other non-recurring sources that new services have developed for ethnic and cultural minorities.

That part of the voluntary sector dealing with the needs of ethnic and cultural minorities is covered in detail in Chapter 9. It identified the short-term funding of much of the black voluntary sector's work and in some cases its cessation. Exactly the same analysis can be applied, however, to funding in the statutory sector, where much of service provision built up for and attuned to the needs of ethnic and cultural minority patients is sustained by short-term funding.

Evolution of Health Authorities: Benefit to Minorities

As health authorities understand their role more and distinguish between what they do well and what can be better done by primary care groups and Trusts, so their role becomes more strategic and long term. In this context the potential for public health and needs-led assessment of ethnic and minority cultural mental health issues can achieve higher status.

Through this approach, while purchasing around individual patients is delegated to primary care-led teams and local authority care managers, longer-term changes can occur which bring black and minority mental health issues into mainstream thinking. In turn these changes improve the orientation in the provision of service by specialist mental health Trusts and primary care-based services.

The health authority will move from the annual contracting cycle dealing with changes at the margin of services (which can sometimes improve matters for ethnic and cultural minority patients) to a three-year service agreement which looks at the wider system and how it impacts on ethnic and cultural minorities and maintains or reduces inequalities. Service agreements will develop within the health improvement programmes.

These changes require regular and structured meetings and information giving/receiving events with individual service users, carers, and black and minority community associations. The process may take time to create trust and openness. Once information and feedback is flowing both ways, the commissioner will face the difficult task of absorbing it all. How to weight information from black service users and groups compared to professional views and financial uncertainties is subtle and so far unclear.

As part of this longer term work, health authorities will help primary care groups to identify and to work with ethnic and cultural minority communities and to engage them in local and health authority plans for mental health (and other) services. At the same time the national recognition of the invaluable role of carers needs further refinement to understand and act upon issues relating to families and carers within ethnic and cultural minority communities. In particular, authorities need to support primary health care teams, through the development of skills and knowledge, to adjust their services to the ethnic and cultural diversity of the local population. Even with a resourced and sustained effort, this process could take several years. It should be started with enthusiasts and opinion formers in primary care.

The rigours of clinical-effectiveness and cost-effectiveness measures, which have been applied most thoroughly so far in surgical specialties of the acute sector, will need to be applied in mental health. A view will have to be taken as to how relevant these approaches are, given the wide range of outcomes that characterise good mental health services. Close working with professionals providing services to black and cultural minorities, as well as individuals and groups from those minorities, will help put the specific approach of effectiveness in a culturally sensitive context. Difficulties in determining criteria to evaluate the effectiveness of these services may take time to emerge.

Future Developments

Despite the complexity of the mental health system as a whole, and the additional poignancy and sensitivity of issues related to ethnic and minority cultural populations within that system, progress can be made. A hierarchy of action might be at national level:

1. Within the government's wider public health agenda (Our Healthier Nation), the NHS Executive and the Department of Health working explicitly with other departments of State to ensure that a coherent national approach to mental health develops. This approach needs to include action to reduce inequalities and social exclusion of black and ethnic minorities. In time a national mental health strategy would develop but much could be done to improve matters in the meantime.
2. Within a public health framework based on partnerships, maintain the development of a comprehensive mental health system at a local

level as a medium-term priority for the NHS as a whole over the next three to five years.

3. Within the development of a comprehensive mental health system, address the specific needs of ethnic and cultural minorities and demonstrate progress.
4. Health authorities held accountable by the NHS Executive through an improved and evolving performance development process that has a focus on minority mental health needs. The annual review between the NHS Executive and each health authority, the importance regional chairs give to the topic when meeting chairs of health authorities and Trusts, and progress against authorities' own targets would fit easily into the evolving accountability system. Sanctions are limited but requirement for a remedial action plan and close monitoring would have an effect.
5. Clear leadership in primary, secondary and tertiary care to make ethnic monitoring of all patients (through the new NHS numbering scheme) become initially mandatory and then an accepted norm.

At local level the health authority, local authority and the voluntary sector should:

1. prepare joint strategies and approaches based on a shared understanding of local needs and a joint analysis of current service configuration relevant to ethnic and cultural minorities within the health improvement programme;
2. make a strategic commitment over a five-year period to integrate culturally sensitive mental health services, based on a partnership between agencies and sectors;
3. be open to the views and input of ethnic and cultural minorities into the planning, commissioning and provision of mental health services;
4. develop and support forums of black and cultural minority voluntary organisations. The aim is to ensure regular and structured opportunities for minorities to meet commissioning staff and discuss needs and services together. An essential element is for the health authority to feed back to minority forums how their views have influenced policy and commissioning and which elements were not accepted and why.

It is possible for government to set a tone and a framework in which the service at local level is commissioned and provided. To some extent, how importantly the differing needs of ethnic and cultural minorities in mental health are viewed locally depends on how much priority they receive at national level. If they are not seen as central at national level there is a danger they will be seen locally as marginal. Clearly it is open to the local health and social care system to place greater emphasis and priority on these needs. Sustained government leadership around ethnicity and health as part of its social exclusion work would be a positive development.

Key debates – to be handled openly but no doubt at times with difficulty – will be to what extent:

1. can public health approaches develop needs assessment so that there is good information from which to base commissioning decisions for the mental health of ethnic and cultural minorities;
2. can mainstream services be sufficiently sensitive to the mental health needs of ethnic and cultural minorities given that they will continue to receive most of statutory funding;
3. is it appropriate to emphasize the funding of specific and targeted mental health services for ethnic and cultural minorities;
4. will primary care groups be better placed to commission culturally sensitive services than health authorities, bearing in mind the critical mass needed to develop and support specialist services;
5. can primary care be a better route of access for ethnic and cultural minorities into the mental health system, with all the benefits of early diagnosis and prevention.

Conclusion

The informed commissioner needs to have the confidence to lead at a local level. Work will be characterised by partnership with communities, professionals and other agencies within the totality of the resource invested in mental health to achieve culturally sensitive commissioning. The tensions, pressures and dilemmas will not go away. Yet the commissioner who can build trust with local communities, GPs and primary care teams, specialist services, local authorities and the voluntary sector will be able to make progress locally while speaking with united backing and practical experience to influence national policy-making. In this way, partnerships can be built not only locally, but between health authorities and the NHS centrally, and in turn with the other key elements of the State system.

References

Department of Health (1989a) *Working for Patients*, pp. 14–15. London: HMSO.
Department of Health (1989b) *Caring for People: Community Care in the Next Decade and Beyond*, p. 33. London: HMSO.
Department of Health (1997) *The New NHS: Modern. Dependable*, pp. 24–31. London: The Stationery Office Ltd.
NHS Executive (1994) *Collection of Ethnic Group Data for Admitted Patients EL(94)77*, pp. 1–2. London: HMSO.
NHS Executive (1997) *NHS Priorities and Planning Guidance 1998/99 EL(97)35*, pp. 2–8. London: HMSO.

Part V
The Future

19

Transformations and New Beginnings

Kamaldeep Bhui and Dele Olajide

Introduction

It is hoped that this book will generate debate which should lead to action to remedy the identified inadequacies in mental health service provision for ethnic minorities. The contributors have presented a variety of views which are not always compatible. This approach recognises the contributions of other disciplines so as to harmonise efforts to deliver care in accord with truly holistic and humanitarian principles. Mental health services in the UK have undergone dramatic changes in organisational principles, largely driven by a clear message that resources are finite. Ethnic minorities who contribute to the economic and cultural fabric of society have largely been neglected in the planning and provision of mental health services (see Chapter 18). Such a position is untenable. This volume aims to realise excellence in mental health care for all.

The assumed universality of emotional distress discourages a more complete analysis of inter- and intra-cultural diversity (see Chapter 4). The application of new technologies in health reinforces the impression that specific interventions have a similar impact on all people as long as they carry the same psychiatric diagnosis. Fulford (Chapter 3) exposes the complexity of such a process, emphasising, as in Chapter 1, that values and subjective judgements are inextricably entwined with mental health practice despite the effort of the professions to develop a more scientific basis to yield impartial judgements. The dispassionate stance of scientific enquiry has not served ethnic minorities well (Fernando, 1991; Littlewood, 1993; Knowles, 1996). Racism manifest as hate and prejudice is condemned in health services. Such attitudes, where they persist, are sufficiently unfashionable to remain inconspicuous. Equal opportunity policies are established but there is little monitoring of equal opportunity practice (see Chapters 12 and 15). How should individuals and organisations respond to patients who racially abuse and threaten staff? What about staff who mistreat other staff or overlook the needs of certain groups of patients? There are practices carried out nationally, organisationally and individually which serve to disadvantage black and ethnic minority people when they are in need of mental health care. It is the daily rituals carried out in the interest of the sufferer that this book scrutinises. Where such practices inadvertently undermine the effective delivery of high quality care, or potentiate the poorer delivery of care to specific cultural groups, one might conclude that the pragmatic outcome is identical to that entertained by blatant prejudicial attitudes. We have chosen to examine and emphasise the procedural operations responsible for disadvantage rather than bluntly apply the term "racism". Such an approach, we believe, also enables corrective action by identifying a focus for reform. This approach might inadvertently be used to deny that racism is a daily social reality for black and ethnic minorities in the UK. So we emphasise that all policy and service solutions must reflect this reality.

The Context: British Society, Identity and Mental Health Services

The first and most difficult task for the health service and all professionals is that of acknowledgement. The quality of care offered to ethnic minority groups in the UK has been inadequate (Parkman *et al.*, 1997; Chapter 1). There is dissatisfaction with the skills and behaviour of professionals, accessibility of services, efficacy of services and with specific interventions. The research data cited by other contributors support and expand upon these findings.

Organisational silence, procedures and politics can readily act as agents of denial, defensiveness and avoidance of responsibility. Within the professions and in the daily working practices of health services, rules and behaviours are established to support the dominant modes of delivering care. This strengthens our psychological defences and so we believe ourselves to act ethically and we thus avoid reflection on the consequences of our actions (Menzies-Lyeth, 1988). All those working to provide health care also need to become *personally available* to hear and metabolise the communities' dissatisfactions with existing services. Each individual must question their own value system; they can do this constructively only if guided by their respective organisations and only then if their professional bodies recognise such a need. It seems these simple prerequisites are still preventing progress.

Planning and Provision of Services for Ethnic and Cultural Minorities

Who Do We Mean by Ethnic?

Ethnic as a term has been abused to represent just what anyone wishes it to represent. It is a sufficiently broad term to encompass a broad range of health and life-styles, culture and race. Its lack of specificity is recognised but it is still deemed to be an improvement on the use of race categories (Smaje, 1995). Race, after all, has even less validity as a marker of health and life-style independent of other demographic variables. Mixed marriages, the process of younger generation's bi-cultural competence, the merging of cultures to produce new musical sounds, appearances and styles of communication all point to new potentialities in our under-standing of ethnicity and of suffering and its alleviation. "Ethnicity" is impressed upon organisations as a good way of measuring ethnic minority needs but these categories do lack precision (see Chapter 15).

The borders between cultures and races and ethnic groups are constantly revised and re-defined by society (Brah, 1996) yet service planners have to define ethnicity in order to plan for the needs of communities. The research agenda similarly has been slow to formulate ethnicity in a meaningful way (Singh, 1997). It is often assumed that a specific ethnic group contains people with similar cultures and similar attitudes to help seeking. These ethnic categories are presumed to reflect similar vulnerabilities to specific disorders and hence we feel informed about planning. Although this is satisfactory as a short-term programme for the benefit of those groups where culture and ethnicity are closely related with health and life-style, it will not be long before these ethnic categories are meaningless in terms of culture. We will need to understand culture as distinct from ethnicity and we will need to distinguish instances in which ethnicity can or can not act as a proxy for culture. For example, new immigrant communities with distinct cultures will continue to encounter mental health services as migra-tion across the globe escalates. Therefore, not only do local provider units need to consider provision to serve Britain's ethnic minorities now, but any service solution must retain the flexibility to adapt to new ethnicities with their specific service needs. For example, the opening of European borders is one source of further immigration yet this appears to have received very little attention by service providers (McKee, 1997). Similarly the Irish community in Britain suffers the highest rates of suicide and schizophrenia, yet their needs receive scant attention.

Purchasing Services

Commissioners are in a position to ensure that the services reflect what population health requires. They are in a position, therefore, to stipulate the quality of care as well as the type of care. Gluckman (Chapter 18) empha-sises the need for commissioners to be fully aware of ethnic minorities and their unique but complex profile of needs. The recent government White Paper advocates the formation of primary care groups that will now be responsible for commissioning. Yet again a policy is formulated without due attention to detail; hence we see retrospective amendments and graft-ing of ethnic minority issues (Free and McKee, 1998). One significant approach is the use of formulae to calculate the amount of revenue that is required by any health or local authority. These formulae are known to have significant limitations (Johnson *et al.*, 1997) including poor utility as indicators of ethnic minority needs (Glover, 1997). Hence there is a real possibility that such formulae will perpetuate inequity of service provision unless there are adjustments for the extra needs of ethnic minority communities (see Chapter 15). Until this level of precision is reached, local specialised surveys remain essential to generate accurate information grounded in the local culture. Cross-cultural research needs to begin in the community which it is supposed to serve, and be guided by its needs and priorities (Patel and Winston, 1994).

Meaningful Research as a Measure of Need

A great deal of research attention has focused on the "epidemic" of schizophrenia amongst black Caribbean and black British residents in the UK (see Chapter 6). Research in this field has mainly focused on biological formulations rather than the possible role of environmental factors in prevention or intervention. The concerns and favoured hypotheses of individual researchers seem to dictate the research agenda. The NHS research and development programme is helping to redress this imbalance but progress is slow. Paradoxically the preoccupation with biological aetiologies has not resulted in the evaluation of biological treatments (see Chapter 6). There has been no systematic effort at evaluating biological treatments amongst specific ethnic minorities in the UK. Their reactions to medication are assumed to be similar to those of any other ethnic group. Evidence from the United States clearly demonstrates differences in pharmacokinetics, pharmacodynamics and cultural dispositions to using medication (Lin *et al.*, 1995; Chapter 6). Despite the mounting evidence, clinicians may be treating black and ethnic minority patients on the basis of faulty research data. Who should take responsibility for this? We believe that both government, service providers and the pharmaceutical industry should recognise the need to ensure that clinical trials include patients from ethnic minorities.

It is known that black and ethnic minorities participate less often in research and drop out more often. Perhaps the subject matter of the research is labelled by them to be "not relevant, nor validly representing their experience of distress". This in itself warrants understanding rather than being ignored as an irritation or limitation of the research method. If black and ethnic minority groups can really see no benefit to research it is unlikely that they will offer their expertise or participate in research programmes.

Community-based Needs Assessment

Developing an understanding of the needs of new communities takes time and persistence. Several methodologies exist. The most likely problem is that one might explore a template of needs which are commonly found amongst the indigenous majority population but which are not of relevance amongst ethnic minority groups. Needs unique to ethnic minorities are then overlooked. Social adversity, poverty and unemployment, for example, are common to all ethnic groups in inner city areas but they might affect all inner city dwellers. How about racist attacks, bullying of children in school, exploitation at work, favouritism for promotion and new jobs, promotion blocked because of communication skills rather than ability, traumatic separation and isolation from families in other countries and frequent stopping by police? Each of these in itself might be traumatic. How about all of these occurring regularly and persistently? Such minor stressors become major stressors as they all collectively serve to undermine confidence and an individual's sense of belonging. Thus the society in which we live becomes depressogenic (Fernando, 1986). That is to say that the realities faced by ethnic minorities generate states of deprivation, feelings of worthlessness and hopelessness. These feelings are precisely those that are identified in a depressive state. We know that if we challenge these beliefs and feelings in an individual, if they are inappropriate, the distorted beliefs are minimised (this is what cognitive therapy tries to do).

We might anticipate, even though we do not know it as scientific knowledge, that creating a society in which these beliefs are socially generated actually initiates and perpetuates depressive states amongst ethnic minorities. Should mental health services be involved in these issues? If such social events cause, precipitate or perpetuate distress, then yes we should at least consider suitable interventions. Certainly to ignore environmental stressors that affect mental well-being, especially if service users ask for assistance, is simply to ensure dissatisfaction and undermine other therapeutic efforts (Conway *et al.*, 1994). Perhaps **one-stop benefit polyclinics**, dealing with welfare benefits, housing or racial abuse established by local and health authorities will be more effective as an intervention than pharmacological management of common mental disorders.

Epidemiological tools and anthropological methods exist to examine the need of populations; these differ in purpose, process and value to service providers as well as in cost (see Chapters 4 and 18). It is clear that the NHS needs to have a valid procedure by which new information about new populations is acquired quickly. Epidemiological surveys take a long time and there always remains the question of cross-cultural validity (Sashidharan and Francis, 1996). Ethnographic data ensure cultural accuracy and avoid reductionist conclusions but do not allow quantification of need as do epidemiological surveys; the latter enable planning for financial provisions. Our own view is that ethnographic data should always be collected in an ongoing manner; this is not just the role of the health service, commissioner or local authority but also of the service providers and individual teams and their members. It indeed could form part of their "training and cultural awareness" task. Local surveys carried out by those providing a service are more likely to improve clinical practice than remote surveys carried out by independent specialist research departments. There is no single method of collecting community-based needs assessments. Specific models do exist; these involve psychiatric teams in which each member takes responsibility for a single cultural group, acquires information from them, works and spends time with them and informs them of available services. Feedback to other mental health professionals is then continuous. Others have tried to engage and employ local community members who then serve as a channel of mutual education. Another approach is to engage fully with independent and voluntary specialist providers such that these groups can complement, scrutinise, educate and train the statutory sector.

Purchasing conferences attended by the public or service users and their families are one possible mechanism for channelling public views into the planning process. Public meetings might lead to more participation by the public in the development of their mental health service but they might also provide education and liaison with other public services that encounter the mentally ill. In the rush to establish community-based facilities, many planners did not anticipate public fears and reactions which resist open-door policies (Wolff *et al.*, 1996); indeed ethnic minorities appeared to be especially concerned and unlikely to welcome the mentally ill into their neighbourhoods. There is a considerable need to ensure that mental health services are accountable to the public just as their intention is to serve the public (Calnan, 1996). Better liaison with the public can ensure better access to leisure, library, and other local public amenities as well as support from local residents and business. Indeed such links may form the basis for new ideas and developments that benefit the local community as well as the mentally ill from ethnic minorities. Of special importance, of course, is liaison with culturally distinct organisations and charities which already serve ethnic minorities as well as majorities (Chapters 9, 10 and 14). Recovery requires a culturally comprehensive approach which includes existing organisations and the expertise of local populations such that care is culturally competent and grounded in local societies.

Organisational Priorities

Juss and Chandra (Chapters 8 and 17) outline the basic requirements of a culturally competent organisation. If services are truly to address the needs of a less visible ethnic group they have to consider widespread changes in their policies and question how prioritisation and promulgation of their values might oppress and hurt the care of minorities. How might a culturally blind and ignorant organisation seek understanding? There is an immediate conflict if organisations deem themselves not to need intervention or adaptation despite the delivery of poor-quality care to ethnic minorities. Values can be argued upon and markers of efficiency and effectiveness might be considered inadequate and hence incomparable across culture groups. Organisations often respond to change by seeking a process of consultation. This can be useful if there is a willingness to examine options honestly; however, such a process can become a hindrance if its purpose is perceived to be one of maintaining the status quo by reinforcing stereotypes. Sue (1995) outlines an approach to multi-cultural organisation development where attempts to alter teaching, academic courses and entry criteria to suit ethnic minorities better were counter-productive. The lessons learnt included a need for:

- realistic assessment of the level of multi-cultural development;
- interrelationship of subsystems to be understood;
- commitment to come from the top;
- understanding that premature introduction of change may only support the mistaken/biased beliefs of the opposition;
- acknowledgement that white people are also victims and under strong institutional pressures to conform.

Juss (Chapter 8) and Chandra (17) each examine the use of cultural identity theory for organisational development (Cross, 1995; Figure 19.1).

These and other management models of organisational development must be seriously considered within any service before it embarks on radical change; the danger of poorly thought out change is failure which reinforces prejudice or introduces a new system that continues to disadvantage ethnic minorities. Sue (1995) unpacks three types of organisation: monocultural, non-discriminatory and multi-cultural. Progress is marked by three stages of organisational development: (i) the functional focus that the organisation must take – recruitment, policies, training, etc; (ii) multi-cultural competencies needed by the organisation – skills, knowledge, beliefs/attitudes; (iii) barriers to multi-culturalism – fear of differences, discrimination, organisational systems. We strongly recommend all services adopt one or more models from which to fashion the most suitable model for their local population.

Quality criteria are essential to ensure that appropriate services and skills are available and that they are effective. These "qualities" of the service are reflected in policies and procedures, cultural and religious service specifications, user involvement, multi-cultural staffing and the development of more specific quality standards for any new developments (Chapter 15). Two of Chandra's objectives deserve specific attention. Staffing within the health service must provide the choice of ethnic, culture, language and religious matches; this is not to say that matching should be routine, indeed we all have personal experiences of patients who prefer to see someone not from their own religious or ethnic group (see also Chapter 15). It is not clear whether this arises because of fears about broken taboos being morally judged by someone from the same ethnic group, or that white staff are more culturally objective and neutral, or indeed the belief that white staff are more qualified and competent – a form of internalised racism (see Chapter 11).

Nonetheless, values, beliefs and attitudes can change only if they are

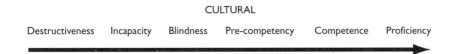

CULTURAL

Destructiveness   Incapacity   Blindness   Pre-competency   Competence   Proficiency

Figure 19.1   Cultural identity theory and organisational development.

represented at all levels of an organisation. The oppression of ethnic minorities working in the NHS is no longer disputed (Chapter 15; Ward, 1996; Littlewood and Lipsedge, 1997). Recruitment and retention of ethnic minority staff forms only the first stage of a lengthy process of changing values and developing a culturally competent workforce. Promotion support, mentoring, access to English classes, career advice are all necessary components. Yet in moves to demonstrate racial equality of an organisation, the actual impact on patient care is rarely examined. The health service prefers to spend money on research and bureaucracy related to race rather than to the conditions experienced by black people as workers or clients (Ward, 1996; see Chapter 15: "the glass ceiling effect"). A programme of action along with cultural and race awareness training for all usually raises concerns amongst staff about scrutiny; yet, as Fulford asserts (Chapter 3), competent cultural psychiatry is good psychiatry just as competent culturally sensitive mental health nursing is good nursing and culturally competent management is good management.

Measuring Outcomes

A valid and broadly agreed measure of charting progress is necessary. Audit tools might be one solution (Sathyamoorthy and Ford, 1997); these can facilitate comparison between voluntary and health service organisations or between different models of mental health service. Such tools must clearly use dimensions of satisfaction as well as clinical and economic outcome. Quality standards encompass aspects of communication, trust, support, being understood, clinical care and satisfaction with each intervention. These criteria can be as specific as required. For example, ensuring physical checks for those with co-morbid physical complaints (cardiovascular disease if of Indian subcontinent origin; sickle cell and hypertension if of Caribbean origin) seems more essential for ethnic minorities in view of their higher risk of developing ischaemic heart disease and other specific physical disorders. Clinical practice guidelines are currently being developed by the research unit of the Royal College of Psychiatrists. Such guidelines are intended to promote best practice and as such could be one source of quality criteria.

Health of the Nation Outcome Scales are also being piloted in many sites. Their value in measuring disabilities and recovery amongst ethnic minority groups is as yet unexplored. Clinical outcome scales are already subject to criticism for not being culturally specific (see Chapter 6 on the PSE). The criteria of a good outcome might differ between users, and voluntary organisations and mental health professionals might value quite different indicators of progress or recovery. Furthermore, critieria based on social service assessments might also be considerably different from the mental health service's self-imposed criteria. The merging of social and health care at the point of delivery should lead to a more shared vision of what constitutes "quality"; however, the voluntary and independent organisations also have a key role here. The majority of the independent and voluntary organisations believe that mental health services can never possibly achieve the cultural and ethnic sensitivities of a small and locally grounded organisation which is expert perhaps in a single cultural or ethnic group. However, if black workers remain at the margins of mental health services they will be unable to influence mainstream services and will fail to challenge existing stereotypes. Hence some mutually informative and advantageous partnerships are essential.

Multi-culturally Effective Mental Health Services

One major oversight in much of the literature about black mental health is that all mental health problems are assumed to be similarly related to service provision problems and service solutions. Hence, schizophrenia services, prevention and treatment programmes for depression, anxiety, substance misuse and psychotherapy may each have to resolve different ethical, clinical and research dilemmas. Each of these services risks theory failure, intervention failure or service structure failure. Theory is informed by both the professional training of the staff and the value attached to specific models of care delivery. Certain models become attractive if they are proven to be effective and popular with patients and providers. The profile of choices and communication issues are likely to differ for each ethnic and cultural group. The special difficulties faced by women, children and adolescents and the elderly each require specific investigation.

Community Mental Health Teams

The nuclear community mental health team includes psychiatrists, psychologists, nurses, occupational therapists and social workers (Figure 19.2). Although these are the core team members, other professions also encounter the mentally ill under certain circumstances. Hence a lawyer may become involved in a mental health tribunal or through the criminal justice system by representing a mentally ill offender. A probation officer likewise might liaise with a pscyhiatrist to secure psychiatric reports and to plan a joint package of care (see Chapter 7). Table 19.1 illustrates the many layers of professions, their associated communication channels and the origins of value systems. It is pertinent that, despite the varied theoretical standpoints of our contributors, we have still managed to represent only a section of those with an interest in improving mental health services for ethnic minorities. Conflicting ideology and miscommunication must be effectively negotiated in order always to secure the most beneficial outcome for any one patient. It is this communication task that poses special problems for the mentally ill and hence the care programme approach (which is also unevaluated across cultural groups) formalises such communication. An

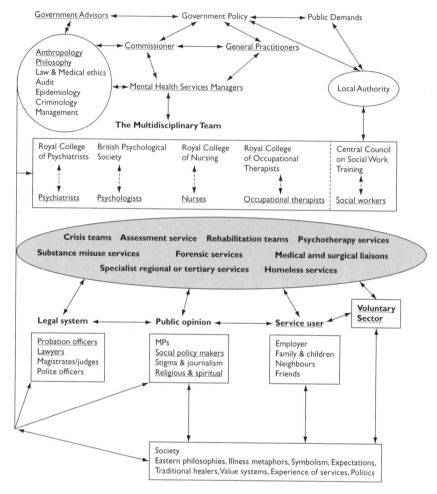

Figure 19.2 Network of services, professions and disciplines which inform delivery of services. Underlined positions are those represented by authors of this book.

added hurdle which is rarely discussed is the value system of each profession; the more socio-centric professions appear more aware of cultural and social issues (see Chapters 4 and 14; Benatar, 1998).

Ethnic minorities in Britain construe misfortune in social and religious terms. Indeed dismissing this as mad or meaningless is characteristic of only a few cultures, including the British one (Littlewood and Lipsedge, 1997; see Chapter 6). Social adversity can be the basis of cultural and social interventions or can make other occupational or pharmacological interventions less likely to succeed (Conway *et al.*, 1994). Marsella (1984, p. 366) emphasises that mental health is not restricted to separate aspects of behaviour and experience but involves harmonious relationships across all areas of functioning. The legacy of our psychiatric concepts arises partly out of Western science and thought which compartmentalises roles,

Table 19.1   Adaptations of a service.

Organisations	Values and mission statements; organisational change; anti-discriminatory policy; joint working policies with other organisations – police, probation, voluntary sector, academic departments, local authority.
Professions	Values, training, continuing education, inter-professional communication; ensure anti-discriminatory practice; acknowledge differences in epistemological and ontological conceptualisation of mental ill-health and its alleviation.
Interventions	Evaluate existing interventions and new ones; if found to be valuable how can interventions be delivered in a culturally syntonic manner: medication, day care, psychotherapy, assessment, support, housing advice, benefits advice, in-patient admission, legal representation.

facilities and knowledge and applies these to the mind, body and spirit separately (Marsella, 1984, p. 365; see Chapter 6). Hence, although a comprehensive mental health service must have all the functional components of any good service, more is required for a multi-culturally effective community service (Table 19.1; Bhui *et al.*, 1995).

If indigenous therapies and healings are requested by ethnic minorities (Mental Health Foundation, 1995) and they have value as interventions, how can we integrate them into a statutory service? Fernando (1991) describes these rich sources of culturally syntonic interventions as "technologies". These must be evaluated firstly from the perspective of the culture of origin before their comparative value is assessed by scientific methodologies which are designed to assess biomedical outcomes. Grafting of one "technology" or healing strategy into another culture's institutions may render the strategy powerless if the ability to effect change is actually embedded in the original culture's beliefs, values and systems of appraising and alleviating distress in its broadest sense. If such technologies (acupuncture, aromatherapy, homeopathy, etc.) can be transported or applied in Western service contexts, how might we evaluate them and resource them? It might be that such technologies have value to other cultures as well as cultures of origin. If we argue for this then we must also explore which Western psychiatric technologies can be of benefit, to which cultural groups, and for which disorders. The reasons for poor adherence to medication regimens might be less to do with biomedical effectiveness than with a failure really to believe in a particular form of healing, and indeed a failure to trust a particular treatment context. Would a South Londoner accept an exorcism for spider phobia? If the practitioner does not believe in the intervention it is unlikely that the service user will have confidence in it. Similarly, if a client requests exorcism what should our response be? Certainly we need to know more before we simply say this is not evidence-based and conclude the client's request to be unreasonable or due to a lack of "insight". Hence, organisation and individuals who have any role in mental health service provision have a duty to equip themselves with adequate knowledge and expertise to make such judgements.

Primary Care

Primary care groups have a greater capacity to link in with local service users and encourage a feeling of ownership of the service amongst service users (see Chapter 13). Indeed GPs as commissioners are in a better position to identify the needs of registered patients in view of their frequent contact with patients and their families. Clearly a plurality of "purchasers" generates complications of communication and conflicting ideology, but these conflicts must be overcome and a collective voice must ensue if there is to be constructive action. Where there is disagreement between professionals about generic mental health issues and concepts, a coherent and co-operative strategy to meet the needs of ethnic minorities is less likely to emerge. Planning must therefore include not only specialist services but a delineation of the role of primary care teams and the criteria by which individuals are cared for by specialist or primary care teams. It is apparent that models of primary care liaison are being implemented but none has taken full account of ethnic minorities' perceptions about who is better suited to manage their emotional distress.

Armstrong (1996) makes a powerful case for the greater validity of the concept of a "psychological problem" as defined by the GP rather than a psychiatrist. Thus psychiatrists tend to report under-detection of psychological problems by GPs as being the level at which practice might be improved (Commander *et al.*, 1997). Certainly there are variations in the detection of psychiatric disorders by GPs. Asian GPs detect less morbidity (Commander *et al.*, 1997); younger GPs, women and multiple partner practices are better at detecting morbidity (Armstrong, 1996; Commander *et al.*, 1997). Perhaps GPs are more attuned to their patients' perceptions and hence their practice is congruent with their patients' preferred treatments rather than those that psychiatrists would recommend. GPs are now at the heart of service developments and, it appears, will take a greater lead (Chapters 13 and 18) in the future planning of mental health services. GPs are, however, responsible for providing care for a variety of other physical conditions and the danger is that mental ill-health will continue to be only biologically conceptualised to the detriment of social and cultural formulations of mental ill-health. Where generic mental health professionals lack expertise in risk assessment and community mental health care, is it not likely that non-specialists are less prepared? If GPs are commissioners of mental health services, they might then prioritise commoner mental disorders such as anxiety and depression. These latter categories show more variability across cultures and hence warrant much greater understanding from a cultural perspective and traditionally have received less attention than psychoses. There is then a risk that the severely mentally ill, amongst whom ethnic minorities are over-represented, are deprived of adequate resources. These tensions must be explicitly debated and resolved.

Voluntary and Independent Providers

The voluntary sector emerged with a great deal of emphasis on providing services to those in the black and ethnic minorities who are invisible to the statutory services until they are admitted in crisis. Voluntary sector services also "prove" their attraction to black and ethnic minority users (Wilson, 1993; Bhui, 1997). Although qualitative studies indicate that voluntary and independent services run by black people are preferred by black patients (see Chapter 9), in this country at least, this has not been proven by quantitative and valid economic and clinical outcomes research which could inform future implementations. Voluntary and independent organisations have the correct philosophy but are not adequately resourced in terms of expertise as well as finance, to carry out evaluations (see Chapter 16). There is a tendency on the part of local authorities to restrict "race relations" initiatives to one-off high-profile measures rather than develop a sustained mainstream-oriented programme of action (Watters, 1996; Chapter 15). "Race" relations may be the wrong context for the development of effective mental health services for ethnic minorities. Ledwith and Husband (Chapter 16) highlight how conflicting policies can each be heralded as innovative solutions. The survival of voluntary sector expertise has therefore suffered; its future in a comprehensive mental health service is uncertain.

Black voluntary organisations nurture cultural and ethnic identity, so that users do not feel disenfranchised and their philosophies of living are understood. Phan and Silove (1997) outline how Vietnamese refugee satisfaction with services specifically for refugees persisted after adjustment for diagnosis, or symptom level. The extent of information provided and the ease of negotiating changes in treatment distinguished between satisfaction levels for specialist and non-specialist services. Hence, each voluntary organisation's success probably has an identifiable aspect of its approach which confers better outcome. If this is understood and can be authentically replicated then there is every possibility that statutory services can learn more effective ways of caring for people with different cultures and world views. Such evaluations are absent in the British literature. Until the statutory sector can learn to provide more effective services for all, the independent and voluntary groups will continue to provide a service.

Indeed it may transpire that statutory sectors find it financially impossible to realise culturally sensitive models. Such a conclusion has not been reached; if it were reached it would condemn all ethnic minorities to receive separate services; such a proposition is not viable economically (see Chapter 18). Hence, an integrated service is a realistic option. Another option is for the voluntary and independent providers to form networks of providers, such that they can be more directly funded and supported to provide culturally specific services (see Chapters 4 and 9). This approach would create competitive tensions between organisations for different clinical populations as well as different ethnic groups (Jennings, 1996).

Criminal Justice System and the Law

There are some pressing issues about the manner in which the criminal justice system handles African-Caribbean mentally disordered defendants (see Chapters 6, 7 and 8; Reed, 1992). Other ethnic and cultural groups are insufficiently prominent to have attracted similar attention. The complexity of relationships between victim and assailant ethnicity, crime, crime reporting and subsequent action must be considered in any explanation (Maden, 1993). Court procedures may act to the disadvantage of black men with schizophrenia just as they act to the detriment of non-mentally ill black men (NACRO, 1989; Hood, 1992). Earlier stages of diversion are also insensitive to the mental health needs of African-Caribbean patients (Guite and Field, 1997). Minor crimes committed by black men are reported more often than if the assailant is white, suggesting that more black men are pursued if they commit a crime (Shah and Pease, 1992; Burney and Pearson, 1995). Although police culture is frequently cited to be hostile to black people (Smith and Gray, 1983) this alone does not explain the findings of black people's over-representation among psychiatric populations where the police do not have a role in admission (Fahy *et al.*, 1987). It appears that African-Caribbean mentally disordered offenders are more firmly engaged with the criminal justice system, and with in-patient and crisis psychiatric services (McGovern and Cope, 1987). This contact may be prolonged by diagnostic confusions or negative stereotyping (Bolton, 1984; Burney and Pearson, 1995). Interestingly African-Caribbeans can avoid police-mediated admission at a first episode of psychosis, if they have a GP or a close friend who facilitates admission (Cole *et al.*, 1995). Hence, effective social networks are crucial to avoid "crisis only" and custodial access to mental health care. The mental health team seems to fail as an effective social network that mediates non-crisis admissions.

The role of the probation service has rarely been considered by mental health multi-disciplinary teams. Bhui (Chapter 7) comprehensively outlines the lack of visible and active joint work in the care of offenders. Partly, there is a lack of understanding of mutual roles, and a notion that collaboration is not easy to achieve. For example, resource limitations are frequently followed by a withdrawal of psychiatric services whenever probation services are actively involved (see Chapter 7). This is paradoxical as sector teams are managing more "risky" people; where there are differences of culture and ethnicity, it is clear that the assessment of psychiatric status and the management options require a more careful appraisal (Bhugra and Bhui, 1997a, 1997b). Creative partnerships with probation officers and the police are essential, yet seem not to have been adequately explored. The reason might again be that mental health services are asking other professions to take a lead in discharging "care programme approach" responsibilities. Other professions might not be prepared to do this because of a lack of familiarity with work with the mentally ill, or indeed simply because this is an additional drain on their scarce resource. Certainly, it seems valuable to ensure that each local mental health team is carefully linked into a named probation officer, police officer and member of the court diversion scheme staff. Jointly agreed policies require careful training to ensure joint policies are followed; culture and race specific issues to do with accurate understanding of intended communication and notions of justice and injustice could be especially productive. Furthermore, the Mental Health Act states that the individual's cultural background be considered, but there is no guidance on how to do this. The Act gives legal sanction to remove civil liberties but neglects guidance on how to minimise unnecessary or prolonged detention. There is no stipulation about the quality of care an individual receives whilst detained. The elderly, the unemployed, the poor, those with little education and those with depression all appear to be more affected by the Act and less likely to challenge its powers by appeal (Bradley *et al.*, 1995; Thomas *et al.*, 1996). Cultural competence in the structure of legislation and its implementation is therefore essential if the law is to be fairly applied (see Chapter 8).

Training and Education

Training and education have been mentioned at an organisation, service and individual level (Chapters 7, 12 and 17; Royal College of Psychiatrists, 1996). Each of the contributors has applauded training as a device for increasing understanding in a non-threatening manner. Professional training requires a great deal of adaptation, but the relevant professions, by their very nature, are inertia ridden. Thus these authors have laid out some of the barriers to, as well as solutions to, the training and education agenda. Clearly there are profession-bounded aspects of training, but there is also potential for shared training objectives. Whether the ambition of multi-professional training can be achieved remains to be seen. Certainly postgraduate courses in anthropology or health service management provide an opportunity for detailed study of culture and its application to mental health service provision. However, formal academic courses may be too detailed or too specific to benefit the local populations to which the student returns. Important principles will certainly be learnt but what the NHS desperately needs is a local system of in-service training (Figure 19.3).

Figure 19.3 outlines some proposed training objectives. Chandra (Chapter 17) emphasises cultural awareness, race awareness and anti-discriminatory training. Each profession has the task of re-visiting potential theory failure, specific intervention failure and service failure. Training at undergraduate

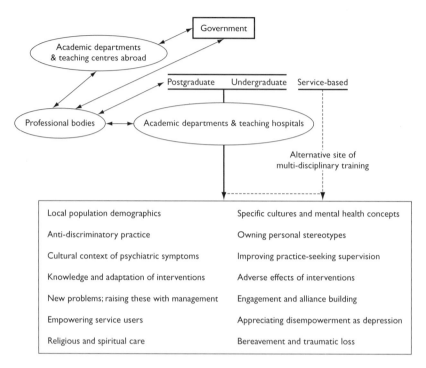

Figure 19.3   Training and education.

and postgraduate level must now reflect that. The volume of the training agenda is becoming even greater as many other professionals now seek expertise in psychiatric practice in view of their greater role in service provision for the severely mentally ill; thus staff of 24-hour supported hostels, social workers who act as keyworkers, the police, independent day care providers, residential wardens or carers, nurses, employers and those in leisure and education who attempt to provide a service to the mentally ill, might all legitimately seek training about mental ill-health and its treatment. Each of these individuals finds themselves with CPA and perhaps supervision register related responsibilities. Does this undermine the principle of normalisation in the least restrictive environment? Here again we have a conflict of policies. We encourage community residence but, to ensure risk minimisation, we inform and indeed train many other professionals to assess risk and to discharge aspects of a care package.

In order to minimise risk, information sharing and education are impera-tive; however, in order to minimise risk, the public and those providing direct care need to be sensitised to risk. For stigmatised minorities who often are invested with behaviours and life-styles to justify their ill treat-ment within a society (Littlewood and Lipsedge, 1997), such sensitisation might give rise to mis-appreciation of risk to the detriment of ethnic minorities. Hence education should not be restricted to clinical and medical matters but should include society, economics, and politics and interactions with health service policy as it affects ethnic minorities in the UK. A shared forum with other non-health professions would also serve a useful purpose.

Conclusions

Passive pondering of national and local data and dense theoretical debate, far removed from the daily lives of the public that we serve, can no longer be offered as a contribution to resolve the inadequacies of mental health service provision for ethnic minorities. We have endeavoured throughout this book to adhere to two principles:

1. Keeping the "person" in mind. This is a difficult yet essential task. No matter how complex the law or the organisation in which each of us works, our joint endeavour is to improve the care and services responsible for delivering that care.
2. The therapeutic relationship must at all times be prioritised and nurtured regardless of changes in policy, practice and organisation.

Local action linked to national and local expertise we see as the pinnacle of effective services. Each team member and each profession have a contribution. We have highlighted the inequalities of opportunity for NHS staff from ethnic minorities who are potential allies in providing culturally sensitive services as well as a culturally competent workforce. Local action can be realised only if there is leadership in the form of specific policies which motivate and organise change (see Chapter 15).

We have raised several weighty subjects which may be sensitive or even given a political slant. Our intention is to focus on inequality of access to care for Britain's multi-cultural society. We recommend the findings of this book to all who share our aims.

References

Armstrong, D. (1996) Construct validity and GPs' perceptions of psychological problems. *Primary Care Psychiatry* **2**: 119–122.

Benatar, S.R. (1998) Social suffering: relevance for doctors. *British Medical Journal* **315**: 1634–1635.

Bhugra, D. and Bhui, K. (1997a) Cross-cultural psychiatric assessment. *Advances in Psychiatric Treatment* **3**: 103–110.

Bhugra, D. and Bhui, K. (1997b) Clinical management of patients across cultures. *Advances in Psychiatric Treatment* **3**: 233–239.

Bhui, K. (1997) Service provisions for London's ethnic minorities. In: Johnson, S. *et al.* (eds) *London's Mental Health*. London: King's Fund Institute.

Bhui, K. *et al.* (1995) Developing culturally sensitive community psychiatric services. *British Journal of Health Care Management* **1**(16): 817–822.

Bolton, P. (1984) Management of compulsorily admitted patients to a high security unit. *International Journal of Social Psychiatry* **30**: 77–84.

Bradley, C., Marshall, M. and Gath, D. (1995) Why do so few patients appeal against detention under section 2 of the Mental Health Act? *British Medical Journal* **310**: 364–367.

Brah, A. (1996) Diversity, difference and differentiation. In: Brah, A. (ed.) *Cartographies of Diaspora. Contesting Identities*. Routledge: London.

Burney, E. and Pearson, G. (1995) Mentally disordered offenders: findings a focus for diversion. *The Howard Journal* **34**(4): 291–313.

Calnan, M. (1996) Why take into account patient views about health care? *British Journal of Health Care Management* **2**(6): 328–330.

Cole, E., Leavey, G., King, M. *et al*. (1995) Pathways to care for patients with first episode psychosis. A comparison of ethnic groups. *British Journal of Psychiatry* **167**: 770–776.

Commander, M.J., Sashi Dharan, S.P., Odell, S.M. and Surtees, P.G. (1997) Access to mental health care in an inner city health district. I: Pathways into and within specialist psychiatric services. *British Journal of Psychiatry* **170**: 312–316.

Conway, A.S., Melzer, D. and Hale, A.S. (1994) The outcome of targeting community mental health services: evidence from West Lambeth schizophrenia cohort. *British Medical Journal* **308**: 627–630.

Cross, W. (1995) The psychology of nigrescence. Revising the Cross model. In: Ponteretto, J.G., Casas, J.M., Suzuki, L.A. and Alexander, C.M. (eds) *Handbook of Multi-cultural Counselling*. Thousand Oaks, California: Sage Publications.

Fahy, T., Bermingham, D. and Dunn, J. (1987) Police admissions to psychiatric hospitals: a challenge to community psychiatry? *Medicine, Science and the Law* **27**: 263–268.

Fernando, S. (1986) Depression in ethnic minorities. In: Cox, J.L. (ed.) *Transcultural Psychiatry*. London: Croom Helm.

Fernando, S. (1991) Technologies for mental health. In: Fernando, S. (ed.) *Mental Health, Race and Culture*, pp. 170–195. London: Mind Publications.

Free, C. and McKee, M. (1998) Meeting the needs of black and minority ethnic groups. *British Medical Journal* **316**: 380.

Glover, G. (1997) Software for Bed Needs: using the new mental illness index. *The Evidence*, Spring 1–2. London: PRISM at Maudsley Hospital and MacMillan Magazines.

Guite, H. and Field, V. (1997) Services for mentally disordered offenders. In: Johnson, S. *et al*. (eds) *London's Mental Health*. London: King's Fund Institute.

Hood, R. (1992) *Race and Sentencing*. Oxford: Clarendon Press.

Jennings, S. (1996) *Creating Solutions. Developing Alternatives in Black Mental Health*. London: King's Fund.

Johnson, S. *et al*. (1997) *London's Mental Health*. London: King's Fund Institute.

Knowles, C. (1996) Racism in psychiatry. *Transcultural Research Review* **33**: 297–318.

Lin, K., Poland, R. and Anderson, D. (1995) Psychopharmacology, ethnicity and culture. *Transcultural Psychiatric Research Review* **32**: 3–40.

Littlewood, R. (1993) Ideology, camouflage or contingency? Racism in British psychiatry. *Transcultural Research Review* **30**: 243–290.

Littlewood, R. and Lipsedge, M. (1997) *Aliens and Alienists. Ethnic Minorities and Psychiatry*. London: Routledge.

McGovern, D. and Cope, R. (1987) The compulsory detention of males of different ethnic groups with special reference to offender patients. *British Journal of Psychiatry* **150**: 505–512.

McKee, M. (1997) The health of gypsies. Lack of understanding exemplifies wider disregard of the health of ethnic minorities. *British Medical Journal* **315**: 1172–1173.

Maden, T. (1993) Crime, culture and ethnicity. *International Review of Psychiatry* **5**: 281–289.

Marsella, A. (1984) Culture and mental health: an overview. In: Marsella, A.J. and White, G.M. (eds) *Cultural Conceptions of Mental Health and Therapy*. Dordrecht: D. Reidal.

Menzies-Lyeth, I. (1988) *Containing Anxiety in Institutions. Selected Essays*. London: Free Association Books.

Mental Health Foundation (1995) *Mental Health in Black and Minority Ethnic People. Time for Action*. The report of a seminar on Race and Mental Health, "Towards a strategy". London: Mental Health Foundation.

NACRO (1989) *Race and Criminal Justice. A Way Forward*. London: National Association for the Care and Resettlement of Offenders.

Parkman, S., Davies, S., Leese, M. *et al*. (1997) Ethnic differences in satisfaction with mental health services among representative people with psychosis in South London: PRISM Study 4. *British Journal of Psychiatry* **171**: 260–264.

Patel, V. and Winston, M. (1994) "Universality of mental illness" revisited assumptions, artefacts and new directions. *British Journal of Psychiatry* **165**: 437–440.

Phan, T. and Silove, D. (1997) The influence of culture on psychiatric assessment: the Vietnamese refugee. *Psychiatric Services* **48**(1): 86–90.

Reed, J. (1992) *Review of Health and Social Services for Mentally Disordered Offenders and Others Requiring Similar Services: Final Summary Report*, p. 3. London: Department of Health and Home Office.

Royal College of Psychiatrists (1996) *Report of the Working Party to Review Psychiatric Practice in a Multi-ethnic Society.* London: Royal College of Psychiatrists.

Sathyamoorthy, G. and Ford, R. (1997) *Audit Tool to Assess the Cultural Sensitivity of Mental Health Services: Staff and User Interview Schedules.* London: The Sainsbury Centre for Mental Health.

Sashidharan, S. and Francis, E. (1996) Epidemiology, ethnicity and schizophrenia. In: Ahmad, W.I.U. (ed.) *Race and Health in Contemporary Britain.* Milton Keynes: Open University Press.

Shah, R. and Pease, K. (1992) Crime, race and reporting to the police. *The Howard Journal* **31**: 192–199.

Singh, S.P. (1997) Ethnicity in psychiatric epidemiology: need for precision. *British Journal of Psychiatry* **171**: 305–308.

Smaje, C. (1995) *Health, Race and Ethnicity. Making Sense of the Evidence.* London: King's Fund Institute.

Smith, D. and Gray, J. (1983) *Police and People in London. The PSI Report.* London: Policy Studies Institute.

Sue, D.W. (1995) Multicultural organisational development: implications for counselling the profession. In: Ponteretto, J.G., Casas, J.M., Suzuki, L.A. and Alexander, C.M. (eds) *Handbook of Multi-cultural Counselling.* Thousand Oaks, California: Sage Publications.

Thomas, P., Romme, M. and Hamelijnck, J. (1996) Psychiatry and the politics of the underclass. *British Journal of Psychiatry* **169**: 401–404.

Ward, L. (1996) Race equality and employment in the National Health Service. In: Ahmad, W.I.U. (ed.) *Race and Health in Contemporary Britain.* Milton Keynes: Open University Press.

Watters, C. (1996) Representations and realities: black people, community care and mental illness. In: Ahmad, W.I.U. and Atkin, K. (eds) *Race and Community Care.* Buckingham, Philadelphia: Open University Press.

Wilson, M. (1993) *Britain's Black Communities.* London: NHS Management Executive, Mental Health Task Force and King's Fund Centre.

Wolff, N. *et al.* (1996) Public education for community care. *British Journal of Psychiatry* **168**: 441.

Index

Numbers in **bold** refer to main discussion